Joelle Thirsk Fathi • Meg Fay Mortman
Editors

Lung Cancer Navigation and Care

A Comprehensive Guide for Navigators and Allied Health Professionals

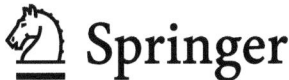

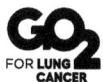

Editors
Joelle Thirsk Fathi
GO2 for Lung Cancer
Washington, DC, USA

Meg Fay Mortman
GO2 for Lung Cancer
Washington, DC, USA

Department of Biobehavioral Nursing
and Health Informatics
University of Washington
Seattle, WA, USA

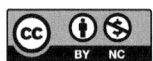

ISBN 978-3-032-02199-1   ISBN 978-3-032-02200-4 (eBook)
https://doi.org/10.1007/978-3-032-02200-4

This work was supported by GO2 for Lung Cancer.

© The Editor(s) (if applicable) and The Author(s) 2026. This book is an open access publication.

Open Access This book is licensed under the terms of the Creative Commons Attribution-NonCommercial 4.0 International License (http://creativecommons.org/licenses/by-nc/4.0/), which permits any noncommercial use, sharing, adaptation, distribution and reproduction in any medium or format, as long as you give appropriate credit to the original author(s) and the source, provide a link to the Creative Commons license and indicate if changes were made.

The images or other third party material in this book are included in the book's Creative Commons license, unless indicated otherwise in a credit line to the material. If material is not included in the book's Creative Commons license and your intended use is not permitted by statutory regulation or exceeds the permitted use, you will need to obtain permission directly from the copyright holder.

This work is subject to copyright. All commercial rights are reserved by the author(s), whether the whole or part of the material is concerned, specifically the rights of translation, reprinting, reuse of illustrations, recitation, broadcasting, reproduction on microfilms or in any other physical way, and transmission or information storage and retrieval, electronic adaptation, computer software, or by similar or dissimilar methodology now known or hereafter developed. Regarding these commercial rights a non-exclusive license has been granted to the publisher.

The use of general descriptive names, registered names, trademarks, service marks, etc. in this publication does not imply, even in the absence of a specific statement, that such names are exempt from the relevant protective laws and regulations and therefore free for general use.

The publisher, the authors and the editors are safe to assume that the advice and information in this book are believed to be true and accurate at the date of publication. Neither the publisher nor the authors or the editors give a warranty, expressed or implied, with respect to the material contained herein or for any errors or omissions that may have been made. The publisher remains neutral with regard to jurisdictional claims in published maps and institutional affiliations.

This Springer imprint is published by the registered company Springer Nature Switzerland AG
The registered company address is: Gewerbestrasse 11, 6330 Cham, Switzerland

If disposing of this product, please recycle the paper.

Lung Cancer Navigation and Care

Preface

Over a decade ago—before we'd even met—when we were both working in thoracic oncology at large health systems on opposite sides of the country, we would never have dreamed of having the privilege and opportunity to write this comprehensive book to help support our colleagues across all disciplines and around the globe in our collective efforts to improve lung cancer care. Reflecting on that time—when the NELSON trial was well underway, the NLST results were "hot off the press," and lung cancer screening was just becoming a recommendation of the US Preventive Services Task Force—it was a pivotal moment in the field. Precision medicine, radiation oncology, and minimally invasive surgery were rapidly transforming the landscape of cancer care, offering more personalized, targeted treatment options and reducing the physical burden of surgery. These innovations have not only improved clinical outcomes but also enhanced the overall patient experience, setting a new standard for how lung cancer is diagnosed and treated. Since then, the progress in awareness, research, targeted treatment, and patient and family support has been nothing short of astronomical. We believe the time is right for a comprehensive, evidence-based guide that synthesizes the latest best practices to equip lung cancer navigators with a clear, practical roadmap to support patients across the continuum of care—from screening through survivorship.

As the readers of this book well know, lung cancer is the leading cause of cancer-related deaths in the United States and worldwide, over breast, colon, and prostate cancers combined. Lung cancer disproportionately affects those who are impacted most by social determinants of health and historically marginalized communities, including Black, Indigenous, and People of Color. These communities are at greater risk of lung cancer with poorer treatment outcomes. Better understanding of cancer biology and new advances in lung cancer treatment, including biomarker testing, promise to save even more lives from lung cancer through advancements in technology, early detection of oncogenes, and targeted therapies. And we all know that this highly stigmatized disease is preventable and curable when people receive timely, evidence-based, efficient, high-quality care.

As the field continues to evolve with advancements, lung cancer navigators are uniquely positioned to bridge the gap between innovation and implementation. The concept of leveraging nurses, social workers, community health workers, and a cadre of Allied Health Professionals to successfully screen and support high-quality lung cancer care delivery to people at risk and experiencing this deadly disease is a well-accepted practice and steadily gaining ground. Not only does a growing body of evidence demonstrate the value of integrating patient navigation across the care continuum for improved outcomes, but those of us on the front lines delivering this care for many years have seen first-hand that the only way to be successful in this complex endeavor is to have ALL these members of our healthcare teams be informed and engaged, have the proper resources and tools for success, and to truly believe that each one of them plays a crucial role in our efforts to improve health outcomes and save lives. And we also know the patient's journey, viewpoints, and experiences, always at the forefront of navigation, inform our collective learnings and practices.

This site-specific, comprehensive guide for Lung Cancer Navigators and Allied Health Professionals who care for and help guide patients across the entire lung cancer continuum is the first of its kind. This clinical companion aims to introduce and provide Lung Cancer Navigators and Allied Health Professionals with end-to-end foundational knowledge, best practices, and critical resources needed to elevate the standard of care and equitable health outcomes through care navigation for people at risk and living with lung cancer. Each chapter is authored by subject matter and navigation experts, offers an in-depth content review, and a vignette structured to illustrate how each content area may be implemented in direct patient navigation across lung cancer care. It concludes with additional relevant key takeaways, best practices, recommended readings, and relevant resources.

It is an honor to work with all of you, to learn with you and from you, and we are forever indebted to all our colleagues, mentors, and team members with whom we have had the privilege of collaborating for many years—you are too numerous to mention. We also wish to sincerely thank our families and Sarah Weston for their patience and steadfast support in the development of this text. Our hope is that our community finds this book helpful and thought-provoking, and we look forward to advancing our shared goals even further in the future together.

Seattle, WA, USA Joelle Thirsk Fathi
Arlington, VA, USA Meg Fay Mortman

Contents

1. **The Stigma of Lung Cancer** 1
   Heidi A. Hamann

2. **Advocacy for People at Risk or Living with Lung Cancer and Their Caregivers Across the Care Continuum** 13
   Danielle Hicks and Maureen Rigney

3. **Navigation in Lung Cancer Prevention, Detection, and Care** 23
   Meg Fay Mortman, Angela Gonnella, and Linda Fleisher

4. **Multi-, Interdisciplinary, and Patient-Centric Team-Based Lung Cancer Care** 35
   Laura Pachella and Loril Garrett

5. **Determinants of Lung Cancer, Disease Development, and Risk Assessment** 49
   Nicholas C. Love and Arpan A. Patel

6. **Critical Role of Genomics for Directed Therapeutic Management of Lung Cancer** 59
   Courtney A. Granville and Jaclyn LoPiccolo

7. **Essential Components for the Development of an Early Lung Cancer Detection Program** 75
   Joelle Thirsk Fathi, Jonathan T. Hontzas, and Sarah A. Weston

8. **Imaging for Screening, Diagnosis, and Staging of Lung Cancer** 91
   Debra S. Dyer

9. **Lung Cancer Screening and Early Detection** 105
   Mary Pasquinelli and Linda Dowling

10. **Tobacco Dependence Treatment and Lung Cancer Control** 119
    Chris Kotsen and Lisa Carter-Bawa

11. **Clinical Manifestations and Presentations of Lung Cancer** 135
    Martina Block

12	**Classification and Staging of Lung Cancer** .... Nicholas C. Love and Arpan A. Patel	149
13	**Surgical Interventions and Care for Lung Cancer Control** .... Keith D. Mortman and Bitana Saintilma	163
14	**Biomarker-Directed Precision Medicine for Lung Cancer Control** .... Parth Desai and Hossein Borghaei	175
15	**Biology and Treatment Options for Non-small Cell Lung Cancer** .... Kimberly Kish	189
16	**Biology and Treatment Options for Small Cell Lung Cancer and Other Lung Neuroendocrine Neoplasm** .... Lei Deng	205
17	**Clinical Trials in Lung Cancer**............................. Andrew Ciupek and Brittney Nichols	215
18	**Evaluation and Management of Lung Cancer and Treatment-Related Side Effects and Symptoms** .... Christopher R. Pallas and Kathryn F. Mileham	227
19	**Supportive, Palliative, and Hospice Care** .... Jennifer E. Jacky and Angie Larsh	255
20	**Best Practice Standards and Models of Care for High-Quality Survivorship**.............................. Christina R. Crabtree-Ide and Tessa Flores	269
21	**Integrative, Complementary, and Alternative Therapies in Lung Cancer Care** .... Rose Wai-Yee Fok and Gary Deng	283
22	**Policy and Advocacy in Lung Cancer** .... Angela M. Barry and Laurie Fenton Ambrose	301

The Stigma of Lung Cancer

Heidi A. Hamann

Contents

Navigation Vignette.. 2
Introduction.. 2
The Importance of Lung Cancer Stigma... 3
Addressing Lung Cancer Stigma.. 4
Conclusion.. 6
Key Takeaways... 7
Key Readings and Resources.. 8
References.. 8

Abbreviations

ACS	American Cancer Society
IASLC	International Association for the Study of Lung Cancer
Kentucky LEADS	Kentucky Lung (cancer) Education Awareness Detection Survivorship
MBS	Mindfulness-based stress reduction
mHealth	Mobile health
MSC	Mindful self-compassion
NLRCT	National Lung Cancer Roundtable
NSCLC	Non-small cell lung cancer

H. A. Hamann (✉)
University of Arizona, Tucson, AZ, USA
e-mail: Heidihamann@arizona.edu

© The Author(s) 2026
J. T. Fathi, M. F. Mortman (eds.), *Lung Cancer Navigation and Care*,
https://doi.org/10.1007/978-3-032-02200-4_1

Navigation Vignette

A 64-year-old married man (Mr. S.) presents for treatment planning after a recent diagnosis of Stage III non-small cell lung cancer (NSCLC). Mr. S. attends the appointment alone, asks minimal questions, and does not appear interested in clinical trial options. When asked if he would like any support services or tobacco cessation resources during treatment, he declines and tells the clinician, "The damage is done. I need to live with the consequences." The busy clinician does not probe any further; this clinician does not feel well equipped to address psychosocial issues and the next patient is waiting. The appointment ends with a treatment plan summary.

Mr. S. attends his first two treatment sessions but then starts missing appointments. As the team contacts the patient to reschedule, his diagnosis and treatment are reviewed in multidisciplinary case conference. After the attending clinician describes this "unengaged and noncompliant patient," a fellowship trainee asks how the stigma surrounding lung cancer may be affecting Mr. S. and the context of his treatment decision. This fellowship trainee has read recent studies describing the broad impact of stigma on lung cancer care, along with recommendations for clinicians to empathically address stigma with their patients. After a brief discussion, the treatment team decides to integrate a discussion of stigma and other treatment barriers with Mr. S. at his next appointment. This discussion helps the clinical team learn about Mr. S.'s feelings of guilt and shame and how they have negatively affected the relationship with his family and his perspective about treatment and behavior change. Mr. S. agrees to engage in psychosocial support services to address stigma; in subsequent appointments, the clinical team notes increased engagement in treatment, including interest in potential treatment trials and focus on functional rehabilitation.

Introduction

This navigation vignette represents stories all too familiar in lung cancer treatment settings when stigma is a barrier to optimal care. Advances in early detection, treatment, and symptom management have generated significant excitement and brought increased visibility to lung cancer care [1–6]. These advances have been accompanied by an unprecedented shift in optimism among thoracic oncology treatment specialists. For example, a 2018 survey found that 67% of oncologists reported adequate treatment options for advanced NSCLC patients, compared to 36% in 2008 [7]. In addition, a dedicated group of lung cancer advocates are highlighting survivorship, supporting research and evidence-based care and promoting policy change [8]. Despite these promising advances, there have been substantial barriers to fully realizing comprehensive lung cancer care [9–11]. A significant percentage of lung cancer patients do not receive molecular testing and evidence-based anticancer treatment [11, 12, 13]. As shown in the Mr. S. vignette, individuals with lung cancer are also less likely to engage in clinical trials, participate in supportive care, and seek rehabilitation services [10, 14–16]. Survey respondents diagnosed with lung cancer report increasing social exclusion as well, with 69% agreeing that those diagnosed are treated differently in society, compared to 51% endorsement 10 years prior [7]. Finally, despite recent improvements, the funding landscape for lung cancer continues to lag behind other cancers, with fewer opportunities for federal research and nonprofit organization funding [17].

The following sections address these barriers to fulfilling the promise of reduced lung cancer burden through the lens of *lung cancer stigma*, defined as the experience and internalization of negative appraisal and devaluation from others [18]. The sections expand upon these concepts, summarizing contemporary research focused on understanding and addressing lung cancer stigma. The last section includes take-home messages and recommendations for continued research, clinical, and policy efforts.

The Importance of Lung Cancer Stigma

The study of lung cancer stigma has been heavily influenced by the work of Goffman, who connected stigma to "discrediting" attributes [19]. Researchers have extended Goffman's focus on stigma to address disease-specific markers and the impact of stereotypes. Measurement of disease-focused stigma has addressed public attitudes and discriminatory actions (e.g., social and enacted stigma), along with the impact of this devaluation on affected individuals (e.g., perceived and internalized stigma) [20]. In the case of lung cancer, a focus on the causal influence of tobacco use, although critical for tobacco control efforts, may have unintended consequences that generate blaming responses and biased negative perceptions toward individuals with lung cancer [21–23]. Lung cancer stigma is common; recent work suggests that over 70% of individuals with lung cancer report clinically significant levels of stigma [24–26]. Previous work has identified three primary elements of lung cancer stigma from the patient perspective: (1) perceived stigma (evaluating what others think and say); (2) internalized stigma (how perceived stigma can affect patients through self-blame and guilt); and (3) constrained disclosure (the way stigma limits discussions of lung cancer with others) [27]. Attention to patient-centered measurement of stigma has resulted in multiple assessment tools specific to lung cancer, including the *Cataldo Lung Cancer Stigma Scale* and the *Lung Cancer Stigma Inventory* [28, 27].

Research has demonstrated pervasive negative consequences of lung cancer stigma, including reduced involvement in early detection interventions, negative psychosocial impact, impaired communication and self-advocacy, inadequate access to diagnosis and treatment, and limited public support for lung cancer research and care [29–34]. As noted in the vignette, the role of stigma in reduced adherence to treatment is particularly impactful; a stigma-related theme identified through quantitative and qualitative research has centered on patients' feelings of unworthiness for medical care and hesitancy in discussing treatment options and medical concerns. Individuals with lung cancer have described how fears of being judged and blamed have limited their ability to effectively communicate with family, friends, and clinical care providers [18, 24, 31, 35, 36]. Although earlier studies of lung cancer primarily focused on cross-sectional relationships between stigma and negative outcomes, more contemporary work has shown the effects of lung cancer stigma to be long-lasting; recent investigations have demonstrated that stigma persists through survivorship and can predict higher levels of psychosocial distress months after initial measurement [30, 37].

Addressing Lung Cancer Stigma

Mitigating the negative impact of lung cancer stigma is an important step in fulfilling the promise of reduced lung cancer burden. As noted in the case of Mr. S., the effective use of stigma awareness, education, and other evidence-based interventions play important roles in addressing lung cancer stigma and improving clinical care. In an effort to best understand modifiable targets for intervention, research has focused on the mechanisms of lung cancer stigma and ways to address it, including focus on the individual, lung cancer clinicians, and larger societal messages. Effectively reducing stigma in these contexts holds promise to improve symptom recognition, earlier diagnosis, and enhanced clinical care outcomes.

Individual Level Approaches

At the individual level, two primary approaches—education and psychosocial interventions—have shown preliminary efficacy in reducing stigma and psychosocial distress. For example, one study focused on developing and testing an interactive mHealth tool to address stigma by coaching patients toward assertive communication with healthcare clinicians. Initial testing with eight patients supported its feasibility and acceptability in practice [38]. A two-arm study from China tested a "self-confidence cultivation" intervention combined with family collaborative nursing and demonstrated significant reductions in lung cancer stigma [39]. A single-arm, open trial tested an acceptance-focused cognitive behavioral intervention with 14 patients and demonstrated feasibility and initial efficacy with decreases in stigma, cancer distress, and depression [40]. Another acceptance-focused intervention, a six-session module specifically tailored for lung cancer stigma, was also shown to be feasible and acceptable in a multi-site sample of 22 individuals with lung cancer [25]. In this study, decreases in internalized stigma and constrained disclosure were associated with the intervention, suggesting preliminary efficacy of the approach. Two studies have focused on mindfulness-based approaches to address lung cancer stigma. In the first, a 4-week mindfulness-based stress reduction (MBSR) intervention was tested compared to a control condition, showing significant decreases in stigma from baseline to 3-month follow-up measurements [41]. A second approach addressed feedback from stakeholders to develop a mindful self-compassion (MSC) intervention to bolster self-compassion and reduce lung cancer stigma. In this report, respondents noted the need to address stigma in a sensitive manner [42].

Clinician-Focused Approaches

Interpersonal approaches to reduce stigma have focused on lung cancer clinicians, as well as caregivers and family members. As noted in the vignette, clinicians may face challenges communicating effectively and empathically with lung cancer patients, especially with busy clinic schedules and limited training. Even clinicians with strong focus on patient-centered care may find it difficult to communicate in a way that empowers patients without exacerbating feelings of self-blame and guilt [43–45]. Empathic patient-clinician communication has been associated with lower levels of stigma, but healthcare clinicians may miss empathic opportunities in lung cancer care [46]. Clinician-focused interventions have incorporated communication skills training, demonstrating feasibility, acceptability, and effectiveness across clinical settings. In one study, 30 lung cancer clinicians who participated in 2.25 hours of didactic communication training reported increased self-efficacy in communicating empathically with individuals diagnosed with lung cancer [47]. In patient encounters, clinicians who participated in the training demonstrated improvement in empathic communication and stigma-mitigating skills; patients also reported higher satisfaction with clinician communication [48]. This empathic communication skills training module has been adapted for community-based settings, including Nigeria, in which 30 physicians and nurses reported higher self-efficacy and demonstrated more empathy and less blame toward lung cancer patients after the intervention [49]. An ongoing study will expand understanding of the intervention through comparison with usual care across a variety of US community oncology settings [50].

Caregiver-Focused Approaches

Caregivers and family members of individuals diagnosed with lung cancer also struggle with stigma and its consequences, including guilt, blame, and limited disclosure. Caregiver- and family-based interventions in the context of advanced lung cancer have shown promise in improving well-being, reducing distress, and reducing caregiving burden [51]. A family-centered approach was incorporated into modules of the Kentucky LEADS Collaborative Lung Cancer Care Survivorship Program, addressing lung cancer-specific stress and social support for caregivers and including activities that explored efforts to respond to stigmatizing comments and behaviors [52]. Early results demonstrated the feasibility of supporting caregivers with the interventional components, with over half of lung cancer survivors including caregivers (e.g., spouses, adult children, siblings) in their sessions; caregivers also participated in their own sessions focused on mitigating stigma and reducing caregiving stress [52]. GO2 for Lung Cancer also supports loved ones of individuals with lung cancer by offering educational and peer support resources focused on coping with stigma [53].

Societal Approaches

Effective large-scale and societal interventions are critical in the efforts to mitigate lung cancer stigma. Social stigma has a powerful influence on structural forces that shape lung cancer care, including advocacy, research funding, and health care policy. As lung cancer treatment has advanced and a growing community of survivors are joining advocacy movements, public awareness of lung cancer has also improved; data from 2018 indicated public awareness and media visibility of lung cancer had significantly increased since 10 years prior [7]. Large-scale advocacy has also included the Stigma and Nihilism Task Group of the American Cancer Society (ACS) National Lung Cancer Roundtable (NLRCT) [54]. This organization, comprised of multidisciplinary lung cancer researchers, clinicians, and patient advocates, is focused on developing and utilizing evidence-based strategies to mitigate social stigma. One initiative, the NLCRT Campaign to End Lung Cancer Stigma, has enacted media training for advocates to enhance lung cancer awareness and disseminated an online version of the training [54, 55]. The Campaign has also developed a Communications Assessment Tool to assist content developers with non-stigmatizing and non-blaming language, images, and context [56]. Finally, driven by advocates, the International Association for the Study of Lung Cancer (IASLC) published guidance on preferred language for oral and written communications [57]. This guide includes a focus on non-stigmatizing language, with encouraging rates of adaptation among conference presenters [58]. Other large-scale efforts have included anti-stigma media campaigns, including Lung Foundation Australia "Free from Stigma!" effort, as well as Lung Cancer Canada's "Stop Asking the Wrong Question" campaign focused on reducing blame and increasing compassion for individuals diagnosed with lung cancer [59, 60].

Conclusion

The hypothetical vignette of Mr. S. helps to illustrate the deleterious consequences of lung cancer stigma, but it also highlights the importance of effective stigma-reduction efforts. Recent years have demonstrated immense progress in addressing lung cancer stigma, but more work is needed. Figure 1.1 illustrates key interventional needs across multiple levels. In particular, it will be important for larger-scale studies to extend pilot findings of stigma-reducing interventions and demonstrate utility across multiple clinical care and behavioral outcomes [61]. Reviewing effective social stigma reduction campaigns in other health domains is also useful for establishing best practices for clinical care and interventions. Finally, expanding and supporting the efforts of multiple stakeholders in lung cancer care, including survivors, families, clinicians, researchers, policymakers, communicators, and other advocates, are crucial components of future success. Ultimately, it takes a coordinated effort to effectively address stigma and reduce the burden of lung cancer.

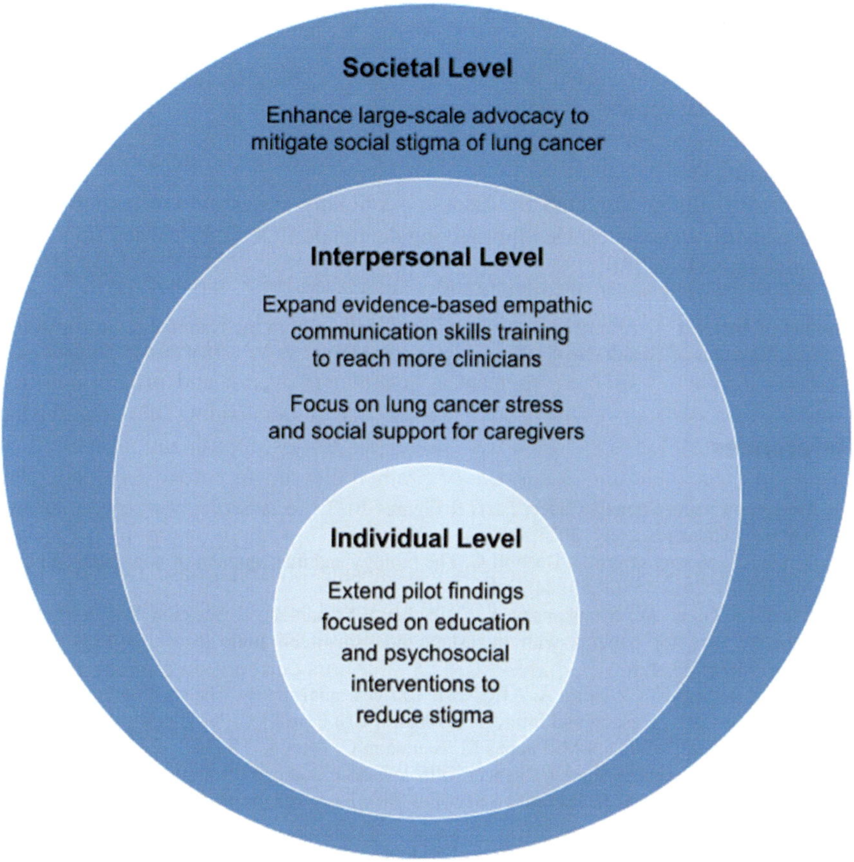

Fig. 1.1 Key interventional needs to address lung cancer stigma across individual, interpersonal, and societal levels

Key Takeaways

- Recent years have ushered in substantial advances in lung cancer detection, treatment, and supportive care. However, the promise of reduced lung cancer burden cannot be fully realized until barriers to care are addressed.
- Lung cancer stigma, the experience and internalization of negative appraisal and devaluation from others, is a significant barrier to optimal lung cancer care.
- Important efforts to reduce lung cancer stigma focus on intrapersonal, interpersonal (family, clinicians), and societal levels.
- Expanded efforts in research, clinical care, and policy are needed to further address lung cancer stigma.

Key Readings and Resources

- A 10-year cross-sectional analysis of public, oncologist, and patient attitudes about lung cancer and associated stigma [7]
- Multilevel opportunities to address lung cancer stigma across the cancer control continuum [18]
- Reducing stigma triggered by assessing smoking status among patients diagnosed with lung cancer: De-stigmatizing do and don't lessons learned from qualitative interviews [36]

Conflict of Interest Dr. Hamann receives research funding from the National Cancer Institute/National Institutes of Health. No Conflict of Interest reported.

References

1. American Cancer Society. Cancer Facts & Figures 2023: special section: lung cancer. Atlanta: American Cancer Society; 2023.
2. Herbst RS, Morgensztern D, Boshoff C. The biology and management of non-small cell lung cancer. NPJ. 2018;553(7689):446–54.
3. Temel JS, Greer JA, Muzikansky A, Gallagher ER, Admane S, Jackson VA, et al. Early palliative care for patients with metastatic non–small-cell lung cancer. N Engl J Med. 2010;363(8):733–42.
4. Vachani A, Sequist LV, Spira A. AJRCCM: 100-year anniversary. The shifting landscape for lung cancer: past, present, and future. Am J Respir Crit Care Med. 2017;195(9):1150–60.
5. Humphrey LL, Deffebach M, Pappas M, Baumann C, Artis K, Mitchell JP, Zakher B, Fu R, Slatore CG. Screening for lung cancer with low-dose computed tomography: a systematic review to update the U.S. Preventive Services Task Force recommendation. Ann Intern Med. 2013;159(6):411.
6. Gandhi L, Rodríguez-Abreu D, Gadgeel S, Esteban E, Felip E, De Angelis F, Domine M, Clingan P, Hochmair MJ, Powell SF, Cheng SY, Bischoff HG, Peled N, Grossi F, Jennens RR, Reck M, Hui R, Garon EB, Boyer M, Rubio-Viqueira B, Novello S, Kurata T, Gray JE, Vida J, Wei Z, Yang Z, Raftopoulos H, Garassino MC. Pembrolizumab plus chemotherapy in metastatic non–small-cell lung cancer. N Engl J Med. 2018;378:NEJMoa1801005.
7. Rigney M, Rapsomaniki E, Carter-Harris L, King JC. A 10-year cross-sectional analysis of public, oncologist, and patient attitudes about lung cancer and associated stigma. J Thorac Oncol. 2021;16(1):151–5.
8. Gilchrist A, Joszt L, Kennelty G, Shaffer AT, Urciuoli B. Lending a hand: lung cancer advocacy groups help those in need. 2016. https://www.curetoday.com/publications/cure/2016/lung-2016-2/lending-a-hand-lung-cancer-advocacy-groups-help-those-in-need. Accessed 25 Feb 2018.
9. Jemal A, Fedewa SA. Lung cancer screening with low-dose computed tomography in the United States-2010 to 2015. JAMA Oncol. 2017;3(9):1278–81.
10. Yates P, Schofield P, Zhao I, Currow D. Supportive and palliative care for lung cancer patients. J Thorac Dis. 2013;5(Suppl 5):S623–8.
11. Ganti AK, Hirsch FR, Wynes MW, Ravelo A, Ramalingam SS, Ionescu-Ittu R, Pivneva I, Borghaei H. Access to cancer specialist care and treatment in patients with advanced stage lung cancer. Clin Lung Cancer. 2017;18(6):640–650.e2.
12. Lim C, Tsao MS, Le LW, Shepherd FA, Feld R, Burkes RL, Liu G, Kamel-Reid S, Hwang D, Tanguay J, da Cunha Santos G, Leighl NB. Biomarker testing and time to treatment decision in patients with advanced non small-cell lung cancer. Ann Oncol. 2015;26(7):1415–21.

13. Gutierrez ME, Choi K, Lanman RB, Licitra EJ, Skrzypczak SM, Pe Benito R, Wu T, Arunajadai S, Kaur S, Harper H, Pecora AL, Schultz EV, Goldberg SL. Genomic profiling of advanced non–small cell lung cancer in community settings: gaps and opportunities. Clin Lung Cancer. 2017;18(6):651–9.
14. Lond B, Dodd C, Davey Z, Darlison L, McPhelim J, Rawlinson J, Williamson I, Merriman C, Waddington F, Bagnallainslie D, Rajendran B, Usman J, Henshall C. A systematic review of the barriers and facilitators impacting patient enrolment in clinical trials for lung cancer. Eur J Oncol Nurs. 2024;70:102564. https://doi.org/10.1016/j.ejon.2024.102564.
15. Kumar P, Casarett D, Corcoran A, Desai K, Li Q, Chen J, Langer C, Mao JJ. Utilization of supportive and palliative care services among oncology outpatients at one academic cancer center: determinants of use and barriers to access. J Palliat Med. 2018;18(6):651–9.
16. Cheville AL, Rhudy L, Basford JR, Griffin JM, Flores AM. How receptive are patients with late stage cancer to rehabilitation services and what are the sources of their resistance? Arch Phys Med Rehabil. 2017;98(2):203–10.
17. Kamath SD, Kircher SM, Benson AB. Comparison of cancer burden and nonprofit organization funding reveals disparities in funding across cancer types. J Natl Compr Canc Netw. 2019;17(7):849–54.
18. Hamann HA, Ver Hoeve ES, Carter-Harris L, Studts JL, Ostroff JS. Multilevel opportunities to address lung cancer stigma across the cancer control continuum. J Thorac Oncol. 2018;13(8):1062–75.
19. Goffman E. Stigma; notes on the management of spoiled identity. Englewood Cliffs: Prentice Hall; 1963.
20. Man Brakel WH. Measuring health-related stigma-a literature review. Psychol Health Med. 2006;11(3):307–34.
21. Hamann HA, Howell LA, McDonald JL. Causal attributions and attitudes toward lung cancer. J Appl Soc Psychol. 2013;43(S1):E37–45. https://doi.org/10.1080/13548500600595160.
22. Bell K, Salmon A, Bowers M, Bell J, McCullough L. Smoking, stigma and tobacco "denormalization": further reflections on the use of stigma as a public health tool. A commentary on Social Science & Medicine's Stigma, Prejudice, Discrimination and Health Special Issue (67: 3). Soc Sci Med. 2010;70(6):795–9. https://doi.org/10.1016/j.socscimed.2009.09.060.
23. Bayer R, Stuber J. Tobacco control, stigma, and public health: rethinking the relations. Am J Public Health. 2006;96(1):47–50. https://doi.org/10.2105/AJPH.2005.071886.
24. Hamann HA, Ostroff JS, Marks EG, Gerber DE, Schiller JH, Lee SJC. Stigma among patients with lung cancer: a patient-reported measurement model. Psychooncology. 2014;23(1):81–92. https://doi.org/10.1002/pon.3371.
25. Kaplan DM, Hamann HA, Price SN, Williamson TJ, Ver Hoeve ES, McConnell MH, Duchschere JE, Garland LL, Ostroff JS. Developing an ACT-based intervention to address lung cancer stigma: stakeholder recommendations and feasibility testing in two NCI-designated cancer centers. J Psychosoc Oncol. 2023;41(1):59–75. https://doi.org/10.1080/07347332.2022.2033377.
26. Bédard S, Sasewich H, Culling J, Turner SR, Pellizzari J, Johnson S, Bédard ELR. Stigma in early-stage lung cancer. Ann Behav Med. 2022;56(12):1272–83. https://doi.org/10.1093/abm/kaac021.
27. Hamann HA, Shen MJ, Thomas AJ, Lee SJC, Ostroff JS. Development and preliminary psychometric evaluation of a patient-reported outcome measure for lung cancer stigma: the lung cancer stigma inventory (LCSI). Stigma Heal. 2017;
28. Cataldo JK, Slaughter R, Jahan TM, Pongquan VL, Hwang WJ. Measuring stigma in people with lung cancer: psychometric testing of the Cataldo lung cancer stigma scale. Oncol Nurs Forum. 2011;38(1):E46–54. https://doi.org/10.1188/11.ONF.E46-E54.
29. Carter-Harris L, Davis LL, Rawl SM. Lung cancer screening participation: developing a conceptual model to guide research. Res Theory Nurs Pract. 2016;30(4):333–52. https://doi.org/10.1891/1541-6577.30.4.333.

30. Rose S, Boyes A, Kelly B, Cox M, Palazzi K, Paul C. Lung cancer stigma is a predictor for psychological distress: a longitudinal study. Lung cancer stigma is a predictor for psychological distress. Psychooncology. 2021;30(7):1137–44. https://doi.org/10.1002/pon.5665.
31. Price SN, Shen M, Rigney M, Ostroff JS, Hamann HA. Identifying barriers to advocacy among patients with lung cancer: the role of stigma-related interpersonal constraint. Oncol Nurs Forum. 2022;49(6):553–63. https://doi.org/10.1188/22.ONF.553-563.
32. Dirkse D, Lamont L, Li Y, Simonič A, Bebb G, Giese-Davis J. Shame, guilt, and communication in lung cancer patients and their partners. Curr Oncol. 2014;21(5):718. https://doi.org/10.3747/co.21.2034.
33. Carter-Harris L, Hermann CP, Schreiber J, Weaver MT, Rawl SM. Lung cancer stigma predicts timing of medical help seeking behavior. Oncol Nurs Forum. 2014;41:E203–10. https://doi.org/10.1188/14.ONF.E203-E210.
34. Weiss J, Stephenson BJ, Edwards LJ, Rigney M, Copeland A. Public attitudes about lung cancer: stigma, support, and predictors of support. J Multidiscip Healthc. 2014;7:293–300. https://doi.org/10.2147/JMDH.S65153.
35. Shen MJ, Hamann HA, Thomas AJ, Ostroff JS. Association between patient-provider communication and lung cancer stigma. Support Care Cancer. 2016;24(5):2093–9. https://doi.org/10.1007/s00520-015-3014-0.
36. Ostroff JS, Banerjee SC, Lynch K, Shen MJ, Williamson TJ, Haque N, Riley K, Hamann HA, Rigney M, Park B. Reducing stigma triggered by assessing smoking status among patients diagnosed with lung cancer: de-stigmatizing do and don't lessons learned from qualitative interviews. PEC Innov. 2022;1:100025. https://doi.org/10.1016/j.pecinn.2022.100025.
37. Williamson TJ, Garon EB, Shapiro JR, Chavira DA, Goldman JW, Stanton AL. Facets of stigma, self-compassion, and health-related adjustment to lung cancer: a longitudinal study. Health Psychol. 2022;41(4):301–10. https://doi.org/10.1037/hea0001156.
38. Brown-Johnson CG, Berrean B, Cataldo JK. Development and usability evaluation of the mHealth tool for lung cancer (mHealth TLC): a virtual world health game for lung cancer patients. Patient Educ Couns. 2015;98(4):506–11. https://doi.org/10.1016/j.pec.2014.12.006.
39. Ye F, Wu Y. Impacts of self-confidence cultivation combined with family collaborative nursing on the hope level, stigma and exercise tolerance in patients undergoing radical resection of pulmonary carcinoma. Front Surg. 2023;10 https://doi.org/10.3389/fsurg.2023.1095647.
40. Chambers SK, Morris BA, Clutton S, Foley E, Giles L, Schofield P, O'Connell D, Dunn J. Psychological wellness and health-related stigma: a pilot study of an acceptance-focused cognitive behavioural intervention for people with lung cancer. Eur J Cancer Care (Engl). 2015;24(1):60–70. https://doi.org/10.1111/ecc.12221.
41. Tian X, Liao Z, Yi L, Tang L, Chen G, Jiménez Herrera MF. Efficacy and mechanisms of 4-week MBSR on psychological distress in lung cancer patients: a single-center, single-blind, longitudinal, randomized controlled trial. Asia Pac J Oncol Nurs. 2023;10(1):100151.
42. Williamson TJ, Brymwitt WM, Gilliland J, Carter-Bawa L, Mao JJ, Lynch KA, Emard N, Omachi S, Jacobs RL, Tefera MY, Reese MT, Ostroff JS. Mindful self-compassion for lung cancer (MSC-LC): incorporating perspectives of lung cancer patients, clinicians, and researchers to create an adapted intervention to reduce lung cancer stigma. Transl Behav Med. 2025;15(1):ibae074. https://doi.org/10.1093/tbm/ibae074.
43. Warren GW, Ward KD. Integration of tobacco cessation services into multidisciplinary lung cancer care: rationale, state of the art, and future directions. Transl Lung Cancer Res. 2015;4(4):339–52. https://doi.org/10.3978/j.issn.2218-6751.2015.07.15.
44. Stiefel F, Bourquin C. Adverse effects of "teachable moment" interventions in lung cancer: why prudence matters. J Thorac Oncol. 2018;13(2):151–3. https://doi.org/10.1016/j.jtho.2017.10.018.
45. Dresler C, Warren GW, Arenberg D, Yang P, Steliga MA, Cummings KM, Stone E, Jassem J. "Teachable moment" interventions in lung cancer: why action matters. J Thorac Oncol. 2018;13(5):603–5. https://doi.org/10.1016/j.jtho.2018.02.020.

46. Morse DS, Edwardsen EA, Gordon HS. Missed opportunities for interval empathy in lung cancer communication. Arch Intern Med. 2008;168(17):1853–8. https://doi.org/10.1001/archinte.168.17.1853.
47. Banerjee SC, Haque N, Bylund CL, Shen MJ, Rigney M, Hamann HA, Parker PA, Ostroff JS. Responding empathically to patients: a communication skills training module to reduce lung cancer stigma. Transl Behav Med. 2021;11(2):613–8.
48. Banerjee SC, Haque N, Schofield EA, Williamson TJ, Martin CM, Bylund CL, et al. Oncology care provider training in empathic communication skills to reduce lung cancer stigma. Chest. 2021;159(5):2040–9.
49. Banerjee SC, Asuzu C, Mapayi B, Olunloyo B, Odiaka E, Daramola OB, Gilliland J, Owoade IA, Kingham P, Alatise OI, Fitzgerald G, Kahn R, Olcese C, Ostroff JS. Feasibility, acceptability, and initial efficacy of empathic communication skills training to reduce lung cancer stigma in Nigeria: a pilot study. J Natl Cancer Inst Monogr. 2024;2024(63):30–7.
50. Banerjee SC, Malling CD, Schofield EA, Carter-Bawa L, Bylund CL, Hamann HA, et al. Empathic communication skills training to reduce lung cancer stigma: study protocol of a cluster randomized control trial. Contemp Clin Trials. 2024;145:107669.
51. Sun V, Grant M, Koczywas M, Freeman B, Zachariah F, Fujinami R, Del Ferraro C, Uman G, Ferrell B. Effectiveness of an interdisciplinary palliative care intervention for family caregivers in lung cancer. Cancer. 2015;121(20):3737–45. https://doi.org/10.1002/cncr.29567.
52. Studts J, Burris J, Andrykowski M, Schapmire T, Head B, Rigney M, Criswell A, Arnold S, Yates A, Blair C, Christian A. MA17.02 Early accrual to a precision lung cancer survivorship intervention: The Kentucky LEADS Collaborative Lung Cancer Survivorship Care Program. J Thorac Oncol. 2018;13(10):S415.
53. GO2 for Lung Cancer. Emotional support. 2025. https://go2.org/resources-and-support/emotional-support/. Accessed 16 Feb 2025.
54. Studts, JL, Carter-Bawa, L, Hamann, HA, Smith, RA, Kazerooni, EA, Rosenthal, LS. The changing lung cancer story: addressing survivorship, stigma, and nihilism to facilitate transformation. [Unpublished manuscript].
55. National Lung Cancer Roundtable. Campaign to end lung cancer stigma. 2022. https://nlcrt.org/wp-content/uploads/Campaign-to-End-LC-Stigma-Overview_Final-Draft_2022.pdf. Accessed 17 Mar 2025.
56. Carter-Bawa L, Ostroff JS, Hoover K, Studts JL. Effective communication about lung cancer screening without iatrogenic stigma: a brief report case study using the lung cancer stigma communications assessment tool of *LungTalk*. JTO Clin Res Rep. 2023;4(11):100585. https://doi.org/10.1016/j.jtocrr.2023.100585.
57. International Association for the Study of Lung Cancer. Language guide. 2021. https://www.iaslc.org/IASLCLanguageGuide. Accessed 12 Mar 2025.
58. Lockstadt C, Feldman J, Studts JL, Ostroff JS, Liu L, Pasquinelli MM, Feldman LE. OA10.06 recognizing early adopters of non stigmatizing language at IASLC WCLC 2022. J Thorac Oncol. 2023;18(11):S67. https://doi.org/10.1016/j.jtho.2023.09.063.
59. Global Lung Cancer Coalition. Lung Foundation Australia launches new anti-stigma campaign. 2019. https://www.lungcancercoalition.org/2019/08/07/lung-foundation-australia-launches-new-anti-stigma-campaign/https://www.lungcancercoalition.org/2019/08/07/lung-foundation-australia-launches-new-anti-stigma-campaign/. Accessed 16 Feb 2025.
60. Lung Cancer Canada. Home—The wrong question. https://thewrongquestion.ca/. Accessed 16 Feb 2025.
61. Yamazaki-Tan J, Harrison NJ, Marshall H, Gartner C, Runge CE, Morphett K. Interventions to reduce lung cancer and COPD-related stigma: a systematic review. Ann Behav Med. 2024;58(11):729–40. https://doi.org/10.1093/abm/kaae048.

Open Access This chapter is licensed under the terms of the Creative Commons Attribution-NonCommercial 4.0 International License (http://creativecommons.org/licenses/by-nc/4.0/), which permits any noncommercial use, sharing, adaptation, distribution and reproduction in any medium or format, as long as you give appropriate credit to the original author(s) and the source, provide a link to the Creative Commons license and indicate if changes were made.

The images or other third party material in this chapter are included in the chapter's Creative Commons license, unless indicated otherwise in a credit line to the material. If material is not included in the chapter's Creative Commons license and your intended use is not permitted by statutory regulation or exceeds the permitted use, you will need to obtain permission directly from the copyright holder.

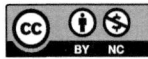

Advocacy for People at Risk or Living with Lung Cancer and Their Caregivers Across the Care Continuum

2

Danielle Hicks and Maureen Rigney

Contents

Navigation Vignette	13
Introduction	14
History of Lung Cancer Advocacy	14
The Role of Individual Advocacy in the Lung Cancer Journey	15
Key Points in the Lung Cancer Experience	16
How Navigators Can Foster Individual Advocacy	17
Practical Ways to Help	17
Role of Advocacy in Collaboration and Conflict	18
Education and Other Resources for the Lung Cancer Community	19
Conclusion	20
Key Takeaways	21
Key Readings and Resources	21
References	21

Navigation Vignette

In January 2013, a patient was incidentally diagnosed with Stage IV non-small cell lung cancer (NSCLC), specifically EGFR-mutated adenocarcinoma. Early on, they connected with the Bonnie J. Addario Lung Cancer Foundation, now GO2 for Lung Cancer, where they received essential patient navigation services, including

D. Hicks (✉)
GO2 for Lung Cancer, San Carlos, CA, USA
e-mail: dhicks@go2.org

M. Rigney
GO2 for Lung Cancer, Washington, DC, USA
e-mail: Mrigney@go2.org

© The Author(s) 2026
J. T. Fathi, M. F. Mortman (eds.), *Lung Cancer Navigation and Care*,
https://doi.org/10.1007/978-3-032-02200-4_2

one-on-one support, oncology consultation guidance, monthly educational programming through the Lung Cancer Living Room series, and evidence-based, easy to understand educational treatment resources. Following a positive therapeutic response, the patient transitioned into advocacy, serving as a peer support mentor in the Phone Buddy Program, a scientific reviewer for the Department of Defense Lung Cancer Research Program, and an advisor for palliative care initiatives, healthcare professionals, and industry partners. Additionally, they shared their personal experience through print and video across varying platforms and led veteran outreach efforts for lung cancer screening. Key factors in their long-term survival included active engagement in treatment planning, participation in clinical trials, a multidisciplinary care approach, and ongoing patient education. Their case highlights the vital role of patient empowerment, psychosocial support, and peer connections in improving outcomes for advanced lung cancer. More than a decade post-diagnosis, they remain a powerful example of extended survival and the importance of comprehensive patient support. Their continued advocacy demonstrates the profound impact of education and community on people diagnosed with lung cancer, offering hope and improving engagement in the treatment decision-making process. Patient navigation played a central role in facilitating timely access to care, demystifying complex treatment options, and sustaining the patient's long-term engagement throughout their cancer journey.

Introduction

Individual advocacy is a testament to human resilience, compassion, and collective action. For decades, the lung cancer community has faced a disease fraught with medical complexity [1], social stigma [2], and emotional challenges [3]. From such personal struggles and collective determination, individual advocacy in lung cancer was born.

Despite great treatment advances that allow people to live with lung cancer longer than ever before [4], medical nihilism persists [5]. Too often marginalized by societal perceptions that closely link lung cancer to cigarette smoking [6], those diagnosed can face a variety of additional challenges as well [7]. However, dedicated individuals have long refused to accept the lung cancer status quo. Through educating themselves, creating networks of support, and driving research funding and advancements in early detection and treatment, advocates have transformed the lung cancer experience.

History of Lung Cancer Advocacy

At one time, lung cancer was a rare disease [8]. Even as incidence increased, lung cancer was no more stigmatized than other types of cancer. The 1964 Surgeon General's report, *Smoking and Health* [9], which definitively linked tobacco use to an increased risk for lung cancer, changed that. Subsequent public health efforts to highlight the dangers of cigarettes, decrease initiation of smoking, and encourage cessation were successful but also had unintended consequences [10].

Even as tobacco companies employed strategies to increase the addictiveness of cigarettes and targeted vulnerable populations [11], tobacco control efforts, like public smoking bans, fostered negative assumptions about those who smoked [10]. With the close link between smoking history and the development of lung cancer, those diagnosed also came to be viewed negatively and often blamed for causing their disease [5].

Chapter 1 on stigma explores the full impact of lung cancer stigma in more depth, including reluctance to disclose the diagnosis and isolation. Coupled with decades of low survival rates, stigma-related factors have had profound effects on advocacy, both individual and public health (Chap. 22) in lung cancer. The breast cancer community shaped early advocacy efforts. As notable women began to speak out about breast cancer, organizations spearheaded work to destigmatize the words "cancer" and "breast." Championing early detection, increasing research funding, and highlighting survivorship led to awareness, more treatment options, and improved survival rates [12].

Similar to other cancer communities, the lung cancer community began to coalesce. By the late 1990s, organizations such as the Lung Cancer Alliance and the Bonnie J. Addario Lung Cancer Foundation (now GO2 for Lung Cancer) [13] proved foundational in challenging public perceptions of the disease. As advocacy efforts worked to shift the lung cancer experience from one of shame and blame to compassion [14], there was also a focus on fostering a better understanding of the disease and finding new, innovative treatments. Other critical inflection points in the lung cancer movement included the validation of decreased disease mortality through the use of low-dose CT scans to screen for lung cancer [15] and the Medicare coverage decision in 2015 that expanded access to lifesaving screening [16]. As public health advocates raised awareness, demanded increased research funding, and brought people together, those living with and at risk for lung cancer and their loved ones became empowered to learn more, connect more, and expect more. Individual advocacy is an important vehicle for making "more" happen.

The Role of Individual Advocacy in the Lung Cancer Journey

Advocacy serves as a bridge between the unknown and the known. It extends far beyond understanding the disease and treatment options and can transform the lung cancer experience. From recognition of risk and adoption of screening through diagnosis, treatment and survivorship, individual advocacy can help meet the often complex physical, emotional, and practical needs of the lung cancer community. It can also create order and provide direction in the midst of often overwhelming situations [17]. Across the spectrum, key points often evoke strong emotional reactions. It is critical that those affected understand their options for psychosocial support as well.

Key Points in the Lung Cancer Experience

Critical points in lung cancer risk, diagnosis, and treatment experience require navigation skills. Initially, understanding risk, current screening criteria, physician referral, the scan process, and interpreting results is important. When nodules are found, individuals need to be aware of the need for ongoing monitoring and follow-up. The diagnostic process requires numerous tests and scans, bringing the need to understand complex medical information and results. Upon diagnosis, comprehending potential treatment options, including clinical trials, possible biomarker testing and results, is critical to making informed decisions. Throughout treatment, patients benefit from recognizing the value of palliative care for symptom management and adapting to potential treatment changes as their situation evolves. As treatment continues or concludes, managing the late and long-term effects becomes increasingly important for quality of life. Finally, patients and families may need to understand and access end-of-life services and support, requiring thoughtful consideration of preferences, values, and available resources. Barriers and motivators to individual advocacy are outlined in Tables 2.1 and 2.2.

Table 2.1 Potential barriers to becoming an individual lung cancer advocate

Barrier	Description
Limited health literacy	Difficulty understanding medical terminology and concepts necessary for effective advocacy
Cultural differences	Differing perspectives on cancer, treatment, and communication styles and methods
Emotional distress	Psychosocial effects of diagnosis and survivorship
Stigma	Reluctance to disclose diagnosis and withdrawal from others due to perceived judgment
Survivor guilt	Minimization of personal experiences with cancer when compared to others
Healthcare system navigation	Difficulty managing complex healthcare processes and systems
Financial and insurance burden	Managing practical effects of a cancer diagnosis and treatments

Table 2.2 Personal motivators to individual advocacy in lung cancer

Motivator	Description
Direct experience	Personal diagnosis or close relationship with someone affected by lung cancer
Family history	Genetic predisposition or multiple family members affected by lung cancer
Professional experience	Healthcare professionals with experience working with the lung cancer community
Policy background	Experience in health policy and an understanding of systemic issues
Altruistic drive	Desire to improve others' lives through volunteering, public health advocacy, and sharing stories of hope

How Navigators Can Foster Individual Advocacy

The journey to becoming an individual advocate is deeply personal, motivated by individual experiences, and driven by compassion. It is often the result of the powerful intersection of personal passion, medical understanding, and community support.

Respecting personal autonomy means honoring individual choices, preferences, and personal boundaries. While not everyone has the interest or capacity to advocate in all aspects of their care or that of a loved one, all can be empowered to do so in the ways most meaningful to them. Lung cancer navigators are critical partners in the advocacy journey.

Through empowering individuals to become educated on lung cancer, navigate the healthcare system, communicate effectively, and access support and education, navigators can help transform people with lung cancer and their loved ones into strong advocates who can influence not only their own outcomes but those for the broader lung cancer community.

The goal of this section is to provide tools to help support self-advocacy

Practical Ways to Help

Lung Cancer Education

The areas of lung cancer risk, early detection, diagnosis and treatment options are increasingly complicated, and it would be unrealistic to expect a lay person to understand it all. However, individual advocacy does require a basic understanding of lung cancer.

Support can be provided by distributing reader-friendly educational materials that address informational needs across the disease spectrum from GO2 for Lung Cancer and other organizations.

Advocacy Skills Development and Education

Navigators can create lists of training opportunities to provide advocates. Non-profit organizations such as the Patient Advocacy Foundation (PAF) and the National Coalition for Cancer Survivors (NCCS) may be helpful for general patient advocacy training. Major universities and cancer centers also may offer in-person and virtual self-advocacy and navigation training. For those serious about becoming certified advocates, see the Patient Advocate Certification Board and the Association of Oncology Nurse and Patient Navigators (AONN+).

Specialized advocacy trainings are also available, such as the financial advocacy boot camp training offered by the Association of Cancer Care Centers (ACCC) and research training opportunities provided by Friends of Cancer Research (FCR) and the American Association for Cancer Research (AACR).

Engagement Opportunities

Connecting with others affected by lung cancer and advocacy organizations is a great way to help with self-advocacy. Through these connections, individuals impacted by lung cancer can become more educated and find emotional support. Some will benefit from multiple types of connections, while others may have no interest or find one type to be enough. Recognizing and respecting individual differences is key.

Engagement Activity Examples

- Attending or starting in-person or virtual lung cancer-specific support groups
- Attending conferences, such as those from the World Conference on Lung Cancer (sponsored by the International Association for the Study of Lung Cancer), the American Society of Clinical Oncology, and the American Cancer Society's National Lung Cancer Roundtable that include patient-centered content and training.
- Participating in lung cancer awareness events, virtually and in-person
- Sharing their stories online and at events
- Volunteering to connect with and support others through online platforms and 1:1 mentoring programs

By addressing these multifaceted needs, advocacy transforms the lung cancer patient's journey from an isolating medical challenge to a supported, empowered experience of comprehensive care and hope. As a navigator, you serve as both a resource for available services and programs as well as a role model others can follow.

Role of Advocacy in Collaboration and Conflict

Individual lung cancer advocacy plays a crucial role in working toward resolving systemic conflicts through collaborations. In collaboration, advocates can work to alleviate conflict by bridging the gaps between patients, healthcare providers, researchers, policymakers, and support organizations, fostering collaboration to improve access to care, research funding, public awareness, and reducing stigma. By sharing first-hand experiences and raising their voices, they help remove conflicts and align efforts across different sectors, ensuring that patient-centered perspectives are considered in decision-making.

Funding Disparities

Lung cancer patients and caregivers play a vital role in advocating for increased federal funding for research by sharing their individual experiences, engaging with policymakers, and raising public awareness. Their unique perspectives and first-hand experiences make a powerful case for why more funding is needed. This can be accomplished by sharing those experiences, meeting with lawmakers, and participating with advocacy organizations to lobby for increased federal funding and policy changes.

Stigma Public Perception

Lung cancer patients and caregivers can also play a crucial role in reducing the stigma associated with the disease by raising awareness, challenging misconceptions, and fostering a more compassionate and informed public perspective. Again, by sharing personal stories and lived experiences, advocating for public awareness, engaging with media and healthcare providers, supporting others diagnosed with lung cancer, and challenging misinformation, can humanize the disease, breakdown stereotypes, and inspire greater understanding and empathy within their communities.

Access to Quality Treatment and Trials

Lung cancer patients and caregivers can advocate for access to quality care by taking an active role in influencing healthcare policies, raising awareness, and ensuring that all patients receive timely, effective, and compassionate treatment. This can again be accomplished by educating and empowering others in your community, speaking to elected officials and policymakers, holding healthcare systems accountable by speaking up about delays in diagnosis, lack of access to biomarker testing, and limited treatment options, and providing lived experience feedback about gaps in care.

Through these efforts, lung cancer patients can play a powerful role in changing the narrative, promoting compassion, and ensuring that all individuals, regardless of income, location, or background, have access to the highest quality care possible and receive the support and respect they deserve.

Education and Other Resources for the Lung Cancer Community

GO2 for Lung Cancer offers a wide variety of educational materials and support programs for people living with and at risk for lung cancer, which you can review at go2.org. We often field inquiries from people in need of practical resources. Our top

Table 2.3 Financial and practical resources for lung cancer patients

Need category	Resource	Description
Insurance issues	Patient Advocate Foundation	Provides case management services and financial aid to Americans with chronic, life-threatening, and debilitating illnesses
Legal and practical concerns	Triage Cancer	Offers education on legal and practical issues that may impact individuals diagnosed with cancer
Employment issues	Cancer and Careers	Empowers and educates people with cancer to thrive in their workplace by providing expert advice, interactive tools, and educational events
Co-pay assistance	Fundfinder	A resource to find financial assistance and to receive alerts when a copayment assistance fund opens up
Transportation assistance	Mercy Medical Angels	Offers medical transportation assistance by air and ground to patients in financial need
Mortgage or rental assistance	Varies	If available, operates at the city, county, or state level
	United Way	Helps people across the USA and Canada find local resources, including housing assistance programs
Energy assistance	Low Income Home Energy Assistance Program (LIHEAP) Clearinghouse	Helps keep families safe and healthy through initiatives that assist families with energy costs

referrals are listed in Table 2.3. If you need more information, or we can help in any way, please call our helpline at 800-298-2436 or email support@go2.org.

A well-established and growing body of professional and patient advocacy organizations, like the American Cancer Society, American Lung Association, and LUNGevity, and specific genetic mutation advocacy groups, also provide support and resources for lung cancer patients.

Conclusion

Individual advocacy for lung cancer represents a powerful force for change that evolves from personal struggles and collective determination. It bridges the gaps between support, knowledge and action, empowering individuals to take control of their health, access critical resources, and demand systemic change. Through education, support, and persistent engagement with healthcare providers, healthcare systems, and policymakers, advocates have transformed the lung cancer experience despite persistent stigma and historical challenges. As navigators empower patients and caregivers with knowledge, skills, and connections, they help create advocates who can influence their own outcomes as well as the outcomes of those in the broader lung cancer community. By addressing funding disparities, challenging public misconceptions, and working to ensure access to quality care for all, individual advocates serve as bridges between patients, healthcare providers, researchers, and policymakers. This collaborative approach to advocacy continues to drive progress in research, treatment options, and supportive services, offering hope to all those affected by lung cancer regardless of their background or circumstances.

Key Takeaways

- Navigators serve critical roles as guides, champions, role models, and facilitators to people affected by lung cancer.
- Navigators are invaluable in providing the education, support, and resources needed by lung cancer community members to become self-advocates.
- Patient advocates improve their own outcomes and future outcomes for anyone diagnosed with this disease.

Key Readings and Resources

- Becoming a Self-Advocate [18].
- Oncology Nurses' Role in Promoting Patient Self-Advocacy [19].
- Seasoned Navigator: A Case Study on Patient Advocacy/Patient Empowerment [20].
- Self-Advocacy Skills for Patients [21].

Conflict of Interest No Conflicts of Interest

References

1. Connor SR, Pyenson B, Fitch K, Spence C, Iwasaki K. Comparing hospice and nonhospice patient survival among patients who die within a three-year window. J Pain Symptom Manag. 2007;33(3):238–46.
2. Hamann HA, Williamson TJ, Studts JL, Ostroff JS. Lung cancer stigma then and now: continued challenges amid a landscape of progress. J Thorac Oncol. 2021;16(1):17–20.
3. Zabora J, BrintzenhofeSzoc K, Curbow B, Hooker C, Piantadosi S. The prevalence of psychological distress by cancer site. Psychooncology. 2001;10(1):19–28.
4. Vavala T, Rigney M, Reale ML, Novello S, King JC. An examination of two dichotomies: women with lung cancer and living with lung cancer as a chronic disease. Respirology. 2020;25(Suppl 2):24–36.
5. Chambers SK, Dunn J, Occhipinti S, Hughes S, Baade P, Sinclair S, et al. A systematic review of the impact of stigma and nihilism on lung cancer outcomes. BMC Cancer. 2012;12:184.
6. Stuber J, Galea S, Link B G. Stigma and smoking: the consequences of our good intentions. Soc Serv Rev. 2009;83(4):585–609.
7. Sanders SL, Bantum EO, Owen JE, Thornton AA, Stanton AL. Supportive care needs in patients with lung cancer. Psychooncology. 2010;19(5):480–9.

8. Witschi H. A short history of lung cancer. Toxicol Sci. 2001;64(1):4–6.
9. United States Department of Health Education and Welfare. Smoking and health: report of the advisory committee to the surgeon general. Washington: U.S. Government Printing Office, 1964.
10. Kim SH, Shanahan J. Stigmatizing smokers: public sentiment toward cigarette smoking and its relationship to smoking behaviors. J Health Commun. 2003;8(4):343–67.
11. United States Public Health Service. Office of the Surgeon General. How tobacco smoke causes disease: the biology and behavioral basis for smoking-attributable disease: a report of the Surgeon General. Rockville/Washington, DC: U.S. Dept. of Health and Human Services, Public Health Service For sale by the Supt. of Docs., U.S. G.P.O.; 2010. p. 704.
12. Braun S. The history of breast cancer advocacy. Breast J. 2003;9(s2):S101–S3.
13. Ambrose LF. History of Lung Cancer Alliance (LCA) 2019. Available from: https://go2.org/about-us/our-history/history-of-lung-cancer-alliance/.
14. Elliott S. Cancer campaign tries using shock to change attitudes. The New York Times. 7/9/2012.
15. Aberle DR, Adams AM, Berg CD, Black WC, Clapp JD, Fagerstrom RM, et al. Reduced lung-cancer mortality with low-dose computed tomographic screening. N Engl J Med. 2011;365(5):395–409.
16. Centers for Medicare and Medicaid Services. Screening for Lung Cancer with Low Dose Computed Tomography (LDCT). 2015. Available from: https://www.cms.gov/medicare-coverage-database/view/ncacal-decision-memo.aspx?proposed=N&ncaid=274.
17. Hagan TL, Donovan HS. Self-advocacy and cancer: a concept analysis. J Adv Nurs. 2013;69(10):2348–59. U.S Department of Health Education and Welfare, Public Health Service.
18. National Coalition for Cancer Survivorship. Becoming a Self-Advocate. 2025. Available from: https://canceradvocacy.org/resources/publications/self-advocacy/becoming-a-self-advocate/.
19. Alsbrook KE, Donovan HS, Wesmiller SW, Hagan TT. Oncology nurses' role in promoting patient self-advocacy. Clin J Oncol Nurs. 2022;26(3):239–43.
20. Bellomo C, Christensen D, Strusowski T. Seasoned navigator: a case study on patient advocacy/patient empowerment. J Oncol Navig Surviv [Internet]. 2016;7(8). Available from: https://www.jons-online.com.
21. Oncology Nurses Society. Episode 235: self-advocacy skills for patients 2025. Available from: https://www.ons.org/education-hub/oncology-nursing-podcast/episode-235-self-advocacy-skills-patients.

Open Access This chapter is licensed under the terms of the Creative Commons Attribution-NonCommercial 4.0 International License (http://creativecommons.org/licenses/by-nc/4.0/), which permits any noncommercial use, sharing, adaptation, distribution and reproduction in any medium or format, as long as you give appropriate credit to the original author(s) and the source, provide a link to the Creative Commons license and indicate if changes were made.

The images or other third party material in this chapter are included in the chapter's Creative Commons license, unless indicated otherwise in a credit line to the material. If material is not included in the chapter's Creative Commons license and your intended use is not permitted by statutory regulation or exceeds the permitted use, you will need to obtain permission directly from the copyright holder.

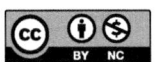

Navigation in Lung Cancer Prevention, Detection, and Care

3

Meg Fay Mortman, Angela Gonnella, and Linda Fleisher

Contents

Navigation Vignette	24
Introduction	24
History of Nurse and Patient Navigation and Where We Are Today	25
Navigation Across the Care Continuum	26
Community Outreach and Engagement	28
Conclusion	30
Key Takeaways	31
Key Readings and Resources	31
References	31

Abbreviations

CHW	Community health worker
LCS	Lung cancer screening
NSCLC	Non-small cell lung cancer
SCLC	Small cell lung cancer

M. F. Mortman (✉) · A. Gonnella
GO2 for Lung Cancer, Washington, DC, USA
e-mail: mmortman@go2.org; agonnella@go2.org

L. Fleisher
Fox Chase Cancer Center, Philadelphia, PA, USA
e-mail: linda.fleisher@fccc.edu

© The Author(s) 2026
J. T. Fathi, M. F. Mortman (eds.), *Lung Cancer Navigation and Care*,
https://doi.org/10.1007/978-3-032-02200-4_3

Navigation Vignette

Mrs. E. is a 64-year-old woman with a 25-pack-year history (smoked one pack per day for more than 25 years) and quit 10 years ago. She began exercising regularly at the local community center and attended a health information session provided by a local community health worker (CHW). Based on many conversations with the CHW, she decided to contact her primary care physician about lung cancer screening (LCS). She received an order and called the local hospital's LCS program, where she spoke with the LCS program navigator. The LCS navigator assisted Mrs. E. with her appointment and discussed the risks and benefits of screening, her medical history, and the overall screening process. Mrs. E. was provided information about what to expect during the scan, the possible results, and potential next steps if anything was found on the exam. A 1 cm irregular nodule was found. Mrs. E. received a call from the LCS program navigator to assist in scheduling appointments with her primary care physician and an interventional pulmonologist, who oversees the screening program. Mrs. E. was referred for several tests, and the LCS program navigator supported her through the diagnostic work-up, educating her about each test, and facilitated her appointment scheduling. Ultimately, Mrs. E. was scheduled for surgery, and she received a diagnosis of Stage IA2 non-small cell lung cancer. Based on biomarker testing, she also learned that she had an EGFR mutation. As a result, she was referred to a medical oncologist for targeted medical therapy. Mrs. E.'s LCS program navigator connected her with the thoracic oncology navigator, who works with the medical oncologist. Mrs. E. was overwhelmed by the sheer number of appointments and tests required. The time spent waiting for results was especially anxiety-inducing. She had difficulty keeping track of her appointments and frequently called the navigator for clarification and reassurance. Mrs. E. felt valued and safe knowing she could call the navigator directly for any questions, from transportation concerns to test results to billing issues. The navigators always knew the answer or knew who to call. Mrs. E. is now 6 months out from surgery and is taking her targeted therapy at home. She follows her survivorship plan and knows that she will continue to be able to connect with her navigator regularly.

Introduction

Lung cancer remains the leading cause of cancer-related deaths, surpassing breast, colon, and prostate cancers combined, with an estimated 234,580 new cases in 2024 (116,310 in men and 118,270 in women) and approximately 125,070 deaths (65,790 in men and 59,280 in women) [1]. There are significant population-based inequities in access and uptake of LCS and unequal burden of lung cancer that impact treatment and survival outcomes among underserved (racial, ethnic, and geographic) and higher-risk populations (e.g., occupational exposure) [2].

Lung cancer disproportionately affects those who are impacted most by social determinants of health and historically marginalized communities, including Black, indigenous, and people of color. These communities are at greater lung cancer risk and have poorer treatment outcomes. Although Black men are 12% more likely to develop lung cancer compared to White men, they are less likely to be diagnosed with small cell lung cancer [1]. Despite this, Black men face a 40% higher mortality rate than White men, and Black populations overall experience disproportionately higher lung cancer mortality rates compared to other racial groups [2]. Black patients are less likely to be eligible for and receive LCS genetic testing for mutations, high-cost and systemic treatments, and surgical intervention compared to White patients [2]. While lung cancer rates have been dropping among men for decades, similar declines in women have only been observed more recently.

Hispanic and American Indian populations also experience higher lung cancer rates, often compounded by limited access to quality healthcare and socioeconomic barriers [3]. Individuals in low-income communities encounter numerous barriers to optimal lung cancer care, including reduced access to preventive screenings, limited healthcare resources, increased exposure to environmental carcinogens, less comprehensive health insurance coverage, and delays in diagnosis and treatment [4]. As such, rural and economically disadvantaged areas demonstrate markedly different lung cancer landscapes. Areas with higher concentrations of industrial and agricultural activities often report elevated lung cancer rates, reflecting prolonged environmental exposure to hazardous substances [5].

People at high risk for lung cancer and who have experienced lung cancer would benefit from working with a navigator. Navigation has emerged as one of the most promising interventions for addressing disparities in health care, with growing evidence to support its impact [6–10]. Navigators, whether a nurse, social worker, or patient, can eliminate barriers to screening [10], reduce time to diagnosis [11], and improve outcomes [8, 10]. Lung cancer, a highly stigmatized disease, is preventable and curable when people receive timely, evidence-based, high-quality care.

History of Nurse and Patient Navigation and Where We Are Today

In the late 1980s, Dr. Harold Freeman championed the *American Cancer Society's National Hearings on Cancer in the Poor* [12] to better understand underserved patients' challenges. Through his practice treating breast cancer in Harlem, Dr. Freeman listened to the challenges his patients faced and, in 1990, the first patient navigation program providing free and reduced-cost screening and one-to-one navigation services. The principles that guided Dr. Freeman's navigation program guide key principles for navigation today (Table 3.1) [13].

From this early pioneering work of Dr. Freeman and over three decades of peer-reviewed research, program evaluation, and policy advocacy, patient navigation in oncology care has become an evidence-based asset to address cancer disparities across the continuum [14]. Today, oncology navigation is a recognized profession which serves a critical role in addressing barriers and facilitating the highest quality of care [15, 16]. Numerous collaborative initiatives [17] have been launched to support the professionalization of oncology navigation, including professional

Table 3.1 Navigation Principles

1. *Patient navigation is a patient-centric healthcare service delivery model.*
2. *Patient navigation serves to virtually integrate a fragmented healthcare system for the individual patient.*
3. *The core function of patient navigation is the elimination of barriers to timely care across all segments of the healthcare continuum.*
4. *Patient navigation should be defined with a clear scope of practice that distinguishes the role and responsibilities of the navigator from that of all other providers.*
5. *Delivery of patient navigation services should be cost-effective and commensurate with the training and skills necessary to navigate an individual through a particular phase of the care continuum.*
6. *The determination of who should navigate should be determined by the level of skills required at a given phase of navigation.*
7. *In a given system of care there is the need to define the point at which navigation begins and the point at which navigation ends.*
8. *There is a need to navigate patients across disconnected systems of care, such as primary care sites and tertiary care sites.*
9. *Patient Navigation systems require coordination.*

Printed with permission from Freeman and Rodriguez [13]

standards [18], role delineation [19], competencies and workforce training, and evaluation metrics [20, 21]. It is a recommended intervention by professional organizations. To guide the delineation of types of navigators, the Professional Oncology Navigation Task Force created consensus-driven standards providing definitions and scope of work for nurse, social work, and patient navigators [19, 22]. Key metrics for program evaluation [20, 21, 23] and more recent efforts for reimbursement are additional foundations to ensure the sustainability of oncology navigation [24–26].

Navigation Across the Care Continuum

Navigation can be integrated across the care continuum, including prevention, screening, diagnosis, treatment, and survivorship, with approaches tailored to meet the needs at each stage. This may be delivered by different professionals identifying and fulfilling the navigator role. Such professional types who serve in this navigator role may include CHWs, patients, nurses, social workers, advanced practice providers, and other allied health professionals. Some navigation programs incorporate multiple navigation roles, recognizing the distinct skills and responsibilities required at different points along the care continuum. For example, CHWs from diverse communities may assist community members in understanding the value of tobacco cessation, LCS, and help them access cessation and screening services. Patient navigators might focus on assisting patients in scheduling their screening appointments and addressing barriers to care, such as transportation or language barriers.

Nurse, advanced practice provider, and social work navigators might focus on ensuring patients have diagnostic work-up as quickly as possible and ensuring patients understand the importance of follow-up of abnormal results and navigating them through treatment, survivorship, and end-of-life.

Standards of Navigation

Navigator practice is guided by professional standards that define their role and direct training requirements. For oncology navigation, the *Professional Oncology Navigation Standards* provide detailed guidance on the training and roles and responsibilities [15, 17, 18]. In many states, CHWs must be certified through standard training. In addition, as navigation has grown and solidified as a profession, there are sub-specialties, such as financial and clinical trial navigation.

A key challenge in navigating the lung cancer care continuum is that screening, diagnostic evaluation, and treatment services are often provided at different locations and frequently by various organizations. This calls for navigators to collaborate closely with multidisciplinary teams, including community outreach programs, tobacco cessation specialists, and many clinical treatment teams. Clearly defining navigation goals at each stage of the care continuum is essential to designing an effective program with well-defined navigation roles and measurable outcomes (Fig. 3.1).

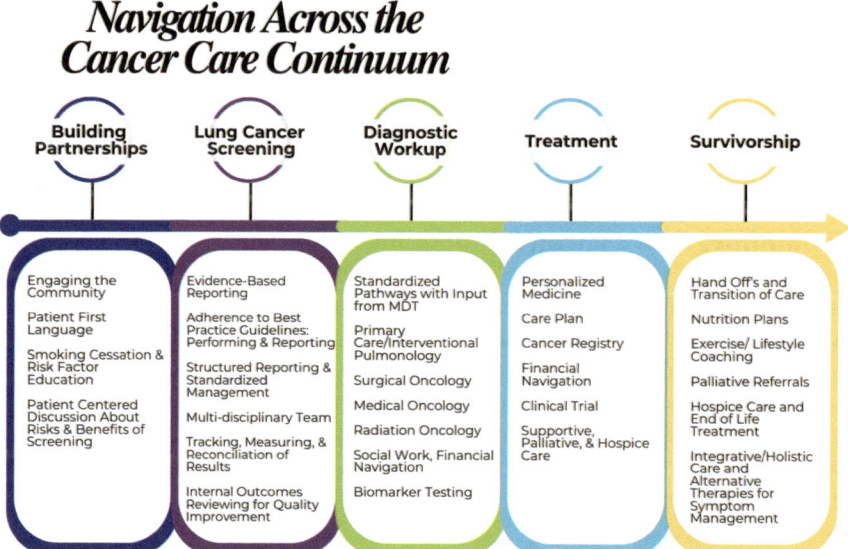

Fig. 3.1 Lung cancer navigation across the continuum

Building Trust

The navigator interacts with the patient at every point along their continuum of care, from providing education in the community, providing access to LCS, along the diagnostic process, and throughout the treatment, survivorship, palliative, and end-of-life experience (Fig. 3.1). Opportunities to improve patient outcomes exist at every stage of the continuum [6–9]. From the first interaction, whether the navigator role is in the community or a cancer center, they are uniquely positioned to connect with and assist the patient in a way that no other role on the multidisciplinary team is able. "Patient navigation services have been shown to foster trust, which is particularly critical for Black patients given their experiences of mistreatment and disrespect by health providers" [7]. Studies have also shown that patient navigation successfully increases the rate of cancer screenings in vulnerable populations [27]. Through trusted, continuous engagement, the navigator serves as a consistent point of support, bridging gaps in care, fostering meaningful connections, and ultimately improving outcomes for patients at risk of or living with lung cancer.

Connecting in the Community

It is crucial to recognize that care extends beyond the walls of hospitals and clinics. The community context plays an important role in an individual's well-being. This is where CHWs help patients understand and access the complex healthcare system and connect them with local resources and support networks. These CHWs are uniquely positioned to bridge the gap between clinical care and patients' everyday lives. Patients live and work in communities that can shape their journey. With a focus on a community-based approach, CHWs and lung cancer navigators can help guide patients through a seamless continuum of care that expands to embrace the broader support system necessary for long-term health.

Community Outreach and Engagement

Lung cancer continues to be one of the leading causes of cancer-related deaths, with disparities in care and outcomes influenced by factors such as socioeconomic status, race, and geographic location. Barriers, including financial and cultural influences, shape these disparities. Addressing these barriers is crucial to improving patient outcomes in cancer care, as these obstacles often hinder timely diagnosis, treatment, and prevention [28]. Community outreach and engagement can help address these disparities and improve the patient experience and lung cancer outcomes.

Barriers in Lung Cancer Prevention, Early Detection, and Care

Barriers to quality care in lung cancer are multifaceted and include financial and economic factors.

- *Socioeconomic Status*—Patients with a lower socioeconomic background may have difficulty paying for care and cannot afford treatment, medications, and diagnostic services [29, 30].
- *Linguistic and Cultural Differences*—Heterogeneous communities behold linguistic and cultural diversity. This diversity may converge and contribute to healthcare ecosystems where underrepresented groups experience lower early detection rates, diagnoses, and treatment [28]. Lung cancer navigators and allied health professionals must develop awareness and appropriate knowledge and skills necessary to meet the needs of all their patients, including those who have immigrated or are limited in English proficiency. Actively identifying related needs of patients assists in avoiding discrimination or bias within the healthcare system and society.
- *Social Constraints*—Distance to specialized cancer centers, inadequate transportation access, childcare needs, or the inability to take time off work are socially driven barriers to care [28]. Such constraints can delay and prevent patients from seeking care and hinder their ability to fulfill recommended treatment plans and follow-up visits. These social limitations may be accentuated depending on the geographic location of patients' residence and their proximity to oncology services, including screening, early diagnosis, treatment, or palliative care services.

Navigation in the Community

CHWs often serve a key role in overcoming patients' cultural, social, and logistical challenges. They not only focus on cancer prevention and early detection but also work to educate communities about cancer screening guidelines, reduce fears and myths about cancer, and build trust within the community [31]. A key aspect of community outreach is the ability to meet the needs of specific populations. The work of CHWs must reflect the needs of the communities they serve, focusing on creating customized navigation programs for the unique challenges faced by different communities [31]. For example, outreach efforts in rural areas may focus on addressing transportation barriers and providing logistical support. In contrast, urban outreach programs may address issues such as language barriers, healthcare mistrust, or fragmented care systems.

Education and Advocacy

In many communities, knowledge gaps remain regarding smoking cessation, LCS, and lung cancer. These gaps are fueled and exacerbated by stigma and misconceptions about treatment and the disease. Navigators serve a crucial role in educating about lung cancer prevention, early detection, and the importance of screening through dispelling myths, addressing fears, and providing accurate information about the risks and benefits of early detection.

Given the diversity of patient populations, one-size-fits-all approaches are insufficient in addressing the barriers to care. Navigation programs must be tailored to the specific needs of the communities they serve. This includes understanding the local healthcare landscape and available resources while identifying and acknowledging the cultural values, social norms, and challenges that different populations may face [31]. CHWs and navigators who are members of the communities they serve—or who share similar cultural, linguistic, or lived experiences—are better equipped to deliver culturally competent, trusted, and comprehensive care coordination [31].

Community Partnerships

Community-based outreach relies on strong collaborative partnerships within the community. Trained navigators are essential in identifying and fostering these partnerships. Community partnerships [31] can include relationships with:

- Healthcare providers
- Neighborhood associations
- Churches
- Community health centers
- Senior centers and others
- Local community-based organizations (CBOs)

These partnerships help to build trust and credibility, allowing navigators to connect with individuals who might otherwise be hesitant to seek care, and help to create a network of support that can assist both navigators and patients with the logistical challenges of accessing care, such as transportation to appointments or providing information on available resources. These social networks serve as sources of support and information within communities and underserved populations.

Conclusion

Lung cancer disproportionately impacts marginalized populations, with social determinants of health contributing to disparities in screening, treatment access, and survival outcomes. Patient navigation has shown promise in addressing these inequalities by helping to reduce barriers to care and supporting more timely access to high-quality, evidence-based treatment. Dr. Freeman's pioneering work laid the foundation for patient navigation to address cancer disparities, evolving into a recognized profession with defined standards, competencies, and training. Navigators address barriers across the lung cancer care continuum and ensure patients receive timely, coordinated care from screening through treatment and survivorship. Community-based navigators are essential in addressing lung cancer disparities by educating communities about cancer prevention and screening, reducing barriers to care, and fostering trust through tailored outreach programs. Collaborative community partnerships with local organizations further enhance these efforts, building support networks that address logistical and cultural challenges while improving patient access to timely, quality care. In every role across the care continuum, the lung cancer navigator is uniquely positioned to identify and address barriers to care, ensuring patients receive comprehensive support and an optimal care experience.

Key Takeaways

- Navigation is an evidence-based intervention to address and impact health disparities in lung cancer across the cancer continuum from prevention, screening, to diagnosis and survivorship.
- There are various models of navigation, and professional standards ensure the quality of navigation provided by a variety of professionals.
- Community outreach and navigation in the community requires strong partnerships and understanding the unique needs of underserved and high-risk populations.
- Navigators can be integrated at every phase of the continuum of care.

Key Readings and Resources

- Academy of Oncology Nurse & Patient Navigators (AONN+) [32].
- American Cancer Society (ACS) National Navigation Roundtable (NNRT) [33].
- American Cancer Society (ACS) Types of Patient Navigation [34].
- Early Lung Cancer Detection Network (ELCDN), LUNGevity [35].
- GO2 for Lung Cancer Lung Cancer Navigator Workshop [36].
- GO2 for Lung Cancer Global Knowledge Center [37].
- Guide to Community Preventive Services Task Force [38].
- National Association of Community Health Workers (NACHW) [39].
- Oncology Nursing Society (ONS) [40].
- Oncology Navigation Standards of Practice [22].

Conflicts of Interest Authors report no conflicts of interest

References

1. American Cancer Society Lung Cancer Statistics | How Common is Lung Cancer? 2024; Available at: https://www.cancer.org/cancer/types/lung-cancer/about/key-statistics.html. Accessed 17 Jan 2025.
2. American Lung Association State of Lung Cancer | Key Findings. 2024; Available at: https://www.lung.org/research/state-of-lung-cancer/key-findings. Accessed 17 Jan 2025.
3. Dwyer LL, Vadagam P, Vanderpoel J, Cohen C, Lewing B, Tkacz J. Disparities in lung cancer: a targeted Literature review examining lung cancer screening, diagnosis, treatment, and survival outcomes in the United States. J Racial Ethnic Health Disparities. 2024;11(3):1489–500.

4. Stein JN, Rivera MP, Weiner A, Duma N, Henderson L, Mody G, Charlot M. Sociodemographic disparities in the management of advanced lung cancer: a narrative review. J Thorac Dis. 2021;13(6):3772–800.
5. Zou K, Sun P, Huang H, Zhuo H, Qie R, Xie Y, , Luo, J, Li, N, He, J, Ashebrook-Kilfoy, B, Zhang, Y. Etiology of lung cancer: evidence from epidemiologic studies. J Natl Cancer Center 2022;2(4):216–225. https://pdf.sciencedirectassets.com/778499/1-s2.0-S2667005422000667-main.pdf.
6. Oh J, Ahn S. Effects of nurse navigators during the transition from cancer screening to the first treatment phase: a systematic review and meta-analysis. Asian Nurs Res. 2021;15(5):291–302.
7. Charlot M, Stein JN, Damone E, Wood I, Forster M, Baker S, Emerson M, Samuel-Ryals C, Yongue C, Eng E, Manning M, Deal A, Cykert S. Effect of an antiracism intervention on racial disparities in time to lung cancer surgery. J Clin Oncol. 2022;40(16):1755–62.
8. Kline RM, Rocque GB, Rohan EA, Blackley KA, Cantril CA, Pratt-Chapman ML, Burris HA, Shulman LN. Patient navigation in cancer: the business case to support clinical needs. J Oncol Pract. 2019;15(11):585.
9. Chan RJ, Milch VE, Crawford-Williams F, Agbejule OA, Joseph R, Johal J, Dick N, Wallen MP, Ratcliffe J, Agarwal A, Nekhlyudov L, Tieu M, Al-Momani M, Turnbull S, Sathiaraj R, Keefe D, Hart NH. Patient navigation across the cancer care continuum: an overview of systematic reviews and emerging literature. CA Cancer J Clin. 2023;73(6):565–89.
10. Nelson HD, Cantor A, Wagner J, Jungbauer R, Fu R, Kondo K, Stillman L, Quiñones A. Effectiveness of patient navigation to increase cancer screening in populations adversely affected by health disparities: a meta-analysis. J Gen Intern Med. 2020;35(10):3026–35.
11. Zhang J, IJzerman MJ, Oberoi J, Karnchanachari N, Bergin RJ, Franchini F, Druce P, Wang X, Emery JD. Time to diagnosis and treatment of lung cancer: a systematic overview of risk factors, interventions and impact on patient outcomes. Lung Cancer. 2022;166:27–39.
12. A summary of the American Cancer Society report to the nation: cancer in the poor. CA Cancer J Clin. 1989;39(5):263–5.
13. Freeman HP, Rodriguez RL. The history and principles of patient navigation. Cancer. 2011;117(15):3539–42. https://acsjournals.onlinelibrary.wiley.com/doi/10.1002/cncr.26262. Accessed 5 Jan 2025
14. Paskett ED, Battaglia T, Calhoun EA, Chappell MC, Dwyer A, Fleisher LG, Greenwald J, Wells KJ. Isn't there enough evidence on the benefits of patient navigation? CA Cancer J Clin. 2023;73(6):562–4.
15. Cancer: a decade later: the state of patient navigation in cancer. Cancer. 2022;128(S13):2553–9.
16. Dwyer AJ, Wender RC, Weltzien ES, Dean MS, Sharpe K, Fleisher L, Burhansstipanov L, Johnson W, Martinez L, Wiatrek D, Calhoun E, Battaglia T. Collective pursuit for equity in cancer care: the National Navigation Roundtable. Cancer. 2022;128(Suppl 13):2561–7.
17. Varanasi AP, Burhansstipanov L, Dorn C, Gentry S, Capossela MA, Fox K, Wilson D, Tanjasiri S, Odumosu O, Saavedra Ferrer EL. Patient navigation job roles by levels of experience: Workforce Development Task Group, National Navigation Roundtable. Cancer. 2024;130(9):1549–67.
18. Berberena L. Oncology Navigation Standards of Professional Practice - Academy of Oncology Nurse & Patient Navigators (AONN+). Available at: https://aonnonline.org/oncology-navigation-standards-of-professional-practice. Accessed 4 Jan 2025.
19. Franklin EF, Dean MS, Johnston DM, Nevidjon BM, Burke SL, Simms Booth LM. Solidifying roles, responsibilities, and the process of navigation across the continuum of cancer care: the Professional Oncology Navigation Task Force. Cancer. 2022;128(Suppl 13):2669–72.
20. Battaglia TA, Fleisher L, Dwyer AJ, Wiatrek DE, Wells KJ, Wightman P, Strusowski T, Calhoun E. Barriers and opportunities to measuring oncology patient navigation impact: results from the National Navigation Roundtable survey. Cancer. 2022;128(Suppl 13):2568–77.

21. Wiatrek D, Johnston D. AONN+ & the American Cancer Society 2020 Navigation Metrics Toolkit. 2020. Available: https://aonnonline.org/images/resources/navigation_tools/2020-AONN-Navigation-Metrics-Toolkit.pdf. Accessed 15 Jan 2025.
22. Oncology navigation standards of professional practice. Clin J Oncol Nurs. 2022;26(3):E14–25.
23. Strusowski T, Stapp J. Patient navigation metrics: measuring the impact of your patient navigation services. Oncol Issues. 2016;31(1):62–9.
24. Scott CW, Dharmarajan K, Robert JG, Sachdeva K, Johnstone D, Hershman DL. Reduction in cancer spending due to patient navigation. JCO Oncol Pract. 2023;19(11):557.
25. Worland SC, Albin M, Dorsey B, Fosnocht K, Gomez J, Johnstone D, Kirayoglu A, Licitra E, Parikh RB, Sachdeva K, Thompson K, Voigt S, Woerner S, Green RJ. Evaluating the effect of a scalable cancer-navigation program on total cost of care. J Clin Oncol. 2022;40(28 Supplement)
26. Dwyer AJ, Weltzien ES, Harty NM, LeGrice KE, Pray SLH, Risendal BC. What makes for successful patient navigation implementation in cancer prevention and screening programs using an evaluation and sustainability framework. Cancer. 2022;128(Suppl 13):2636–48.
27. Shusted CS, Barta JA, Lake M, Brawer R, Ruane B, Giamboy TE, Sundaram B, Evans NR, Myers RE, Kane GC. The case for patient navigation in lung cancer screening in vulnerable populations: a systematic review. Popul Health Manag. 2019;22(4):347–61.
28. Rivera MP, Katki HA, Tanner NT, Triplette M, Sakoda LC, Wiener RS, Cardarelli R, Carter-Harris L, Crothers K, Fathi JT, Ford ME, Smith R, Winn RA, Wisnivesky JP, Henderson LM, Aldrich MC. Addressing disparities in lung cancer screening eligibility and healthcare access. An Official American Thoracic Society Statement | American Journal of Respiratory and Critical Care Medicine. Am J Respir Crit Care Med. 2020;202(7):95–112.
29. Freeman HP, Chu KC. Determinants of cancer disparities: barriers to cancer screening, diagnosis, and treatment. Surg Oncol Clin N Am. 2005;14(4):655–69.
30. Carter-Harris L, Gould MK. Multilevel barriers to the successful implementation of lung cancer screening: why does it have to be so hard? Ann Am Thorac Soc. 2017;14(8):1261–5.
31. Wallington S, Oppong B, Dash C, Coleman T, Greenwald H, Torres T, Iddirisu M, Adams-Campbell LL. A community-based outreach navigator approach to establishing partnerships for a safety net mammography screening center. J Cancer Educ. 2018;33(4):782–7.
32. Academy of Oncology Nurse & Patient Navigators (AONN+) Admin A. Home - (AONN+). 2025; Available at: https://aonnonline.org/. Accessed 4 Jan 2025.
33. National Navigation Roundtable (NNRT). Available at: https://navigationroundtable.org/. Accessed 30 Jan 2025.
34. American Cancer Society (ACS) Types of Cancer Navigators | Patient Navigation. Available at: https://www.cancer.org/cancer/patient-navigation/types-of-cancer-navigators.html. Accessed 6 Feb 2025.
35. Early Lung Cancer Detection Network. 2025; Available at: https://elcdn.org/. Accessed 3 Mar 2025.
36. GO2 for Lung Cancer Lung Cancer Navigator Workshop | GO2 Healthcare Provider Portal. Available at: https://hcp.go2.org/navigator-workshop/. Accessed 4 Jan 2025.
37. GO2 for Lung Cancer, GO2 Global Knowledge Center (GKC) for Lung Cancer. Available at: https://gkc.go2.org/. Accessed 4 Jan 2025.
38. National Navigation Roundtable (NNRT) Guide to Community Preventive Services. 2025; Available at: https://navigationroundtable.org/resource/guide-to-community-preventive-services/. Accessed 6 Feb 2025.
39. National Association of Community Health Workers (NACHW). Home NACHW. 2025; Available at: https://nachw.org/. Accessed 05 May 2025.
40. Oncology Nursing Society (ONS) The Professional Home for Oncology Nurses. 2025; Available at: https://www.ons.org/. Accessed 4 Jan 2025.

Open Access This chapter is licensed under the terms of the Creative Commons Attribution-NonCommercial 4.0 International License (http://creativecommons.org/licenses/by-nc/4.0/), which permits any noncommercial use, sharing, adaptation, distribution and reproduction in any medium or format, as long as you give appropriate credit to the original author(s) and the source, provide a link to the Creative Commons license and indicate if changes were made.

The images or other third party material in this chapter are included in the chapter's Creative Commons license, unless indicated otherwise in a credit line to the material. If material is not included in the chapter's Creative Commons license and your intended use is not permitted by statutory regulation or exceeds the permitted use, you will need to obtain permission directly from the copyright holder.

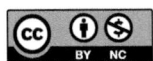

Multi-, Interdisciplinary, and Patient-Centric Team-Based Lung Cancer Care

4

Laura Pachella and Loril Garrett

Contents

Navigation Vignette	36
Introduction	36
Patient- and Family-Centered Care	37
Multidisciplinary and Interdisciplinary Approach to High-Quality Care and Health Outcomes	37
Members of the Interdisciplinary Team	38
Collaborative Practice Improves Patient Experience	45
Conclusion	46
Key Takeaways	46
Key Readings and Resources	46
References	47

Abbreviations

APP	Advanced practice provider
CT	Computed tomography
GOC	Goals of care
LC	Lung cancer
MDC	Multidisciplinary care
PN	Patient navigator
QOL	Quality of life
SBRT	Stereotactic body radiation therapy
TB	Tumor board

L. Pachella (✉) · L. Garrett
Rutgers Cancer Institute/RWJ Barnabas Health, New Brunswick, NJ, USA
e-mail: Lap253@cinj.rutgers.edu; lg874@cinj.rutgers.edu

© The Author(s) 2026
J. T. Fathi, M. F. Mortman (eds.), *Lung Cancer Navigation and Care*,
https://doi.org/10.1007/978-3-032-02200-4_4

Navigation Vignette

JP is a 68-year-old gentleman with an 80-pack-year smoking history who presented to his primary care provider with a non-productive cough 6 weeks ago. JP reported weight loss over the last 2 months. A chest x-ray identified a lung mass. JP was referred for a chest CT scan, which confirmed a lung mass with adenopathy in the hilar lymph nodes. JP was referred to pulmonary for endobronchial ultrasound with navigational bronchoscopy and biopsy, where mediastinal lymph nodes were also biopsied to stage his disease.

The pathology of the lung mass revealed adenocarcinoma consistent with a primary LC. JP was referred to the thoracic multidisciplinary care (MDC) clinic for evaluation. The nurse navigator called the patient to review current testing and provide anticipatory guidance to ensure JP would know what to expect at the appointment. The nurse navigator recognized that social support would be important for JP. He was encouraged to have a family member or friend accompany him to the appointment.

JP consulted with the thoracic surgeon, who reviewed his imaging reports and pathological findings from his biopsies. The surgeon advised JP that his cancer outcomes and overall health would benefit from smoking cessation and referred him to a smoking cessation specialist. The medical and radiation oncologists also met with JP to review the treatment plan. They recommended surgical excision of his tumor, followed by reevaluation and consideration for adjuvant systemic therapy based on final surgical pathology. After his oncology workup and visit, the patient navigator contacted JP to offer support and answer questions.

Introduction

Lung cancer screening (LCS), lung cancer (LC) detection, diagnostic workup, cancer diagnosis, treatment, and disease surveillance are all complex endeavors. This work involves multiple healthcare disciplines across the LC care continuum to practice in parallel (interdisciplinary) and collaboratively (multidisciplinary) for optimal patient and family-centered care and health outcomes. Each professional discipline and the importance of their roles in LC care will be described in detail. The LC navigator serves as the point person for patients and helps them understand their next steps as the treatment plan unfolds. In the setting of annual LCS and even at the time of LC diagnosis, it is important for patients to know and understand their current health status or diagnosis and treatment options and to learn about those options from a team of trusted LC specialists [1]. The ideal LC care plan involves all necessary specialties and incorporates the needs of patients and families while pursuing treatment goals of care (GOC).

Patient- and Family-Centered Care

Bidirectional communication between the patient and family support system and the multidisciplinary team will support the goal of adherence to the treatment plan while maintaining patient autonomy. When patients are diagnosed with LC, they bring with them a variety of backgrounds, life experiences, socioeconomic situations, and previous experiences with the healthcare system that can influence their response to treatment discussions and decisions. Patient- and family-centered care is an approach to planning, delivering, and evaluating health care grounded in mutually beneficial partnerships among health care providers, patients, and families [2].

At the time of LC diagnosis, patients and families can become confused regarding the need for multiple appointments with specialists to determine a treatment plan. The navigator provides a layer of support to guide the process and ensure appropriate testing and consultations are performed. Patients can find themselves repeating the same story of symptoms and diagnosis to multiple providers. Navigators can help patients streamline this clinical history, including the onset of symptoms, diagnostic workup, and treatment to date, to make encounters more productive.

It is helpful for family members to accompany patients to appointments to provide emotional support and assist patients and family members in better understanding the care plan. Quality of life (QOL) should be a priority in discussions at the time of LC diagnosis and when determining treatment to understand the patient and family GOC [3]. The path to treatment is often not straightforward or clear and can include multiple acceptable options. Patient autonomy is established, upheld, and maintained when they are provided the opportunity to review and better understand their options, the potential risks, benefits, and side effects of therapeutic interventions, and the opportunity to engage in conversation and ask questions. It is best practice for members of MDC teams to undergo communication skills training to improve communication among peers, colleagues, patients, and families [4].

Multidisciplinary and Interdisciplinary Approach to High-Quality Care and Health Outcomes

The need for MDC was recognized in the 1980s to bring together cancer experts in multiple modalities to create a non-biased treatment plan for the patient while adhering to recognized treatment guidelines [5]. An interdisciplinary care team is composed of individual members who bring specific knowledge to a patient's care. MDC represents the collaborative approach to making clinical decisions and creating a care plan. This is typically achieved in settings where many healthcare professionals meet to share knowledge and collaborate on behalf of the patient for optimal health outcomes. An example would be tumor board (TB) discussions; each specialty team member contributes their expert knowledge and opinion in this meeting. As a result, a consensus decision is achieved to present the best possible treatment option. Interdisciplinary care teams are characterized by five common elements:

shared decision-making, partnership, interdependency, balanced power, and process/use of protocols [6]. Achieving multidisciplinary coordinated LC care is imperative because of the volume of patients, lethality of disease, and well-described disparities in quality and patient outcomes [1].

TB discussions with the MDC team contribute to constructive revisions of LC diagnoses and treatment plans, reflective of expert multidisciplinary input, in new cancer cases, better adherence to evidence-based guidelines, improved consideration for inclusion in clinical trials, and more accurate staging and treatment, resulting in increased survival rates [7]. Barriers to effective MDC team discussions exist, including poor attendance, inadequate patient information, lack of technical or administrative support, inadequate communication, unequal participation in decision-making, hierarchical boundaries, and unskilled leadership. Each must be overcome to have effective patient discussions and optimize the value of the MDC approach [5].

When a cancer diagnosis is in the process of being established, the sheer volume of testing to diagnose, stage, and treat LC can be overwhelming, in addition to patients and families needing to attend multiple appointments with varying specialists. MDC clinics coordinate scheduling to ease the burden for patients being seen by numerous disciplines within the same visit or trip to the medical center, rather than meeting with each provider individually on discordant days and times. This MDC care model allows the individual providers of the MDC team the opportunity in person to review the patient's case together and proceed with a plan of care. The MDC clinic is a streamlined approach that requires great coordination, with which a patient navigator can assist. Alternatively, patient navigators can assist the patient in setting up multiple appointments with specialists.

Members of the Interdisciplinary Team

Patient Navigator

Patient navigators are an integral member of the interdisciplinary care team. They assist patients within their scope of practice or professional role and can be clinically or non-clinically focused. Clinically based navigators (nurses, advanced practice nurses, and others) often participate in screening programs, attend TBs, educate patients, mitigate barriers to care, advocate on a patient's behalf, and provide anticipatory guidance throughout the care trajectory. They serve as a key point of contact and support for patients and are often seen as disease site experts. Additionally, they facilitate care team communication and ensure resources and appropriate supportive care services have been activated. Non-clinically based navigators perform much of the same, focusing primarily on reducing barriers to care by utilizing system and community resources and addressing practical concerns such as financial toxicity or timely access to care. Please see Chap. 3 for a more detailed description of patient navigation. The remainder of this section will focus on additional care team members. Please see Table 4.1 for a synopsis of the disciplines and their timing in the patient's cancer care continuum.

Table 4.1 Timing and role of interdisciplinary care team in the cancer care continuum

Team member	Key responsibility	Description of role
Pulmonologist	Screening/diagnosis	Oversee screening program and tumor boards. Monitor, manage, and work up concerning thoracic findings (i.e., lung nodules and lung masses)
Interventional pulmonologist	Diagnosis/treatment/survivorship	Use imaging and minimally invasive equipment to diagnose, treat, and manage lung cancer non-surgically
Radiologist	Screening/diagnosis/treatment/survivorship	Review and interpret imaging and make recommendations for follow-up imaging across the lung cancer continuum
Interventional radiologist	Diagnosis	Collect tissue (biopsy) through transthoracic techniques using imaging guidance
Pathologist	Diagnosis	Through molecular and histological analyses of tissue, diagnose lung cancer, classify and stage tumors, and inform treatment decisions
Thoracic surgeon	Diagnosis/treatment/survivorship	Diagnose and surgically treat lung cancer and provide disease surveillance
Medical oncologist	Treatment/survivorship	Diagnose and treat lung cancer with systemic therapies and disease surveillance
Radiation oncologist	Treatment/survivorship	Treat and palliate lung cancer with radiation treatment modalities
Advanced practice provider (nurse practitioner or physician assistant)	Screening/diagnosis/treatment/survivorship	Provide comprehensive cancer care, patient education, and support in collaboration with physicians and other MDC team members
RN clinic coordinator	Screening/diagnosis/treatment/survivorship	Coordinate care and provide education and clinic support
Patient/oncology navigator	Screening/diagnosis/treatment/survivorship	Eliminate barriers to care, oversee the continuum of care, and offer support and guidance
Nutritionist	Treatment/survivorship	Assess and monitor nutritional status. Educate patients and treat nutritional deficiencies
Rehabilitation specialist	Treatment/survivorship	Assess mobility, support pretreatment, and treatment optimization
Research nurse	Treatment	Provide education, facilitate access to research studies, and provide patient support throughout the study period

(continued)

Table 4.1 (continued)

Team member	Key responsibility	Description of role
Social worker	Screening/diagnosis/treatment/survivorship	Provide psychosocial support and resources throughout the continuum of care
Tobacco treatment specialist	Screening/diagnosis/treatment/survivorship	Provide smoking cessation education, counseling, pharmacotherapy, and ongoing support
Palliative care	Treatment/survivorship/end of life	Provide symptom management, promote quality of life, and guide care decisions with MDC team
Chaplain	Diagnosis/treatment/survivorship/end of life	Provide spiritual support, help find meaning and cope with the disease and offer grief support

Pulmonologist

Pulmonologists are critical to the team because they are responsible for ensuring an appropriate diagnosis for the patient. Patients are referred to pulmonology for diagnostic workup when concerning findings, like lung nodules and masses, are identified on imaging. Pulmonologists are equipped to perform diagnostic and staging bronchoscopies or engage interventional radiology services to perform CT-guided biopsies. Pulmonologists often see patients in MDC clinics and present them at TBs, facilitating the value of the entire TB MDC, reviewing and weighing in with their expert opinions in determining the best approach to nodule management.

Interventional Pulmonologist

Interventional pulmonologists are consulted for complex diagnostic and staging needs. In addition to having general pulmonology expertise, they are specifically trained in bronchoscopy, endobronchial ultrasound, and the use of minimally invasive technologies such as navigational or robotic bronchoscopy. These interventionalists are adept at obtaining tissue through these various technological approaches, including lymph node sampling, and treating airway obstructions. They regularly participate in TB discussions. Technologies are currently being developed to treat lung cancer during robotic bronchoscopy, where patients could be diagnosed and treated during the same procedure. Interventional pulmonologists will be instrumental in utilizing and optimizing such technology and the novel clinical opportunities it will bring.

Radiologist

Radiologists are responsible for interpreting imaging studies and providing guidance and recommendations for additional imaging that may be needed. They are important partners in LCS through structured reading and reporting by the Lung-RADS (Lung Imaging Reporting and Data System) classification system, which drives lung nodule management. Radiologists also participate in TBs by reviewing and presenting relevant imaging to date and recommending any additional imaging that may be needed. Their expertise is also critical in LC staging and management, and in the setting of disease progression.

Interventional Radiologist

Interventional radiologists perform biopsies using imaging guidance along with performing minimally invasive procedures such as inserting a port to receive systemic treatment (intravenous chemotherapy or immunotherapy). During TB discussions, interventional radiologists review images to determine the best approach for performing biopsies essential to diagnosing, staging, and confirming metastatic disease. They also perform biopsies during the TB so that needed testing can be ordered following the TB conference to expedite care.

Pathologist

Pathologists are responsible for interpreting tissue (from biopsies) under the microscope and determining if cancer is present, the cancer type, and the extent of disease. Knowing the type of cancer and location of the cancer guides treatment planning and options. During TB discussions, pathologists present the histological findings, cancer diagnosis, and explain why the specific diagnosis was made. They also report any inconsistencies with pathology and recommend additional biopsies if needed to confirm a diagnosis or complete staging. Pathologists also have a key role in molecular testing and identification of driver mutations, which are critical to targeted therapies.

Thoracic Surgeon

Thoracic surgeons are responsible for surgical resection/excision of thoracic malignancies, including lung cancers (see Chap. 13). They perform lobectomies, wedge resections, and other surgical procedures, including mediastinoscopies, as indicated, for lymph node collection and dissection for cancer staging and control, respectively. During TB, thoracic surgeons offer expert insight into surgical options and the risks and benefits of surgical approaches for various cancer stages. Occasionally, if cancer is suspected and a biopsy cannot be performed via usual minimally invasive techniques, surgery may be instrumental in the diagnostic, curative, and cancer control settings.

Medical Oncologist

Medical oncologists are responsible for determining and recommending guideline-directed systemic treatment options based on cancer type and stage, as well as the presence or absence of specific tumor markers and driver mutations influencing targeted therapy options. Medical oncologists share which systemic treatment(s) they recommend to patients during TB discussions, including those with evidence of LC recurrence or disease progression, to determine the best next steps for effective LC treatment.

Radiation Oncologist

Radiation oncologists evaluate a patient's candidacy for radiation therapy and provide expert recommendations regarding the most appropriate treatment approach, including whether radiation should be administered alone or in combination with systemic therapy (see Chaps. 15 and 16). For patients with early-stage LC who are not candidates for surgery, radiation therapy, such as stereotactic body radiation therapy (aka SBRT), may be considered as a curative alternative. Radiation oncologists also prescribe radiation to treat cancer metastases with a palliative rather than a curative intent. Radiation oncologists collaborate with other providers in TB discussions to ensure radiation options are understood.

Advanced Practice Provider

Nurse practitioners and physician assistants (aka advanced practice providers (APP)) play a key role in the care and management of LC patients. They actively participate in TB and MDC team care as they work independently, side-by-side, and collaboratively with physician colleagues and others. They are often trained as tobacco treatment specialists, possess leadership roles in lung cancer screening programs, provide oversight and management of lung nodules, and independently manage and follow patients across the LC continuum, including in the treatment, surveillance, survivorship, palliative, and end-of-life phases of care.

MDC Clinic Registered Nurse

Registered nurses in the MDC clinic serve as the key point of contact for patients for clinic-related concerns and provide education, support, and care coordination for patients. Clinic nurses often fulfill many roles, including that of a lung cancer navigator, ensuring patients know their next steps and are available for questions. Nurses attend TB to share and ensure patient-specific concerns are addressed and needs are met. Following the TB, nurses ensure orders are entered and completed while advocating for patients and expediting scheduling needs.

Dietitian

Dietitians play an integral role in ensuring the nutritional status of patients is optimized following an LC diagnosis and during treatment. They are especially helpful if patients are experiencing symptoms interrupting nutritional needs and unexpected weight loss, especially in later LC stages. Patients receiving radiation therapy or chemoradiation (concurrent treatment) are at a higher risk of needing interventions to maintain adequate nutritional status. Dietitians work with patients to develop strategies to overcome side effects and supplement their nutritional intake.

Cancer Rehabilitation Specialist

Cancer rehabilitation specialists are essential to optimizing patients' energy levels and overall functional status before, during, and after treatment. Rehabilitation specialists attending TB discussions identify patients who would benefit from rehabilitation services. This is especially helpful for patients needing a surgical intervention for early-stage LC, as prehabilitation can help optimize patients for surgery. Rehabilitation is also important during systemic treatment and can help patients maintain strength and improve QOL.

Research Nurse

Research nurses are familiar with LC research and the clinical trials available to patients in their area or health system. Research nurses review the office or MDC clinic schedule and attend TB discussions to inform providers if research studies are available for their patients and if they meet the eligibility criteria for participating in a clinical trial. If a study is identified as a potential match for a patient, nurses can meet with patients at the time of the MDC clinic appointment.

Medical Social Worker

Medical social workers are experts with psychosocial support and resources for overcoming barriers to accessing care. Medical social workers frequently participate in MDC clinic visits and attend TB discussions to offer insight into patient experiences, provide support, identify basic needs, and offer patient resources. Medical social workers also assist with distress tool screening and suicide assessments, if indicated, at the time of the clinic visit and help mitigate financial and psychosocial concerns.

Tobacco Treatment Specialist

Tobacco treatment specialists specialize in smoking cessation-related behavioral counseling and pharmacotherapy treatment while determining a personalized cessation plan (see Chap. 10). A tobacco treatment specialist is an important member of the MDC team. Tobacco treatment specialists attending TB discussions develop awareness of the patient's treatment plan and leverage this knowledge to determine the most effective and personalized therapeutic approach.

Palliative Care

Palliative care specialists are integral to the care of LC patients to support symptom management and promote the best QOL possible. Palliative care providers are instrumental in discussing GOC and end-of-life planning. Many LC programs have recognized the importance of early interventions from palliative care but have found it difficult to provide due to physician staffing. The ideal state is to have palliative care team members attending TB discussions and being part of the patient's plan of care beginning at diagnosis.

Chaplain

Chaplains are considered key members of the MDC team and are frequently consulted to provide comfort, support, and spiritual guidance to patients, family members, and caregivers. They assist with spiritual coping and counseling, as well as GOC discussions. They are especially helpful during end-of-life and hospice discussions and family conferences, for related grief support, and in helping process spiritual needs. Chaplains may also provide supportive resources and assist with complicated decision-making and ethics consultations.

Collaborative Practice Improves Patient Experience

Multidisciplinary care has been noted to improve physician collaboration, decrease patient anxiety, and prevent the need for multiple appointments. Patients experiencing MDC report feeling more confident and satisfied with their care when multiple physicians assess their treatment needs and address their concerns [1]. Quality of care with improvement in following diagnostic and treatment guidelines has been seen in adherence to MDC [8]. MDC has been shown to decrease the time from diagnosis to treatment and is associated with improved clinical outcomes and patient satisfaction [9]. Compared to serial care, patients randomized to receive MDC were more likely to undergo appropriate, guideline-directed invasive and mediastinal staging confirmation. Additionally, patients on the multidisciplinary arm were more likely to receive stage-appropriate treatment [3].

It is important to recognize that not all patients live within an area with an MDC facility for LC care. Patients without access to a comprehensive cancer center face barriers to screening and treatment [5]. In the United States, when specifically looking at tobacco use as a risk factor for developing LC, smoking is more prevalent among rural residents than urban dwellers [10]. Comprehensive cancer centers with full MDC care are more likely to be located in large metropolitan areas. This discordance in access to MDC care outside comprehensive cancer centers may contribute to treatment disparities and potential challenges for patient navigation in rural settings.

MDC team discussions are essential to patient-focused care characterized by collaboration, communication, and streamlining diagnostics and treatment [11]. There is no substitute for bringing a team of LC specialists together to form an MDC team to make diagnostic and treatment recommendations. The Commission on Cancer recognizes TBs (a prime example of MDC in action) as a powerful tool and key to developing a unique care plan, specific to each patient. Each specialty contributes their knowledge and expertise, and the patients benefit from the net effect of the treatment discussion.

As the complexity of LC care increases, so does the need for increased collaboration among the treating specialists [12]. The MDC team interprets the National Cancer Comprehensive Network and other diagnostic and staging guidelines to ensure patients are staged appropriately. They evaluate patient candidacy for the various treatment modalities available, such as neoadjuvant systemic therapy or the local treatment of oligometastatic disease. Without the collaboration of the MDC team, these approaches and others could be missed, or patients could not be identified for treatment [6].

Collaboration is also required to ensure a patient-centered care approach [12]. MDC team treatment recommendations may need to be modified, and a new consensus achieved to meet the needs of patients and their GOC. Additionally, close communication and care coordination are needed to navigate patients and families through the healthcare system and to ensure optimal care, utilizing appropriate supportive care team members. The MDC approach also allows for consistent messaging between providers and patients across the continuum of lung cancer (see Table 4.1: Timing and role of interdisciplinary care team in the cancer care continuum).

Conclusion

MDC is the foundation of LC care [11] and the most patient-centered approach. Collaboration among team members is necessary to accomplish MDC, and interdisciplinary meetings provide the optimal setting for MDC. Navigators play a key role in supporting patients. They are essential members of the MDC team, as they provide education and support to patients and their families and facilitate communication between members of the MDC team [1].

Key Takeaways

- An interdisciplinary approach to diagnosing and treating lung cancer is essential for optimal patient outcomes.
- Multidisciplinary care discussions include interdisciplinary tumor boards, which are essential to determining the best course of action to diagnose, stage, and treat lung cancer patients.
- Multidisciplinary care clinics are an effective strategy to streamline lung cancer diagnosis and treatment and prevent multiple patient appointments.
- Lung cancer treatment decision-making needs to be patient-centered, considering patient preferences and goals of care.

Key Readings and Resources

- Patient and physician perceptions of lung cancer care in a multidisciplinary clinic model [3].
- Multidisciplinary care models for patients with lung cancer [4].
- Prospective Comparative Effectiveness Trial of Multidisciplinary Lung Cancer Care Within a Community-Based Health Care System [8].
- Impact of a specialist clinical cancer pharmacist at a multidisciplinary lung cancer clinic [13].
- Disparities in Cancer Stage Outcomes by Catchment Areas for a Comprehensive Cancer Center [14].
- Multidisciplinary lung cancer clinic: An emerging model of care [15].

Conflicts of Interest Authors report no conflicts of interest

References

1. Osarogiagbon RU, Rodriguez HP, Hicks D, Signore RS, Roark K, Kedia SK, et al. Deploying team science principles to optimize interdisciplinary lung cancer care delivery: avoiding the long and winding road to optimal care. J Oncol Pract. 2016;12(11):983–91.
2. International Palliative Care and Family Caregiver (IPFCC); [updated] 2023. Available from: https://www.ipfcc.org/.
3. Linford G, Egan R, Coderre-Ball A, Dalgarno N, Stone CJL, Robinson A, et al. Patient and physician perceptions of lung cancer care in a multidisciplinary clinic model. Curr Oncol. 2020;27(1):e9–e19.
4. Hardavella G, Frille A, Theochari C, Keramida E, Bellou E, Fotineas A, et al. Multidisciplinary care models for patients with lung cancer. Breathe (Sheff). 2020;16(4):200076.
5. LaVigne AW, Doss VL, Berizzi D, Johnston FM, Kiess AP, Kirtane KS, et al. The history and future of multidisciplinary cancer care. Semin Radiat Oncol. 2024;34(4):441–51.
6. Morabito A, Mercadante E, Muto P, Manzo A, Palumbo G, Sforza V, et al. Improving the quality of patient care in lung cancer: key factors for successful multidisciplinary team working. Explor Target Antitumor Ther. 2024;5(2):260–77.
7. Morabito A, Mercadante E, Muto P, Palumbo G, Manzo A, Montanino A, et al. Risk management activities in a lung cancer multidisciplinary team at a comprehensive cancer center: results of a prospective analysis. JCO Oncol Pract. 2023;19(3):e315–e25.
8. Smeltzer MP, Ray MA, Faris NR, Meadows-Taylor MB, Rugless F, Berryman C, et al. Prospective comparative effectiveness trial of multidisciplinary lung cancer care within a community-based health care system. JCO Oncol Pract. 2023;19(1):e15–24.
9. Stone CJL, Robinson A, Brown E, Mates M, Falkson CB, Owen T, et al. Improving timeliness of oncology assessment and cancer treatment through implementation of a multidisciplinary lung cancer clinic. J Oncol Pract. 2019;15(2):e169–e77.
10. Centers for Disease Control. National Health Interview Survey, 1965–2022. Analysis performed by the American Lung Association Epidemiology and Statistics Unit using SPSS software. 2022. Available from: https://www.cdc.gov/.
11. Bertolaccini L, Mohamed S, Bardoni C, Lo Iacono G, Mazzella A, Guarize J, et al. The interdisciplinary management of lung cancer in the European Community. J Clin Med. 2022;11(15):4326.
12. Heinke MY, Vinod SK. A review on the impact of lung cancer multidisciplinary care on patient outcomes. Transl Lung Cancer Res. 2020;9(4):1639–53.
13. Walter C, Mellor JD, Rice C, Kirsa S, Ball D, Duffy M, et al. Impact of a specialist clinical cancer pharmacist at a multidisciplinary lung cancer clinic. Asia Pac J Clin Oncol. 2016;12(3):e367–74.
14. Desjardins MR, Kanarek NF, Nelson WG, Bachman J, Curriero FC. Disparities in cancer stage outcomes by catchment areas for a comprehensive cancer center. JAMA Netw Open. 2024;7(5):e249474.
15. Saw SPL, Chua KLM, Ong BH, Lim DWT, Lai GGY, Tan DSW, et al. Multidisciplinary lung cancer clinic: an emerging model of care. Ann Acad Med Singap. 2022;51(12):793–5.

Open Access This chapter is licensed under the terms of the Creative Commons Attribution-NonCommercial 4.0 International License (http://creativecommons.org/licenses/by-nc/4.0/), which permits any noncommercial use, sharing, adaptation, distribution and reproduction in any medium or format, as long as you give appropriate credit to the original author(s) and the source, provide a link to the Creative Commons license and indicate if changes were made.

The images or other third party material in this chapter are included in the chapter's Creative Commons license, unless indicated otherwise in a credit line to the material. If material is not included in the chapter's Creative Commons license and your intended use is not permitted by statutory regulation or exceeds the permitted use, you will need to obtain permission directly from the copyright holder.

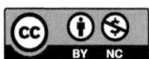

Determinants of Lung Cancer, Disease Development, and Risk Assessment

5

Nicholas C. Love and Arpan A. Patel

Contents

Navigation Vignette	50
Introduction	51
Pathogenesis and Carcinogenesis of Lung Cancer	51
Risk Factors for the Development of Lung Cancer	52
Lung Cancer Screening and Prevention (NSCLC and SCLC)	53
LDCT Classification and Recommended Follow-Up Intervals	54
Therapeutic Treatment Implications of Molecular (Biomarker) Testing	56
Emerging Perspectives and Future Directions	56
Key Takeaways	56
Key Readings and Resources	57
References	57

Abbreviations

CT	Computed tomography
EGFR	Epidermal growth factor receptor
LDCT	Low dose CT
MRI	Magnetic resonance imaging
NSCLC	Non-small cell lung cancer
PET	Positron emission tomography
PM	Pleural mesothelioma
SCLC	Small cell lung cancer

N. C. Love (✉) · A. A. Patel
Wilmot Cancer Institute, University of Rochester Medical Center, Rochester, NY, USA
e-mail: NicholasC_Love@URMC.Rochester.edu; Arpan_patel@URMC.Rochester.edu

© The Author(s) 2026
J. T. Fathi, M. F. Mortman (eds.), *Lung Cancer Navigation and Care*,
https://doi.org/10.1007/978-3-032-02200-4_5

Navigation Vignette

Ms. C., a 62-year-old former administrative assistant with a 40-pack-year tobacco use history, visited her primary care physician complaining of a persistent cough for 3 months with associated fatigue and unexplained 10-pound weight loss over the past 6 months. She quit smoking 15 years ago and had been diligent about getting her annual physical examinations but had never undergone lung cancer screening. During her initial visit, her physician noted that due to her smoking history and age, she would have qualified for annual low-dose CT (LDCT) screening, which, unfortunately, had not been previously discussed with her.

A chest X-ray was ordered for her symptoms, which revealed a concerning 3.2 cm mass in the right upper lobe. This finding prompted an immediate referral for a chest CT scan, which confirmed the presence of the mass and identified enlarged hilar lymph nodes. Given these findings, Ms. C. was referred to a pulmonologist who ordered a CT-guided needle biopsy. The pathology results revealed adenocarcinoma of the lung, classified as non-small cell lung cancer (NSCLC). Her pulmonologist explained that modern lung cancer care requires a multidisciplinary approach and referred her to a comprehensive cancer center. She met with a thoracic surgeon, a medical oncologist, and a radiation oncologist there. The team ordered additional testing, including a positron emission tomography CT (PET-CT) scan for staging and comprehensive molecular (biomarker) testing of her tumor specimen to determine if her lung cancer has a targetable genetic mutation, pulmonary function tests to evaluate her candidacy for surgery, and a magnetic resonance imaging (MRI) of the brain to evaluate for intracranial distant metastatic disease. Coordination of these appointments and the creation of a patient calendar by the clinic nurse navigator was integral to Ms. C's initial workup, given the multitude of imaging appointments, procedures, and consulting services that needed to be involved.

The molecular analysis of her lung cancer revealed an epidermal growth factor receptor (EGFR) mutation, a finding that would significantly impact her treatment options. Her cancer was staged as Stage IIIA due to the primary tumor size and lymph node involvement. The multidisciplinary tumor board discussed her case and recommended a multimodal approach to treatment, including neoadjuvant chemotherapy and immunotherapy, followed by definitive surgery. Ms. C's oncology team explained her treatment options, with the nurse navigator using visual aids and written materials to help her understand the complex decision-making process. They emphasized the importance of the EGFR mutation, explaining that targeted therapy with an EGFR inhibitor would be incorporated into her treatment plan. The treatment schedule was ultimately incorporated into the patient's calendar to help guide the patient through treatment.

Throughout her treatment journey, Ms. C. faced several challenges common to lung cancer patients. She experienced feelings of guilt related to her smoking history, and she connected with local cancer support groups through the clinic nurse navigator. The social worker assisted with transportation to daily radiation treatments.

Three months into treatment, imaging showed a significant response to therapy.

Introduction

Lung cancer is one of the leading causes of cancer-related mortality worldwide, with over two million new diagnoses and 1.8 million deaths annually [1, 2]. There were an estimated 234,580 new cases of lung cancer diagnosed in the United States in 2024, comprising 11.7% of all new cancer cases [3]. This chapter will review the three broad categories of lung cancer: non-small cell lung cancer (NSCLC), small cell lung cancer (SCLC), and mesothelioma. These categories of lung cancer are based on fundamental biological differences that significantly impact both therapeutic approaches and patient outcomes.

The two primary categories of bronchogenic carcinoma (cancer that arises from the epithelial cells that line the airways of the lungs) are non-small cell lung cancer (NSCLC) and small cell lung cancer (SCLC). NSCLC accounts for approximately 80–85% of all lung cancer cases [3, 4] and encompasses several different histological subtypes that demonstrate different patterns of growth and molecular alterations. Adenocarcinoma, the predominant subtype of NSCLC, typically arises from the distal airways and alveolar cells. Adenocarcinoma frequently presents with distinct genetic alterations, particularly in never-smokers. These mutations, if present, can provide a molecular target for therapeutic agents. Squamous cell carcinoma, conversely, generally develops from the proximal airways and is closely associated with a personal history of tobacco use [4, 5].

SCLC comprises approximately 14% of all lung cancer cases [3] and is strongly associated with tobacco exposure, with only a minority of cases occurring in individuals who have never smoked [5]. SCLC is particularly aggressive, with a 5-year relative survival of 9.2% [6], due to rapid cellular proliferation and early metastatic spread (often with distant metastatic disease present at the time of initial diagnosis). In contrast, NSCLC typically follows a more measured progression pattern, with a 5-year relative survival closer to 30% [6], underscoring the greater diversity of NSCLC in its response to environmental factors and therapeutic interventions.

Malignant pleural mesothelioma (PM) represents one of the most challenging thoracic malignancies encountered in clinical practice. As a rare cancer originating in the mesothelial surfaces of the pleura, PM affects almost 3500 individuals annually in the United States. The disease's aggressive nature, combined with its typically late presentation, results in poor outcomes for most patients, with median survival of approximately 1 year after diagnosis and a 5-year overall survival rate of 14.8% [6, 7].

Pathogenesis and Carcinogenesis of Lung Cancer

The development and pathogenesis of lung cancer involve a series of events that occur together to transform normal respiratory epithelium into cancerous tissue (see Chap. 6). This process includes genetic and epigenetic alterations that impact key cellular processes governing growth, survival, and differentiation. These changes may be inherited or acquired through multiple mechanisms, such as direct DNA damage from carcinogens and chronic inflammation [5, 8].

Inherited genetic susceptibility to the development of cancer includes variations in carcinogen metabolism, DNA repair, and immune function, which can compound the risk for developing cancer [8]. Pre-existing respiratory conditions can further increase the risk of developing lung cancer by creating an environment of chronic inflammation and tissue damage, such as is the case with chronic obstructive pulmonary disease (COPD) [9, 10].

Acquired cellular alterations typically include the activation of oncogenes and inactivation of tumor suppressor genes, leading to inhibition of programmed cell death (apoptosis) and essentially infinite survival and proliferative potential [8]. These changes can be accompanied by sustained inflammatory responses, which create a supportive microenvironment for continued tumor growth and progression. The recruitment of inflammatory cells to the tumor microenvironment further propagates cancer growth by releasing growth factors and cytokines and promoting angiogenesis. Chronic inflammation can also promote further genetic damage (and subsequently, mutagenesis) through the production of reactive oxygen free radicals [9]. As the disease progresses, the cancer cells can acquire the ability to infiltrate surrounding tissue and blood vessels, which ultimately causes the cancer to spread elsewhere in the body (i.e., metastasize).

Risk Factors for the Development of Lung Cancer

Environmental exposures play a crucial role in lung cancer development, with tobacco smoke representing the single most significant risk factor [9, 11]. The relationship between exposure to tobacco smoke (both first- and second-hand) and lung cancer development demonstrates clear dose-dependent characteristics, with risk increasing in proportion to both the duration of smoking and the intensity (or amount) of exposure. The carcinogenic effects of tobacco operate through multiple mechanisms, including direct DNA damage, chronic inflammation, and the creation of a pro-tumorigenic microenvironment [5]. Tobacco exposure also causes synergistic effects with other environmental carcinogens (e.g., radiation exposure or radon), which potentiates their harmful impact and can further increase cancer risk [4, 5].

While tobacco smoking remains the predominant risk factor, directly accounting for 85–90% of cases of lung cancer, other environmental exposures play an increasingly recognized role in the development of lung cancer [11, 12]. Occupational exposures contribute to 5–10% of cases, with asbestos exposure accounting for 3–4% of cases [4]. Asbestos exposure demonstrates a particularly concerning synergistic relationship with tobacco smoke, where combined exposure can multiply the risk of lung cancer development significantly above the risk posed by either factor alone by up to 14-fold [4]. PM is closely associated with asbestos exposure. Occupational exposure, particularly in industries such as construction, shipbuilding, and mining, has historically represented the primary risk factor for the development of PM [11]. Despite significant reductions in asbestos use since the 1970s, the United States continues to report the highest number of PM cases and deaths worldwide, a consequence of historical industrial exposure patterns and the disease's long latency period. Increasing incidence rates have been observed in several regions globally, underscoring the significant global health burden associated with asbestos exposure. The mortality burden from asbestos-related diseases has remained stable from 1999 to 2015 despite reductions in asbestos use, suggesting the need for more effective treatments [4].

Environmental pollutants, including urban and indoor air pollution, are increasingly recognized as contributors to lung cancer risk. Particulate matter found in air pollutants from automobile exhaust, factories, or combustion, especially particulate matter less than or equal to 2.5 μm in diameter (PM2.5), has been consistently associated with increased lung cancer incidence, even among never-smokers. The mechanisms through which these pollutants promote carcinogenesis likely involve oxidative stress, direct genetic damage to respiratory epithelial cells, and chronic inflammation [5].

Lung Cancer Screening and Prevention (NSCLC and SCLC)

Early detection screening programs (see Chap. 9) are crucial in reducing the mortality of lung cancer, as the treatment of localized or early-stage lung cancer can potentially be curative, and advanced disease has traditionally poor survival rates. The US Preventive Services Task Force and the Centers for Medicare & Medicaid Services (CMS) recommend that adults aged 50–80 years (CMS recommendations 50–77 years) who have a 20 pack-year smoking history and either currently smoke or have quit within the past 15 years receive annual lung cancer screening with LDCT. This section reviews the data that support these guidelines as per the National Lung Screening Trial [13] and the Randomized Lung Cancer Screening Trial [14].

The results of the NLST demonstrate a reduction in risk of lung cancer mortality in patients assigned to lung cancer screening with LDCT as compared with patients screened with chest radiography. Eligible participants in this trial were 55–74 years of age, had a history of cigarette smoking totaling at least 30 pack-years, and either currently smoked or had quit smoking within the past 15 years. Eligible patients were randomized to receive screening either with LDCT or chest radiography. Those assigned to receive screening with LDCT received three screenings at 1-year intervals. The NLST reported a relative reduction in the mortality rate from lung cancer of 20% (95% CI, 6.8–26.7; $P = 0.004$) in the LDCT screening group compared with the chest radiography screening group at a median duration of follow-up of 6.5 years. The number needed to screen with LDCT to prevent one death from lung cancer was calculated at 320.

The NELSON trial was designed to investigate whether screening for lung cancer using LDCT could reduce 10-year lung cancer mortality in high-risk individuals. The trial defined its target population based on the following criteria: individuals aged 50–75 years, current or former smokers who quit within 10 years, individuals who smoked greater than 15 cigarettes daily for 25 years or more, and those who smoked more than 10 cigarettes daily for greater than 30 years. Individuals who qualified underwent four rounds of LDCT screening for lung cancer at an interval of 1, 2, and 2.5 years. Lung cancer mortality was reduced by approximately 26% in the primary analysis of high-risk men and 61% in the smaller subgroup analysis of high-risk women over a 10-year period. The original trial demonstrated impressive screening performance metrics with a baseline sensitivity of 94.6%, a negative predictive value of 99.7%, a low false-positive rate of 64.3% (compared to >96% in other trials), and an overall lung cancer detection rate of 0.9% [14].

Although the number of women studied was small in the NELSON study, other studies, including an analysis of the NLST stratified by patient demographics, suggested a possible differential benefit to lung cancer screening by sex, which is the subject of ongoing research [15]. Research also indicates that African Americans face disproportionately higher impacts from lung cancer compared to other racial or ethnic groups in the United States [16]. This disparity manifests as elevated incidence and mortality rates, alongside a concerning tendency for later-stage diagnosis, which significantly affects treatment options and survival outcomes [2, 16].

Despite a clear benefit to early detection of lung cancer, screening is often underutilized when compared with other cancer screenings, such as breast, colon, or cervical cancer, particularly in light of these striking results [2]. Further, despite advances in lung cancer screening, lung cancer risk prediction models have not been incorporated into practice guidelines, and these models are not routinely used to guide screening eligibility or in clinical practice. However, a multitude of such models do exist.

LDCT Classification and Recommended Follow-Up Intervals

Radiologists use volumetric measurements rather than traditional diameter-based assessments to classify lung cancer screening findings and guide further screening intervals or diagnostic evaluation. The American College of Radiology Lung CT Screening Reporting and Data System (Lung-RADS) is categorized broadly into four levels (Table 5.1). Lung-RADS 1 is classified as "negative" and Lung-RADS 2 is classified as "benign," both of which warrant no alteration in the 12-month screening LDCT interval. Lung-RADS 3 is classified as "probably benign," with a recommended 6-month follow-up LDCT interval. Lung-RADS 4A is classified as "suspicious," with a recommended 3-month follow-up LDCT interval or followup PET/CT scan. Lastly, Lung-RADS 4B is classified as "very suspicious," and recommended follow-up includes either diagnostic CT chest (with or without contrast), PET/CT, tissue biopsy, or subspecialty referral. Additional modifiers such as "X" or "S" may be used to denote the presence of additional features that increase the concern for lung cancer (e.g., spiculation, evolving ground glass nodules, or enlarged lymph nodes) or clinically significant findings unrelated to lung cancer, respectively. Further specifics that are incorporated into the Lung-RADS classification system can be found in Table 5.1 [17].

Table 5.1 Lung-RADS® v2022 [17]

Lung-RADS	Category Descriptor	Findings	Management
0	**Incomplete** Estimated Population Prevalence: ~1%	Prior chest CT examination being located for comparison (see note 9)	Comparison to prior chest CT;
		Part or all of lungs cannot be evaluated	Additional lung cancer screening CT imaging needed;
		Findings suggestive of an inflammatory or infectious process (see note 10)	1-3 month LDCT
1	**Negative** Estimated Population Prevalence: 39%	No lung nodules OR Nodule with benign features: • Complete, central, popcorn, or concentric ring calcifications OR • Fat-containing	12-month screening LDCT
2	**Benign** - Based on imaging features or indolent behavior Estimated Population Prevalence: 45%	Juxtapleural nodule: • < 10 mm (524 mm³) mean diameter at baseline or new AND • Solid; smooth margins; and oval, lentiform, or triangular shape	
		Solid nodule: • < 6 mm (< 113 mm³) at baseline OR • New < 4 mm (< 34 mm³)	
		Part solid nodule: • < 6 mm total mean diameter (< 113 mm³) at baseline	
		Non solid nodule (GGN): • < 30 mm (< 14,137 mm³) at baseline, new, or growing OR • ≥ 30 mm (≥ 14,137 mm³) stable or slowly growing (see note 7)	
		Airway nodule, subsegmental - at baseline, new, or stable (see note 11)	
		Category 3 lesion that is stable or decreased in size at 6-month follow-up CT OR Category 4B lesion proven to be benign in etiology following appropriate diagnostic workup	
3	**Probably Benign** - Based on imaging features or behavior Estimated Population Prevalence: 9%	Solid nodule: • ≥ 6 to < 8 mm (≥ 113 to < 268 mm³) at baseline OR • New 4 mm to < 6 mm (34 to < 113 mm³)	6-month LDCT
		Part solid nodule: • ≥ 6 mm total mean diameter (≥ 113 mm³) with solid component < 6 mm (< 113 mm³) at baseline OR • New < 6 mm total mean diameter (< 113 mm³)	
		Non solid nodule (GGN): • ≥ 30 mm (≥ 14,137 mm³) at baseline or new	
		Atypical pulmonary cyst: (see note 12) • Growing cystic component (mean diameter) of a thick-walled cyst	
		Category 4A lesion that is stable or decreased in size at 3-month follow-up CT (excluding airway nodules)	
4A	**Suspicious** Estimated Population Prevalence: 4%	Solid nodule: • ≥ 8 to < 15 mm (≥ 268 to < 1,767 mm³) at baseline OR • Growing < 8 mm (< 268 mm³) OR • New 6 to < 8 mm (113 to < 268 mm³)	3-month LDCT; PET/CT may be considered if there is a ≥ 8 mm (≥ 268 mm³) solid nodule or solid component
		Part solid nodule: • ≥ 6 mm total mean diameter (≥ 113 mm³) with solid component ≥ 6 mm to < 8 mm (≥ 113 to < 268 mm³) at baseline OR • New or growing < 4 mm (< 34 mm³) solid component	
		Airway nodule, segmental or more proximal - at baseline (see note 11)	
		Atypical pulmonary cyst: (see note 12) • Thick-walled cyst OR • Multilocular cyst at baseline OR • Thin- or thick-walled cyst that becomes multilocular	
4B	**Very Suspicious** Estimated Population Prevalence: 2%	Airway nodule, segmental or more proximal - stable or growing (see note 11)	Referral for further clinical evaluation
		Solid nodule: • ≥ 15 mm (≥ 1767 mm³) at baseline OR • New or growing ≥ 8 mm (≥ 268 mm³)	Diagnostic chest CT with or without contrast; PET/CT may be considered if there is a ≥ 8 mm (≥ 268 mm³) solid nodule or solid component; tissue sampling; and/or referral for further clinical evaluation Management depends on clinical evaluation, patient preference, and the probability of malignancy (see note 13)
		Part solid nodule: • Solid component ≥ 8 mm (≥ 268 mm³) at baseline OR • New or growing ≥ 4 mm (≥ 34 mm³) solid component	
		Atypical pulmonary cyst: (see note 12) • Thick-walled cyst with growing wall thickness/nodularity OR • Growing multilocular cyst (mean diameter) OR • Multilocular cyst with increased loculation or new/increased opacity (nodular, ground glass, or consolidation)	
		Slow growing solid or part solid nodule that demonstrates growth over multiple screening exams (see note 8)	
4X	Estimated Population Prevalence: < 1%	Category 3 or 4 nodules with additional features or imaging findings that increase suspicion for lung cancer (see note 14)	
S	**Significant or Potentially Significant** Estimated Population Prevalence: 10%	Modifier: May add to category 0-4 for clinically significant or potentially clinically significant findings unrelated to lung cancer (see note 15)	As appropriate to the specific finding

© 2022 American College of Radiology® | All rights reserved

Published in https://www.acr.org/Clinical-Resources/Clinical-Tools-and-Reference/Reporting-and-Data-Systems/Lung-RADS, under CC BY-ND 4.0 license
Printed with permission from the American College of Radiology. Committee on Lung-RADS®. Lung-RADS Assessment Categories 2022. Lung-RADS® v2022

Therapeutic Treatment Implications of Molecular (Biomarker) Testing

Understanding lung cancer's molecular and cellular basis has had profound implications for therapeutic approaches. Identifying specific driver mutations has led to the development of targeted therapies that can effectively "stop" the cancer life cycle [8] (see Chap. 14). This personalized approach to treatment requires that comprehensive molecular testing be performed on the tissue biopsy specimen in order to identify actionable mutations, which can lead to treatment considerations. Therefore, molecular profiling is paramount in guiding treatment and is recommended by national organizations for all stages of lung cancer. Key actionable mutations in adenocarcinoma (NSCLC) of the lung include alterations in the proto-oncogenes *EGFR, ALK, ROS1, BRAF*, and others. These specific cancer alterations have associated targeted therapies, and more therapeutics for other alterations are currently in development. The effectiveness of these targeted approaches has contributed to an improvement in overall survival for patients diagnosed with targetable mutations.

Emerging Perspectives and Future Directions

The field of lung cancer research continues to evolve rapidly, with new insights into disease pathogenesis emerging at an astounding rate. Integrating multiple data types, including genomic, transcriptomic, and proteomic information, provides an increasingly detailed understanding of the complex biology underlying lung cancer development and progression. This knowledge continues to inform the development of novel therapeutic strategies and approaches to patient care.

Future directions in lung cancer research and treatment will likely focus on several key areas, including developing more effective strategies for early detection, identifying new therapeutic targets, and optimizing existing treatment approaches with particular attention to immunotherapy and targetable therapy resistance. The evolution of our understanding of lung cancer biology will undoubtedly lead to further improvements in patient care and outcomes.

Key Takeaways

- Both first- and second-hand exposure to tobacco smoke account for 85–90% of lung cancer cases [4].
- Occupational or environmental exposures have a further synergistic effect on the risk for lung cancer, with asbestos exposure being closely associated with mesothelioma development.
- The pathogenesis of lung cancer involves complex molecular mechanisms driven by both inherited genetic susceptibility and acquired genetic and chronic inflammatory changes.

- Guidelines recommend annual lung cancer screening with low-dose spiral CT for patients aged 50–80 who have a ≥20-pack-year smoking history and who currently smoke cigarettes or have quit within the past 15 years.
- The American College of Radiology Lung CT Screening Reporting and Data System (Lung-RADS) is used to categorize screening low-dose spiral CT findings and stratify further management and screening intervals.

Key Readings and Resources

- American College of Radiology Committee on Lung-RADS®. Lung-RADS Assessment Categories 2022 [17].
- Malignant Mesothelioma Treatment (PDQ®)–Health Professional Version [18].
- Non-Small Cell Lung Cancer Treatment (PDQ®)–Health Professional Version [19].
- Small Cell Lung Cancer Treatment (PDQ®)–Health Professional Version [20].

Conflicts of Interest The authors report no relevant conflicts of interest to disclose.

References

1. Ferlay J, Ervik M, Lam F, Laversanne M, Colombet M, Mery L, Piñeros M, Znaor A, Soerjomataram I, Bray F. Global cancer observatory: cancer today. Lyon: International Agency for Research on Cancer; 2024. Available from: https://gco.iarc.who.int/today. Accessed 16 April 2025.
2. Brock BA, Mir H, Flenaugh EL, Oprea-Ilies G, Singh R, Singh S. Social and biological determinants in lung cancer disparity. Cancers (Basel). 2024;16(3):612. Published 2024 Jan 31. https://doi.org/10.3390/cancers16030612.
3. American Cancer Society: Cancer Facts and Figures 2024. American Cancer Society, 2024 Available from: https://www.cancer.org/content/dam/cancer-org/research/cancer-facts-and-statistics/annual-cancer-facts-and-figures/2024/2024-cancer-facts-and-figures-acspdf. Cited 2025 Jan 25.
4. Corrales L, Rosell R, Cardona AF, Martín C, Zatarain-Barrón ZL, Arrieta O. Lung cancer in never smokers: the role of different risk factors other than tobacco smoking. Crit Rev Oncol Hematol. 2020;148:102895. https://doi.org/10.1016/j.critrevonc.2020.102895.
5. Minna JD, Roth JA, Gazdar AF. Focus on lung cancer. Cancer Cell. 2002;1(1):49–52. https://doi.org/10.1016/s1535-6108(02)00027-2.
6. SEER*Explorer: An interactive website for SEER cancer statistics [Internet]. Surveillance Research Program, National Cancer Institute; 2025 Apr 16. [cited 2025 Apr 16]. Available from: https://seer.cancer.gov/statistics-network/explorer/. Data source(s): SEER Incidence Data, November 2024 Submission (1975–2022), SEER 21 registries (excluding Illinois). Expected Survival Life Tables by Socio-Economic Standards.
7. Beebe-Dimmer JL, Fryzek JP, Yee CL, et al. Mesothelioma in the United States: a Surveillance, Epidemiology, and End Results (SEER)-Medicare investigation of treatment patterns and overall survival. Clin Epidemiol. 2016;8:743–50. Published 2016 Oct 26. https://doi.org/10.2147/CLEP.S105396.
8. Hanahan D, Weinberg RA. Hallmarks of cancer: the next generation. Cell. 2011;144(5):646–74. https://doi.org/10.1016/j.cell.2011.02.013.

9. Brenner DR, McLaughlin JR, Hung RJ. Previous lung diseases and lung cancer risk: a systematic review and meta-analysis. PLoS One. 2011;6(3):e17479. Published 2011 Mar 31. https://doi.org/10.1371/journal.pone.0017479.
10. Caramori G, Casolari P, Cavallesco GN, Giuffrè S, Adcock I, Papi A. Mechanisms involved in lung cancer development in COPD. Int J Biochem Cell Biol. 2011;43(7):1030–44. https://doi.org/10.1016/j.biocel.2010.08.022.
11. Kanwal M, Ding XJ, Cao Y. Familial risk for lung cancer. Oncol Lett. 2017;13(2):535–42. https://doi.org/10.3892/ol.2016.5518.
12. Shankar A, Dubey A, Saini D, et al. Environmental and occupational determinants of lung cancer. Transl Lung Cancer Res. 2019;8(Suppl 1):S31–49. https://doi.org/10.21037/tlcr.2019.03.05.
13. National Lung Screening Trial Research Team, Aberle DR, Adams AM, et al. Reduced lung-cancer mortality with low-dose computed tomographic screening. N Engl J Med. 2011;365(5):395–409. https://doi.org/10.1056/NEJMoa1102873.
14. Ru Zhao Y, Xie X, de Koning HJ, Mali WP, Vliegenthart R, Oudkerk M. NELSON lung cancer screening study. Cancer Imag. 2011;11 Spec No A(1A):S79–84. Published 2011 Oct 3. https://doi.org/10.1102/1470-7330.2011.9020.
15. Pinsky PF, Church TR, Izmirlian G, Kramer BS. The National Lung Screening Trial: results stratified by demographics, smoking history, and lung cancer histology. Cancer. 2013;119(22):3976–83. https://doi.org/10.1002/cncr.28326.
16. Namburi N, Timsina L, Ninad N, Ceppa D, Birdas T. The impact of social determinants of health on management of stage I non-small cell lung cancer. Am J Surg. 2022;223(6):1063–6. https://doi.org/10.1016/j.amjsurg.2021.10.022.
17. American College of Radiology Committee on Lung-RADS®. Lung-RADS assessment categories 2022. Lung-RADS® v2022. Available at: https://www.acr.org/Clinical-Resources/Clinical-Tools-and-Reference/Reporting-and-Data-Systems/Lung-RADS. American College of Radiology. Accessed on 2/11/2025.
18. PDQ® Adult Treatment Editorial Board. PDQ malignant mesothelioma treatment. Bethesda: National Cancer Institute. Updated 04/24/2024. Available at: https://www.cancer.gov/types/mesothelioma/hp/mesothelioma-treatment-pdq. Accessed 04/14/2025. [PMID: 26389420].
19. PDQ® Adult Treatment Editorial Board. PDQ non-small cell lung cancer treatment. Bethesda: National Cancer Institute. Updated 03/21/2025. Available at: https://www.cancer.gov/types/lung/hp/non-small-cell-lung-treatment-pdq. Accessed 04/14/2025. [PMID: 26389304].
20. PDQ® Adult Treatment Editorial Board. PDQ small cell lung cancer treatment. Bethesda: National Cancer Institute. Updated 03/26/2025. Available at: https://www.cancer.gov/types/lung/hp/small-cell-lung-treatment-pdq. Accessed 04/14/2025. [PMID: 26389347].

Open Access This chapter is licensed under the terms of the Creative Commons Attribution-NonCommercial 4.0 International License (http://creativecommons.org/licenses/by-nc/4.0/), which permits any noncommercial use, sharing, adaptation, distribution and reproduction in any medium or format, as long as you give appropriate credit to the original author(s) and the source, provide a link to the Creative Commons license and indicate if changes were made.

The images or other third party material in this chapter are included in the chapter's Creative Commons license, unless indicated otherwise in a credit line to the material. If material is not included in the chapter's Creative Commons license and your intended use is not permitted by statutory regulation or exceeds the permitted use, you will need to obtain permission directly from the copyright holder.

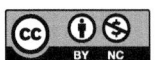

Critical Role of Genomics for Directed Therapeutic Management of Lung Cancer

6

Courtney A. Granville and Jaclyn LoPiccolo

Contents

Navigation Vignette	60
Introduction	61
Genomics and Proteomics	62
Genomic and Proteomic Approaches and Analytic Methods	62
Molecular Genetics of Lung Cancer	65
Benefits and Current Application of Genomics to Lung Cancer Treatment and Care	67
Conclusion	69
Key Takeaways	69
Key Readings and Resources	70
References	70

Abbreviations

AI	Artificial intelligence
ALK	Anaplastic lymphoma kinase
BRAF	V-Raf murine sarcoma viral oncogene homolog B
CDKN2A/B	Cyclin-dependent kinase inhibitor 2A/2B
COE	GO2 center of excellence
DNA	Deoxyribonucleic acid

C. A. Granville (✉)
GO2 for Lung Cancer, Washington, DC, USA

J. LoPiccolo
Department of Medical Oncology, Dana-Farber Cancer Institute, Boston, MA, USA

The Lowe Center for Thoracic Oncology, Dana-Farber Cancer Institute, Boston, MA, USA
e-mail: Jaclyn_LoPiccolo@DFCI.HARVARD.EDU

© The Author(s) 2026
J. T. Fathi, M. F. Mortman (eds.), *Lung Cancer Navigation and Care*,
https://doi.org/10.1007/978-3-032-02200-4_6

EGFR	Epidermal growth factor receptor
FISH	Fluorescence in situ hybridization
GWAS	Genome wide association studies
GO2	GO2 for Lung Cancer
HER2	Human epidermal growth factor receptor 2
IHC	Immunohistochemistry
KRAS	Kirsten rat sarcoma viral oncogene homolog
LUAD	Lung adenocarcinoma
MALDI	Matrix-assisted laser desorption ionization
MET	Mesenchymal-epithelial transition factor
ML	Machine learning
MS	Mass spectrometry
NSCLC	Non-small cell lung cancer
NCCN®	National comprehensive cancer network
NGS	Next-generation sequencing
NRG	Neuregulin
NLP	Natural language processing
PD-L1	Programmed cell death ligand 1
PRS	Polygenic risk score
RET	Rearranged during transfection
RNA	Ribonucleic acid
RNAseq	RNA sequencing
ROS1	ROS proto-oncogene 1, receptor tyrosine kinase
SCLC	Small cell lung cancer
TMB	Tumor mutational burden
TP53	Tumor protein 53
WES	Whole exome sequencing
WGS	Whole genome sequencing

Navigation Vignette

Ms. S. is a 52-year-old female with no known risk factors for lung cancer. During a routine annual exam, she presented to her gynecologist with a persistent and productive cough that had been worsening and was accompanied by white sputum, without fevers or known viral illness. Additionally, she reported feeling short of breath for several weeks prior. Her gynecologist referred her to Dr. J., her primary care physician in the *GO2 Centers of Excellence* network, who ordered a chest X-ray that showed an abnormality in the right upper lobe, followed by a chest CT and biopsy that diagnosed a Stage IIIB non-small cell lung adenocarcinoma. Ms. S. was introduced to a social worker, D.W., MSW, OSW-C, a lung cancer navigator, as a multidisciplinary lung cancer care team member assigned to manage her case. In addition to standard biomarker testing as part of her care, D.W. suggested that Ms. S. participate in an ongoing remote, direct-to-patient clinical research study to have whole genome sequencing of her tumor. D.W. worked with the study team to ensure that part of her tumor biopsy was sent to researchers at *GO2 for Lung Cancer* and the *Addario Lung Cancer Medical Institute* for next-generation sequencing.

Ms. S.'s comprehensive genomic profiling revealed an *EGFR exon 19 deletion*, a driver mutation known to respond well to targeted therapy. Based on these findings, her oncology team recommended initiating treatment with an EGFR tyrosine kinase inhibitor rather than proceeding immediately with conventional chemotherapy or radiation. This targeted approach offered Ms. S. the potential for improved progression-free survival and fewer side effects compared to standard therapies.

Ms. S. began her oral targeted therapy within weeks of diagnosis, supported by regular monitoring and symptom management coordinated by her care team, including social worker D.W., because her treatment was tailored to the specific biology of her cancer, she experienced a rapid reduction in tumor size and improvement in her breathing and energy levels.

Access to genomic testing not only personalized Ms. S.'s treatment but also connected her to a broader community of research and advocacy. The study she joined offered additional support resources and updates on emerging treatments that might benefit her in the future. Ms. S.'s experience underscores the growing impact of precision medicine in lung cancer—providing patients with targeted, effective care based on the unique molecular features of their disease.

Introduction

Lung cancer is a highly heterogeneous disease with the highest mortality rate of any cancer [1]. While data about the role of individual genes and proteins in the development and treatment of lung cancer has become more robust over the past two decades, less is known about how genes may work together to influence lung cancer risk, progression, and response to therapy.

Molecular Biology 101: DNA, RNA, Proteins and Targeted Therapy

The central dogma of molecular biology is that genes, which are encoded by deoxyribonucleic acid (DNA), are transcribed (or copied) to messenger ribonucleic acid (mRNA), which are then translated into proteins that carry out specific functions within the cell. In a normally functioning cell, mRNA and proteins are made in response to specific signals to ensure proper functioning [2].

In cancer, gene mutations or changes in DNA sequence can lead to alterations in gene expression or activity [3]. These changes cause cells to survive, divide, and/or act abnormally. Targeted therapies are very effective at counteracting specific driver mutations, so it is important to understand the molecular biology of a tumor before beginning treatment.

Gene sequencing and immunohistochemistry play critical roles in understanding cancer biology and personalized medicine by detecting mutations driving lung cancer to guide treatment decisions, understand resistance, and develop more effective therapies. This allows for a more precise and individualized approach to cancer care, as opposed to a "one-size-fits-all" treatment strategy.

Many driver mutations can be detected by approaches that look specifically at known alterations (called "targeted" sequencing or detection). However, newer approaches to sequencing allow for a comprehensive look at all genes and proteins simultaneously and have both clinical and exploratory applications.

Genomics and Proteomics

Genomics and proteomics are two approaches to analyzing many genes and the proteins those genes produce and can give information about levels of many genes or proteins simultaneously. Genomic profiling using next-generation sequencing (NGS) is currently the preferred approach for comprehensive biomarker testing in lung cancer per the NCCN Guidelines®, but NGS has applications beyond the identification of tumor biomarkers [4]. For example, the patterns that emerge from looking across groups of genes, proteins, or their expression levels may be most useful to stratify for cancer risk, prognosis, potential response to treatment, or to predict recurrence or resistance to therapy. Polygenic risk scores integrate the effect of multiple genes or gene variants on the risk of developing lung cancer [5–7] but are not currently used in clinical practice.

Key Definitions

- *Genomics*: The simultaneous analysis of multiple genes (DNA) or gene expression (RNA) in a tissue sample. The analysis of multiple RNA molecules is also referred to as *transcriptomics*.
- *Proteomics*: The simultaneous analysis of multiple proteins in a tissue sample.
- *Polygenic risk*: The contribution of several genes together to define risk.

Genomic and Proteomic Approaches and Analytic Methods

DNA and RNA Sequencing and Expression Analysis

There are several complementary methods for analyzing both tumor and normal tissue genomes, including DNA and RNA analysis (Table 6.1). DNA sequencing directly examines the sequence of genes (and, for example, detects mutations and changes in gene copy number), while RNA sequencing examines the expression level of these same genes and can be useful as a complementary method for detecting oncogenic fusions and gene amplifications.

Genomics is a field focused on analyzing the entire genome or all the DNA of a person or a sample (such as a blood or saliva sample, or a tumor biopsy), whereas

Table 6.1 Methods for genomic and proteomic analysis

Method	Target	Features
Genomic and transcriptomic analyses [8–13]		
Next generation sequencing (NGS)	DNA	A set of techniques that rely on massively parallel sequencing and can detect several alterations in a single analysis
Targeted NGS	DNA	Sequences a pre-selected panel of cancer-related genetic alterations, including single nucleotide variants, copy number variations, and rearrangements such as insertions/deletions or fusions
Whole exome sequencing (WES)	DNA	NGS of all exons (protein coding regions) and junctions of intron (non-coding region) and exon; detects mutations, insertions, and deletions
Whole genome sequencing (WGS)	DNA	Sequences entire genome including regions of unknown function or that serve a regulatory function; detects structural variants, regulatory regions, epigenetic changes in addition to mutations, insertions, and deletions
Microarray analysis	RNA	Uses hybridization of probes to identify and quantify gene expression levels
RNA sequencing (RNAseq)	RNA	Uses sequencing to detect and quantify gene expression levels
Proteomic analysis [14, 15]		
2-D gel electrophoresis (2-DE) and mass spectrometry (MS)	Peptides	Uses 2D gel electrophoresis for separation by size and charge; proteins are broken down into smaller pieces and then sequenced using MS
Matrix-assisted laser desorption ionization (MALDI)-MS	Polypeptides	MS sequences whole proteins; used to identify structure and function

genetics is the study of a single gene or group of genes, and focused more on heredity [16]. In genomics, either the DNA or RNA is sequenced and quantified using NGS, or, in the case of RNA, known sequences may be quantified using microarray analysis [8, 9]. Genomic analyses may be useful for identifying variations in one or more genes or understanding gene expression. Gene expression is measured by assessing RNA levels and is also referred to as transcriptomics [10].

The different applications of NGS and RNA sequencing vary in cost and the level of genome coverage [17]. Targeted NGS, for example, looks at a panel of specific genes (also called panel-based NGS), can include anywhere from 20 to 500 genes on more extensive panels, is less expensive and may be quicker, but it may miss some variants. Whole genome sequencing (WGS) and whole exome sequencing (WES) sequence larger areas of the genome and can therefore identify novel variants, but these are often not clinically actionable (meaning there are no identified targeted treatments available for this variant at this time) with current treatments, the analysis is usually more expensive, and the turnaround time is often longer.

Similarly, there are differences in the approaches to analyzing RNA that should be considered. Microarray analysis is high-throughput and relatively quick, but it only analyzes expression of specific targets and lacks precision. At the same time,

RNA sequencing offers broader coverage of the genome and greater precision, but it is more expensive [11]. RNA sequencing is used clinically, while microarray analysis is used more in research settings.

Protein Sequencing and Expression Analysis

Clinically, protein biomarkers are assessed using a targeted approach (i.e., they measure only specific proteins, mainly by immunohistochemistry), and proteomic techniques (such as mass spectrometry, etc.) that assess protein sequences and expression on a global level are more experimental.

Targeted detection of protein overexpression or protein alterations, such as rearrangement and amplification, generally relies on techniques called immunohistochemistry (IHC) and fluorescence in situ hybridization (FISH). These techniques can be used to detect changes in some clinically actionable genes (e.g., *ALK*, *MET*, *ROS1*, *HER2*, and *TRK*). In some cases, IHC is used as a screening assay that requires confirmation by FISH or genomic methods, as well as to detect levels of programmed death-ligand 1 (PD-L1) expression [4].

Proteomics analyzes all proteins in a sample and largely relies on mass spectrometry (MS) for sequencing following separation by gel electrophoresis or digestion by enzymes [14]. In addition to assessing levels of expression, proteomics may also detect levels of activity or structural variability [15]. These assays are more experimental and are not currently applied to guide clinical care.

Proteomics has been used as a research tool for diagnostic purposes, biomarker discovery, and drug development. While it arguably tells us more about how cancer is functioning or what it relies on to survive than genomics or transcriptomics, proteomics is complex because proteins are dynamic and constantly changing. For example, protein expression can differ based on the environmental and cellular conditions, and proteins are often modified post-translationally, giving them an altered function.

Like genomics, approaches to proteomic analysis differ in cost and the type of data revealed. 2-DE coupled with MS is generally useful to identify differences in expression levels between samples and changes to a specific protein. However, while more expensive and labor-intensive, MALDI-MS can identify protein interactions and modifications.

Use of Genomic and Proteomic Data to Estimate Risk

Both genomic and proteomic data can be used to look at specific genes and proteins and identify mutation prevalence [18]. Genome-wide association studies (GWAS) can identify common inherited (also called germline) genetic variants associated with lung cancer development [19, 20]. These studies examine genetic risk of lung cancer but do not give any information on lung cancer once it has developed. GWAS is performed by comparing common variants in the entire genome across two different populations (for example, those with or without lung cancer) and identifies gene variants (or mutations) that differ significantly in number between the two sets of samples to look for associations with a given trait or characteristic. Genes that are identified as associated with lung cancer can then be further investigated to determine the role that they could play in cancer development, maintenance, or progression [21].

Polygenic risk is quantified as a polygenic risk score (PRS), which is calculated as the sum of the number of germline variants associated with lung cancer that an individual carries, in relation to the strength of association each variant has with lung cancer development [22, 23]. PRS can be used to predict the risk of developing lung cancer [24, 25], which has been demonstrated to vary across subpopulations, including race/genetic ancestry [6].

Pattern Detection in Genomic and Proteomic Data

Although identifying single genes that play a role in lung cancer is one application of genomics and proteomics, the large datasets produced from these analyses are more commonly leveraged for patterns that emerge. Bioinformatics and more advanced analytic approaches, such as machine learning and natural language processing, are useful for analyzing the large datasets that emerge from genomic and proteomic assays. Additionally, many software solutions and web-based algorithms are available to aid in the analysis of the large datasets that are produced by genomics and proteomics and can describe clinically relevant endpoints such as tumor mutational burden, mutational signatures, copy number alterations, gene fusions and structural variants, chromosomal instability, and aneuploidy [26].

Molecular Genetics of Lung Cancer

Our understanding of the underlying genetics of NSCLC and SCLC differs. In NSCLC, particularly those that arise in people with little or no tobacco exposure, many genetic alterations have been identified that drive lung cancer and can be targeted with treatment, while in SCLC, the genetics are less well-defined, and biology is thought to be largely tobacco-driven. The American College of Medical Genetics and Genomics and the Association for Molecular Pathology developed consensus guidelines that describe the relative frequency of genetic variants [27]. The utility of these biomarkers is briefly described below and is explained in more detail in Chaps. 14 and 19.

Our knowledge of the genetic landscape and targetable or clinically actionable genomic alterations (also called "biomarkers") in lung cancer largely drives current treatment paradigms. Additionally, genomic and proteomic signatures are emerging for a variety of uses, including risk prediction, prognosis, response to treatment, and guidance for therapy following recurrence, and/or the development of resistance to targeted therapies (Table 6.2).

Table 6.2 Selected investigational gene, gene expression, and protein signatures in lung cancer

Signature type	Methods	Description	Clinical application
NSCLC			
Gene copy number [28]	WGS	Three profiles identified	Potential to inform treatment and provide prognostic info
Gene expression [29]	WES and RNA-Seq	Id driver mutations; "passive smoking" signature identified	Inform treatment
Gene mutation [30]	FoundationOne CDx or FoundationOne liquid CDx (targeted NGS)	Id co-alterations in ALK-rearranged tumors, including CDKN2A/B loss in 18%, which was associated with increased risk of brain metastasis	Prognostic; could guide dosing decisions and brain follow-up
Mutation signatures [31]	CancerVision test (WGS)	Three profiles identified	Signatures could guide treatment selection or exclusion or clinical trial identification
Gene mutation [32–34]	RNA-Seq	Id fusions of RET, ALK, and ROS1	Treatment selection
SCLC			
Gene expression [35]	LC-SCRUM-Asia (targeted NGS)	Five signatures identified	Identified a PI3K/Akt/mTOR pathway mutation subgroup for a phase 2 trial of Gedatolisib
Mutation signatures [31]	WGS	Three signatures identified	Signatures could guide treatment selection or exclusion or clinical trial identification
Protein signatures [36]	Multi-omic	Four signatures identified	Treatment strategies

Non-small Cell Lung Cancer

Current practice and care for patients with non-small cell lung cancer (NSCLC) relies upon assessment of specific tumor biomarkers to inform precision medicine (see Chap. 15). There are currently several well-defined genes and proteins, including mutations (see Abbreviations list above for full names) in *EGFR*, *HER2*, *KRAS*, *MET*, and *BRAF* genes, as well as fusions (also called rearrangements) in *ALK*, *RET*, *ROS1*, *TRK*, and most recently NRG1, that are used to determine the appropriate course of treatment and care. Genomic studies reveal that the prevalence of such biomarkers for which targeted therapies are available in the first line is 68–92% in tumors from people who never smoked [37, 38], and much lower in those with any smoking status. For example, in people who smoke/d, the prevalence of EGFR mutations is between 7% and 18%, and the prevalence of ALK mutations is 0–3% [39]. These targetable alterations are important biomarkers that drive first-line treatment selection in NSCLC (see Chaps. 14, 15, and 18). Additionally, the expression of PD-L1 (a protein expressed on the surface of the tumor cells and immune cells) can be used to guide eligibility and the selection of immunotherapy treatments [40].

Patterns of gene expression also reveal that the underlying molecular genetics of NSCLC are more complex than single-biomarker dependence, and WGS reveals patterns associated with distinct molecular subtypes of lung cancer. One study assessed gene copy number in a set of 232 tumors from patients who had never smoked [28] while another looked at gene expression using WES and RNA-Seq [29]. Both uncovered three distinct profiles; however, the overlap and/or relationship between these profiles is unknown.

Small Cell Lung Cancer

In small cell lung cancer (SCLC), the use of biomarkers to drive precision medicine has not caught up to NSCLC, but molecular classifications derived from genomic analyses have recently been described and may be useful to guide treatment (see Chap. 16). One is the neuroendocrine vs. endocrine classification that was first defined by Gazdar and colleagues in 1985 [43]. Newer classifications build on these two phenotypes and suggest that particular therapeutic approaches may be more useful in each, but there is no guideline-driven consensus at this time [41–43]. Emerging anti-DLL3 therapies (such as the bispecific T-cell engager, tarlatamab) show promise in treating SCLC by targeting the DLL3 protein, which is highly expressed in SCLC cells but minimally present in normal tissue, enabling T-cell-driven tumor destruction.

Benefits and Current Application of Genomics to Lung Cancer Treatment and Care

Genomics and proteomics have applications in both clinical and investigational research settings. Genomic studies, either DNA or RNA sequencing, have revealed a high prevalence of varying driver alterations (cellular DNA changes that contribute to the development and proliferation of cancer) in lung cancer (mutation, rearrangement, or amplification of driver genes), regardless of smoking status, although targetable alterations are enriched in those who have not smoked. This justifies the standard practice to include targeted biomarker testing as part of the diagnostic phase in lung cancer so that treatment can be appropriately matched to the tumor genotype, known as "genotype-directed therapy."

Emerging Applications for Genomics and Proteomics to Inform Treatment

While genomics has current applications for treatment selection, proteomics is less well-developed, largely due to the rapidly changing nature of proteins and issues with protein stability in patient-derived samples. In theory, both genomics and proteomics are equally powerful as research tools by providing a mechanism to identify unique profiles and better understand the molecular mechanisms driving lung cancer development, response to treatment, and progression. Additionally, genomic and, perhaps eventually, proteomic signatures (patterns or characteristic features within genomes unique to individuals) may soon have clinical utility, for example, when:

- targetable mutations are not detected by standard biomarker testing
- progressive disease is observed, and there are no additional standard approaches

One example of how genomics can help inform treatment comes from a recent multi-site cohort study in Latin America. This study identified patients with ALK-rearranged lung cancers and their tumors sequenced using targeted NGS [44]. A variety of concurrent mutations were identified in 72 of 116 cases (62%), including mutations in *TP53* and loss of *CDKN2A/B*. Loss of *CDKN2A/B* was associated with increased frequency of brain metastasis and poorer overall and progression-free survival. The authors of the study suggest that understanding the relationship between co-mutation and prognosis should direct dose optimization as well as follow-up care, including frequency of brain follow-up in cases of co-occurring ALK-rearrangement and *CDKN2A/B* loss.

Additionally, genomics demonstrated that loss of *CDKN2A/B* is frequently accompanied by deletion of methylthioadenosine phosphorylase (MTAP) [45]. MTAP deficiency may serve as a biomarker that can guide treatment because patients who present with loss of MTAP generally do not respond to immune checkpoint inhibitors and do respond to PRMT5 inhibitors currently in clinical trials and development [46].

A small retrospective study using WGS also demonstrated the clinical application of genomic technologies and highlights where deeper sequencing can have clinical utility when targeted NGS is negative [47]. The researchers used a predetermined panel of 323 cancer-related genes to interrogate nine cancer cases, including four lung cancers. Rare targetable fusion mutations were detected in two cases, while both a single nucleotide and a splicing mutation were found in one case, and five single-nucleotide mutations were discovered in the fourth case. In the first three cases, targeted therapies were subsequently used in the treatment of the patients, achieving responses in two. This example also demonstrates the important role of WGS in identifying fusion mutations; its use should be considered especially in young non-smoking patients for whom these mutations are more common when targeted NGS is negative.

Use of Genomics and Proteomics Beyond Targetable Mutations

As described above, analysis of immune markers in the WES study in patients who had not smoked revealed genomic profiles that were described as immune hot, cold, or intermediate. It is possible that these patterns could be used to identify patients who are more or less likely to respond to immunotherapy. However, the hypothesis has not been tested [29], and generally, immunotherapy response in patients without tobacco exposure has been poor.

In addition to identifying targetable mutations, panel-based NGS can quantify the tumor mutational burden (TMB), which can also be used to guide treatment [31]. TMB is a marker for response to immunotherapy—those with a higher mutational burden have better clinical outcomes, including objective response and progression-free survival following treatment with PD-1 inhibitors, than those with lower TMB [48].

Genomics can also be used to describe a person's underlying inherited genetics, which can influence risk for the development of lung cancer and potentially clinical outcomes. Although not in routine clinical use, germline-directed sequencing may be useful for constructing PRS with potential utility in five clinical areas—risk prediction, diagnostics, treatment guidance, clinical trial efficiency, and improving public health [49].

The utility of PRS in informing cancer prognosis is still not well understood. Xi et al. recently demonstrated that PRS does not predict survival in 17 different cancers [50]. They suggest that additional factors may need to be incorporated to produce a score useful for outcome prediction. Finally, current PRSs in lung cancer, which are derived from studies mainly looking at smoking-related lung cancer, are good indicators of risk in those of European or Caucasian descent but are not predictive in the Black population, highlighting the need for additional research to identify and validate genetic risk factors for other ethnic groups [6].

Conclusion

Genomics and proteomics are established tools for understanding the underlying biological processes driving lung cancer. In the clinical setting, NGS, FISH, and ICH are utilized as best practice for detecting specific biomarkers at both diagnosis and the time of disease progression. These biomarkers direct the use of targeted therapies or provide information about prognosis and mechanisms of resistance.

Key Takeaways

- When available, panel-based comprehensive NGS is a best practice for biomarker testing in lung cancer.

- Broader genomic profiling (such as WES and WGS) and proteomics are currently primarily research tools but may have clinical utility when standard results are not straightforward or return negative.
- Polygenic risk scores may be useful to identify high-risk individuals in a research setting, but additional work is needed to make PRS clinically applicable.
- Polygenic risk scores are not currently useful as outcome predictors in lung cancer.

Key Readings and Resources

- Biochemistry, Replication and Transcription [2]
- Cancer Genetics Overview (PDQ®)–Health Professional Version [51]
- Lung Cancer in Patients Who Have Never Smoked—An Emerging Disease [39]
- National Comprehensive Cancer Network (NCCN) Clinical Practice Guidelines in Oncology (NCCN Guidelines®): Non-Small Cell Lung Cancer [4]

Conflict of Interest None.

References

1. Siegel RL, Giaquinto AN, Jemal A. Cancer statistics, 2024. CA Cancer J Clin. 2024;74(1):12–49.
2. Mercadante AA, Dimri M, Mohiuddin SS. Biochemistry, replication and transcription. Treasure Island: StatPearls; 2025.
3. MedLine Plus [Internet]. What is a gene variant and how do variants occur? Genetics: Help Me Understand Genetics: Variants and Health March 25, 2021 [cited 2025 April 20]; Available from: https://medlineplus.gov/genetics/understanding/mutationsanddisorders/genemutation/.
4. National Comprehensive Cancer Network, 2024. NCCN clinical practice guidelines in oncology (NCCN Guidelines®): Non-Small Cell Lung Cancer. V3.2025. Accessed 7 Apr 2025.
5. Boumtje V, Manikpurage HD, Li Z, Gaudreault N, Armero VS, Boudreau DK, et al. Polygenic inheritance and its interplay with smoking history in predicting lung cancer diagnosis: a French-Canadian case-control cohort. EBioMedicine. 2024;106:105234.
6. Trendowski MR, Lusk CM, Wenzlaff AS, Neslund-Dudas C, Gadgeel SM, Soubani AO, et al. Assessing a polygenic risk score for lung cancer susceptibility in non-hispanic white and black populations. Cancer Epidemiol Biomarkers Prev. 2023;32(11):1558–63.
7. Wang X, Zhang Z, Ding Y, Chen T, Mucci L, Albanes D, et al. Impact of individual level uncertainty of lung cancer polygenic risk score (PRS) on risk stratification. Genome Med. 2024;16(1):22.
8. DeRisi J, Penland L, Brown PO, Bittner ML, Meltzer PS, Ray M, et al. Use of a cDNA microarray to analyse gene expression patterns in human cancer. Nat Genet. 1996;14(4):457–60.
9. Frampton GM, Fichtenholtz A, Otto GA, Wang K, Downing SR, He J, et al. Development and validation of a clinical cancer genomic profiling test based on massively parallel DNA sequencing. Nat Biotechnol. 2013;31(11):1023–31.
10. Xu W, Seok J, Mindrinos MN, Schweitzer AC, Jiang H, Wilhelmy J, et al. Human transcriptome array for high-throughput clinical studies. Proc Natl Acad Sci USA. 2011;108(9):3707–12.
11. Wang Z, Gerstein M, Snyder M. RNA-Seq: a revolutionary tool for transcriptomics. Nat Rev Genet. 2009;10(1):57–63.

12. Kohno T. Implementation of "clinical sequencing" in cancer genome medicine in Japan. Cancer Sci. 2018;109(3):507–12.
13. Yoshida T, Yatabe Y, Kato K, Ishii G, Hamada A, Mano H, et al. The evolution of cancer genomic medicine in Japan and the role of the National Cancer Center Japan. Cancer Biol Med. 2023;21(1):29–44.
14. Hanash S. Disease proteomics. Nature. 2003;422(6928):226–32.
15. Al-Amrani S, Al-Jabri Z, Al-Zaabi A, Alshekaili J, Al-Khabori M. Proteomics: concepts and applications in human medicine. World J Biol Chem. 2021;12(5):57–69.
16. Green E. Talking glossary of genomic and genetic terms. National Institutes of Health, National Human Genome Research Institute; 2014. Available from: https://www.genome.gov/genetics-glossary.
17. Abbasi A, Alexandrov LB. Significance and limitations of the use of next-generation sequencing technologies for detecting mutational signatures. DNA Repair (Amst). 2021;107:103200.
18. Li W, Olivier M. Current analysis platforms and methods for detecting copy number variation. Physiol Genomics. 2013;45(1):1–16.
19. Gorman BR, Ji SG, Francis M, Sendamarai AK, Shi Y, Devineni P, et al. Multi-ancestry GWAS meta-analyses of lung cancer reveal susceptibility loci and elucidate smoking-independent genetic risk. Nat Commun. 2024;15(1):8629.
20. Bosse Y, Amos CI. A decade of GWAS results in lung cancer. Cancer Epidemiol Biomarkers Prev. 2018;27(4):363–79.
21. Uffelmann E, Huang QQ, Munung NS, de Vries J, Okada Y, Martin AR, et al. Genome-wide association studies. Nat Rev Methods Primers. 2021;1:59.
22. Klein RJ, Gumus ZH. Are polygenic risk scores ready for the cancer clinic?-a perspective. Transl Lung Cancer Res. 2022;11(5):910–9.
23. Cancer Genetics Overview (PDQ®)–Health Professional Version National Cancer Institute; 2024.
24. Jia G, Lu Y, Wen W, Long J, Liu J, Tao R, et al. Evaluating the utility of polygenic risk scores in identifying high-risk individuals for eight common cancers. JNCI Cancer Spectr. 2020;4(3):pkaa021.
25. Jia G, Wen W, Massion PP, Shu X-O, Zheng W. Incorporating both genetic and tobacco smoking data to identify high-risk smokers for lung cancer screening. Carcinogenesis. 2021;42(6):874–9.
26. Luthra A, Mastrogiacomo B, Smith SA, Chakravarty D, Schultz N, Sanchez-Vega F. Computational methods and translational applications for targeted next-generation sequencing platforms. Genes Chromosomes Cancer. 2022;61(6):322–31.
27. Richards S, Aziz N, Bale S, Bick D, Das S, Gastier-Foster J, et al. Standards and guidelines for the interpretation of sequence variants: a joint consensus recommendation of the American College of Medical Genetics and Genomics and the Association for Molecular Pathology. Genet Med. 2015;17(5):405–24.
28. Zhang T, Joubert P, Ansari-Pour N, Zhao W, Hoang PH, Lokanga R, et al. Genomic and evolutionary classification of lung cancer in never smokers. Nat Genet. 2021;53(9):1348–59.
29. Devarakonda S, Li Y, Martins Rodrigues F, Sankararaman S, Kadara H, Goparaju C, et al. Genomic profiling of lung adenocarcinoma in never-smokers. J Clin Oncol. 2021;39(33):3747–58.
30. Lara-Mejia L, Cardona AF, Mas L, Martin C, Samtani S, Corrales L, et al. Impact of concurrent genomic alterations on clinical outcomes in patients with ALK-rearranged NSCLC. J Thorac Oncol. 2024;19(1):119–29.
31. Kim R, Kim S, Oh BB, Yu WS, Kim CW, Hur H, et al. Clinical application of whole-genome sequencing of solid tumors for precision oncology. Exp Mol Med. 2024;56(8):1856–68.
32. Kohno T, Ichikawa H, Totoki Y, Yasuda K, Hiramoto M, Nammo T. KIF5B-RET fusions in lung adenocarcinoma. Nat Med. 2012;18:375–7.

33. Lipson D, Capelletti M, Yelensky R, Otto G, Parker A, Jarosz M. Identification of new ALK and RET gene fusions from colorectal and lung cancer biopsies. Nat Med. 2012;18:382–4.
34. Takeuchi K, Soda M, Togashi Y, Suzuki R, Sakata S, Hatano S. RET, ROS1 and ALK fusions in lung cancer. Nat Med. 2012;18:378–81.
35. Umemura S, Udagawa H, Ikeda T, Yoh K, Niho S, Goto K. Clinical significance of a prospective large genomic screening for SCLC: the genetic classification and a biomarker-driven phase 2 trial of Gedatolisib. Transl Oncol. 2025;20(2):177–93.
36. Liu Q, Zhang J, Guo C, et al. Proteogenomic characterization of small cell lung cancer identifies biological insights and subtype-specific therapeutic strategies. Cell. 2024;187:184–203. e28.
37. Devarakonda S, Li Y, Rodrigues FM, Sankararaman S, Kadara H, Goparaju C, et al. Genomic profiling of lung adenocarcinoma in never-smokers. J Clin Oncol. 2021;39(33):3747.
38. Zhang T, Joubert P, Ansari-Pour N, et al. Genomic and evolutionary classification of lung cancer in never smokers. Nat Genet. 2021;53:1348–59.
39. LoPiccolo J, Gusev A, Christiani DC, Janne PA. Lung cancer in patients who have never smoked – an emerging disease. Nat Rev Clin Oncol. 2024;21(2):121–46.
40. Ghringhelli F, Bibeau F, Greillier L, Fumet J-D, Ilie A, Monville F, et al. Immunoscore immune checkpoint using spatial quantitative. Lancet. 2023;92:1–12.
41. Rudin CM, Poirier JT, Byers LA, Dive C, Dowlati A, George J, et al. Molecular subtypes of small cell lung cancer: a synthesis of human and mouse model data. Nat Rev Cancer. 2019;19(5):289–97.
42. Gay CM, Stewart CA, Park EM, Diao L, Groves SM, Heeke S, et al. Patterns of transcription factor programs and immune pathway activation define four major subtypes of SCLC with distinct therapeutic vulnerabilities. Cancer Cell. 2021;39(3):346–60. e7.
43. Gazdar AF, Carney DN, Nau MM, Minna JD. Characterization of variant subclasses of cell lines derived from small cell lung cancer having distinctive biochemical, morphological, and growth properties. Cancer Res. 1985;45(6):2924–30.
44. Lara-Mejia L, Cardona AF, Mas L, Martin C, Samtani S, Corrales L, et al. Impact of concurrent genomic alterations on clinical outcomes in patients with ALK-rearranged NSCLC. Non Small Cell Lung Cancer. 2024;19(1):119–29.
45. Su CY, Chang YC, Chan YC, Lin TC, Huang MS, Yang CJ, et al. MTAP is an independent prognosis marker and the concordant loss of MTAP and p16 expression predicts short survival in non-small cell lung cancer patients. Eur J Surg Oncol. 2014;40(9):1143–50.
46. Brune MM, Savic Prince S, Vlajnic T, Chijioke O, Roma L, Konig D, et al. MTAP as an emerging biomarker in thoracic malignancies. Lung Cancer. 2024;197:107963.
47. Kim M, Jeong JY, Park NJ-Y, Park JY. Clinical utility of next-generation sequencing in real-world cases: a single-institution study of nine cases. In Vivo. 2022;36:1397–407.
48. Rizvi NA, Hellmann MD, Snyder A, Kvistborg P, Makarov V, Havel JJ, et al. Cancer immunology. Mutational landscape determines sensitivity to PD-1 blockade in non-small cell lung cancer. Science. 2015;348(6230):124–8.
49. Maamari DJ, Abou-Karam R, Fahed AC. Polygenic risk scores in human disease. Clin Chem. 2025;71(1):69–76.
50. Xing J, Jiang X, Li H, Chen S, Zhang Z, Wang M, et al. Prognostic evaluation of polygenic risk score underlying pan-cancer analysis: evidence from two large-scale cohorts. EBioMedicine. 2023;89:104454.
51. PDQ® Cancer Genetics Editorial Board. Cancer Genetics Overview (PDQ®): Health Professional Version. PDQ Cancer Information Summaries. Bethesda; 2002.

Open Access This chapter is licensed under the terms of the Creative Commons Attribution-NonCommercial 4.0 International License (http://creativecommons.org/licenses/by-nc/4.0/), which permits any noncommercial use, sharing, adaptation, distribution and reproduction in any medium or format, as long as you give appropriate credit to the original author(s) and the source, provide a link to the Creative Commons license and indicate if changes were made.

The images or other third party material in this chapter are included in the chapter's Creative Commons license, unless indicated otherwise in a credit line to the material. If material is not included in the chapter's Creative Commons license and your intended use is not permitted by statutory regulation or exceeds the permitted use, you will need to obtain permission directly from the copyright holder.

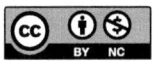

Essential Components for the Development of an Early Lung Cancer Detection Program

7

Joelle Thirsk Fathi ⓘ, Jonathan T. Hontzas ⓘ, and Sarah A. Weston ⓘ

Contents

Navigation Vignette.	76
Introduction.	77
Integrating Centers for Medicare and Medicaid Services Requirements.	77
Lung Cancer Yield in Early Lung Cancer Detection Programs.	78
Essential Operational and Clinical Components of Early Lung Cancer Detection Programs.	78
Start-Up and Sustainability: The Financial Implications of Early Lung Cancer Detection Programs.	81
Deconstructing Discrimination and Structural and Systemic Injustices to Improve Lung Cancer Outcomes.	82
Quality Performance and Improvement Planning for Early Lung Cancer Detection Programs.	83
Adherence as a Quality Measure Critical to Quality Outcomes.	84
Healthcare Effectiveness Data and Information Set (HEDIS) Measures.	84
Growth and Sustainability of Early Lung Cancer Detection Programs.	84
Conclusion.	85
Key Takeaways.	85
Key Readings and Resources.	85
References.	86

J. T. Fathi (✉)
GO2 for Lung Cancer, Washington, DC, USA

Department of Biobehavioral Nursing and Health Informatics, University of Washington, Seattle, WA, USA
e-mail: thirsk@uw.edu

J. T. Hontzas
Cancer Center and Research Institute, University of Mississippi Medical Center, Jackson, MS, USA

Department of Population Health Science, University of Mississippi Medical Center, Jackson, MS, USA

S. A. Weston
GO2 for Lung Cancer, Washington, DC, USA

© The Author(s) 2026
J. T. Fathi, M. F. Mortman (eds.), *Lung Cancer Navigation and Care*,
https://doi.org/10.1007/978-3-032-02200-4_7

Abbreviations

BPA	Best practice advisory
CMS	Centers for Medicare and Medicaid Services
EHR	Electronic health record
ELCD	Early lung cancer detection
IPN	Incidental pulmonary nodule
LCS	Lung cancer screening
LDCT	Low-dose computed tomography
USPSTF	United States Preventive Services Task Force

Navigation Vignette

Nurse Practitioner T. works in a pulmonology clinic, seeing patients with asymptomatic lung nodules detected through chest imaging for any indication requiring further evaluation and diagnostic workup. He is responsible for longitudinal patient panel management to ensure no nodule is left behind. Nurse Practitioner T. frequently sees patients who meet current United States Preventive Services Task Force criteria for lung cancer screening in the clinic. He is aware that millions of people are eligible for lung cancer screening and the absence of a lung cancer screening program in the health system where he works.

Nodule management algorithms and appropriate interval follow-up imaging are frequent topics of conversation with the pulmonology team, with varying management recommendations by his pulmonology colleagues. Over time, Nurse Practitioner T. identified the complexities of lung nodule management, including the need for multidisciplinary, standardized, and guideline-directed input on the more complex cases. With further consideration and research, he identified the opportunity to streamline lung nodule management efforts for people with lung nodule(s) who either do or do not meet screening eligibility. In determining this need and opportunity in his health system, he spearheaded the design and development of an *Early Lung Cancer Detection* program. His initial steps in this process included inquiry into the current evidence and guidelines for lung cancer screening and incidental pulmonary nodules. He utilized the content of this chapter and others to inform himself of the background and critical considerations when leading this effort, to initiate and establish relationships with key stakeholders, and to build a framework for an Early Lung Cancer Detection program aiming to close health disparity and equity gaps. Finally, Nurse Practitioner T. developed a business plan using the GO2 for Lung Cancer *Thoracic Oncology Business Model* to garner clinical and administrative leadership's institutional resources and support, which is necessary to initiate, grow, and sustain a clinical program.

Introduction

For nearly three-quarters of a century, lung cancer has been one of the leading (and is currently the number one) causes of cancer-related morbidity and mortality in the United States and worldwide [1–4]. First-hand cigarette smoke exposure is known to be the primary risk for developing lung cancer ahead of second-hand smoke, radon, and occupational and environmental exposures [5]. Traditionally presenting in later and more advanced stages, the 5-year survival from lung cancer hovered at 11% until recently [5]. Now, the 5-year survival rate has more than doubled, reaching 28.4% [6], largely due to the discovery, development, and frequency of genomic testing, targetable mutation detection, personalized treatment options, and most notably, favorable stage shift appreciated with early lung cancer detection (ELCD) through screening [5].

More than 30 years ago, researchers initiated an investigation into the use of low-dose CT (LDCT) scan for lung cancer screening (LCS) [7] and compared LDCT to chest X-rays to detect lung cancer in earlier stages. Using LDCT, the National Lung Screening Trial (NLST) demonstrated a significant 20% lung cancer mortality reduction [8]. The more recent Nederlands-Leuvens Longkanker Screenings Onderzoek (NELSON) trial showed a 26% mortality benefit with an even greater benefit of LCS in women [9]. Since 2010, lung cancer screening has been a United States Preventive Services Task Force (USPSTF) preventive health recommendation for people at high risk who meet currently accepted criteria [10] and has been recognized as a covered service by the Centers for Medicaid and Medicare (CMS) since 2015 [11]. Since then, LCS rates have been consistently rising (the current national screening average of eligible individuals screened is 16%) [12], but that still leaves the vast majority of eligible individuals, over 12 million people in the United States, unscreened and an additional 1.5 million people with incidental pulmonary nodules (IPN) in need of surveillance [13]. Healthcare teams must rapidly develop and refine early lung cancer detection (LCS and IPN) programs to improve effectiveness and efficiency in identifying lung cancers for a more favorable stage shift. Implementing well-constructed ELCD programs while placing the patients' needs center-stage can significantly improve survival rates through timely diagnosis and intervention, ultimately shifting the prognosis for those who are affected by this disease.

Integrating Centers for Medicare and Medicaid Services Requirements

Thoughtful and intentional development of effective early lung cancer detection programs must incorporate the CMS-required elements, which must be satisfied for reimbursement. They ensure that qualifying criteria are met, shared decision-making occurs, cigarette smoking is addressed, and guideline-directed baseline and follow-up imaging is obtained at appropriate intervals. The CMS National Coverage Determination (CMS-NCD) for LCS includes coverage requirements that must be adhered to when administering lung cancer screening [11]. Current evidence, clinical guidelines, and CMS requirements drive health systems to resource and programmatize LCS. They are also key considerations when determining the needed resources, structure, and operations of an ELCD program(s) to make a strong business case for health systems to invest in these life-saving programs.

Lung Cancer Yield in Early Lung Cancer Detection Programs

The management of incidental pulmonary nodules (lung nodules detected outside the screening setting) is complex and known to yield a higher rate of lung cancer (2–4% detection rate) [14] than those detected in screening programs (1.1–1.6% detection rate) [8, 9, 15]. There are several compelling and prudent reasons to invest in pragmatic ELCD programs, including:

1. Significant false positive rates (3.9% and 24.2%) [8, 9] and over-diagnosis rates (8.9% and 18.4%) [8, 9] observed in the NLST and NELSON trials, respectively
2. Prevalence of incidental findings
3. Potential for screening complications
4. Mortality benefits of early lung cancer detection

Care delivery models must be person-centered and designed to serve the express needs of the 14.5 million people who are at risk and qualify for lung cancer screening [16] and the added 1.5 million people with incidental pulmonary (IPN) nodules detected annually [17].

Essential Operational and Clinical Components of Early Lung Cancer Detection Programs

Critical Engagement of Key Stakeholders for Successful Clinical Programs

The development and growth of ELCD programs are complex, multifaceted, and resource-intensive (see Chap. 9). Key stakeholders, including clinical and organizational/system leadership (C-Suite and others) (see Table 7.1), must be identified and convened early to secure essential buy-in and commitment of resources to build a high-quality program. An initial program development element is deciding which department(s) will be responsible for the program's operation and success and establishing a formal governance structure. These responsibilities and accountabilities for the ELCD program must be clearly outlined for successful development and implementation.

Table 7.1 Key clinical and organizational/system stakeholders

Clinical Leaders
Appropriate clinical/medical staff leadership (primary care, pulmonology, radiology, and oncology (medical, surgical, and radiation), radiology)
Clinic administrative/operational leadership (nursing, medical, program, director, manager)
Community-based organization representing high-risk, diverse populations
Organizational Leaders
Chief Executive Officer
Chief Financial Officer
Chief Information and Technology Officer
Chief Marketing Officer
Chief Medical Officer
Chief Operating Officer

Multidisciplinary Teams in Screening and Nodule Management

Quality care in ELCD programs offers access to guideline-directed screening and follow-up imaging, multidisciplinary review and management of lung nodules and other findings detected, and efficiencies in time to diagnosis and treatment without harm [18]. Studies show that while significant awareness of nodule management guidelines exists, there is a 30–60% variance in adherence to such guidelines among radiologists and community pulmonologists [19–23]. Programs powered by multidisciplinary care teams with pulmonary and oncology specialists that include cancer navigators are more effective in such endeavors [24, 25]. Preliminary data across multiple studies identify some plausible factors for this success, including timeliness and optimization of coordinated care delivery, the ease of scheduling across specialties, provider-to-provider communication in care planning, and preventing patients from being lost to follow-up [25].

Depending on local resources, the design of the program (centralized, decentralized, or hybrid), and the available workforce, the composition of the multidisciplinary ELCD teams and Nodule and Tumor Boards may vary but usually include a combination of specialists (pulmonary, thoracic surgery, medical and radiation oncology, radiology, primary care, cancer navigation, tobacco treatment specialist). Whether housed in a large tertiary–quaternary medical center or a community facility, ELCD programs should identify and fully engage a diverse and multidisciplinary team that adheres to best practice guidelines to meet the programmatic demands and patient needs.

Radiology Partners and Infrastructure Supporting Early Detection Programs

Early lung cancer detection programs must ensure patients receive imaging with radiology partners who adhere to best practice and safety standards. Radiology plays a critical role as a partner in ELCD programs. Engaging a radiology champion

Table 7.2 Radiology requirements for administering lung cancer screening [11, 27–29]

Adherence to low-dose CT imaging for baseline and follow-up lung cancer screenings and incidental pulmonary nodule surveillance when clinically indicated to minimize patient radiation exposure while maintaining appropriate imaging quality for interpretation
Utilization of LCS technical specifications as directed by the American College of Radiology (ACR) including volumetric CT dose index (CTDIvol) of 3.0 milligray (mGy) for standard-sized patients and suitable changes for smaller or larger patients
Standardized interpretation and reporting templates are used by reading radiologists for consistent, imaging-based management of nodules and other findings
Lung CT screening reporting and data system (Lung-RADS) should be used for LDCT LCS imaging reporting
Fleischner society's 2017 guidelines for Management of Incidental Pulmonary Nodules should be used for IPN imaging reporting

early in the program development process for appropriate program implementation is essential to ensure adherence to the approved guidelines and metrics [26] and quality health outcomes. Regardless of program or facility type, a minimum of several radiology-based standards (see Table 7.2) must be applied to provide appropriate, evidence-based, and high-quality management of LCS and IPN patients in an ELCD program. Radiology departments responsible for LDCT imaging are encouraged to adhere to the American College of Radiology adult LCS technical specifications [27].

Technology for Identification and Management of Lung Nodules

Establishing and utilizing technology to optimize quality care delivery and health outcomes is paramount for ELCD programs in the initial phases of program planning and the subsequent growth process. Clinicians can leverage the electronic health record (EHR) to mine discrete data elements and identify people who may be eligible for LCS. LCS best practice advisory (BPA) alerts should be embedded within the clinical decision support system within the EHR [30] and positioned to alert clinicians when engaging a patient eligible for LCS. These improve patient safety and allow for better adherence to the clinical guidelines associated with both groups [30]. Similar EHR-based functionalities and natural language processing software, using artificial intelligence and algorithms, can be harnessed as a quality control measure to identify patients in the health system with IPN imaging findings that require follow-up imaging, for example [31]. Nodule management programs, either EHR-based or third-party software solutions, house dashboards and functionality that aid in customized automation to safely and effectively manage ELCD populations (see Table 7.3).

Table 7.3 Features and functionality of lung nodule management software programs [32, 33]

Clinical Component
Quality dashboard for ELCD quality improvement initiatives, program monitoring, and reporting
Radiology report data extraction for patient and physician letter generation
Integration in electronic health record to facilitate patient tracking through portal alerts, correspondence, results reports, and recommended timed follow-up and reminders to prevent attrition
Worklist generation for patient and results management
Complement staff reminders
Radiology Component
Computer-aided detection (CAD) capability to aid in nodule detection on imaging
Volumetric nodule measurement for size accuracy and nodule comparison over time
Malignancy risk calculators to aid in decision-making
Interoperability in imaging data transmission and sharing with ELCD program EHRs using digital imaging and Communications in Medicine (DICOM)

Integration of Smoking Cessation Services to Save Lives

Offering smoking cessation services to people undergoing LCS is a CMS requirement [11]. Quitting smoking is beneficial for both those at high risk for lung cancer due to a significant first-hand smoke exposure history and those diagnosed with lung cancer. These related health benefits include a reduced chance of developing a second primary lung cancer [34] and better overall survival for people who quit before, at, or around a cancer diagnosis (with a positive correlation between years since quitting and increased survival benefit) [35, 36]. Improved long-term survival can also be appreciated by providing cessation services post-lung cancer diagnosis, especially with successful cessation within 6 months of diagnosis [37, 38]. Integration of smoking cessation services at the time of LCS and IPN evaluation is a crucial component of any ELCD program. The National Institutes of Health Smoking Cessation at Lung Examination Collaborative researchers are now reporting the findings from their clinical trials on the most effective methods for integrating such services in the context of LCS [39, 40]. Finally, GO2 for Lung Cancer's LCS Clinical Workflow Models can help determine where cessation may be included in the workflows of centralized, decentralized, and hybrid LCS care delivery models [41].

Start-Up and Sustainability: The Financial Implications of Early Lung Cancer Detection Programs

When building and growing clinical programs that provide healthcare services, the value of the clinical service, expected program outcomes, and the return on investment, including projected revenue and margin yield from the various funding streams (largely from insurance plans/coverage), are central to committing to such endeavors. The cost-effective and positive contribution of ELCD programs to organizational revenue margins has been shown [42–44]. However, the revenues and expenses incurred in providing ELCD services are a complex process, variable, and depend highly on the cost of care delivery (administrative, staff, equipment, space, etc.) and the health plans or insurance types (payer mix) that cover the population the health system serves. Ultimately, a comprehensive, well-planned ELCD program provides healthcare savings and can be financially beneficial and self-sustaining. These components are needed to develop a sound business proforma that projects future performance based on plausible assumptions.

The GO2 for Lung Cancer Thoracic Oncology Business Model is a simple and free tool that may be customized for ELCD programs and their locally available resources to project the financial performance of LCS and IPN programs year-over-year [45]. This model supports forecasting for fee-for-service and value-based contracts across commercial, Medicare, and Medicaid, health plans. This business model captures billable services related to the early detection process, including those for shared decision-making, navigator services, LDCT and follow-up imaging, downstream revenue for diagnostic workup imaging and procedures, and treatment of lung cancers detected in an ELCD program by stage distribution. Finally, the model produces the necessary outputs (i.e., business proforma, presentation tables, and figures) for review by key leadership members and related discussions and presentations.

Deconstructing Discrimination and Structural and Systemic Injustices to Improve Lung Cancer Outcomes

People who experience discrimination, including those who identify as LGBTQ2IA+, people who are adversely impacted by social determinants of health, and those who experience lower socioeconomic status and rurality, are at higher risk for lung cancer and more likely to suffer from healthcare access issues [46, 47]. Racial and ethnic minorities are less likely to be screened and diagnosed early, receive guideline-concordant care, and experience lower survival rates than White people, with Black men being at the highest risk for lung cancer-related mortality than any other group [48]. To constructively address these health disparities and inequities, ELCD programs must develop strategies within health systems and clinical care pathways and, in partnership with the community, deconstruct structural and systemic barriers affecting the most vulnerable and historically oppressed populations.

To achieve progress in addressing equity and the needs of all people at risk for lung cancer, delivering the right screening and care to those eligible and in need at the right time requires prioritizing the most marginalized and at-risk populations with expedient and action-oriented attention to:

1. Actively and accurately assess the ELCD program's target population and determine their location within the health system's service area to ensure inclusiveness in outreach and engagement;
2. Authentically collaborate with local community health workers and community-based organizations using vetted strategies to bridge medical mistrust and to reach disadvantaged communities and their at-risk members where they are; [49]
3. Collect and track demographic information for people seen in health systems compared to service areas to continuously monitor the current state of individuals served and identify system-based inequalities, direct individual engagement, track health outcomes, measure progress in reaching desired populations, and proactively improve performance; [49, 50]
4. Identify and resolve barriers to accessing and receiving preventive health services and care for all at-risk people needing LCS and IPN care;
5. Advocate for establishing and maintaining telehealth-capable technology, organizational support, and policy to offer screening and care by telehealth and mobile units to reduce health disparities and inequities resulting from stigma and social, employment, financial, and geographic barriers to seeking and achieving access and care; [51, 52]
6. Drive awareness and train clinicians and healthcare staff on the effects of and how to address clinician and staff positionality, privilege, and implicit and explicit biases to mitigate and eliminate prejudice and the stigma of lung cancer; [49]
7. Persistently strive to illuminate areas of opportunity to close health disparity and inequity gaps while informing communities and policymakers through related research, white papers, public service announcements, and advocacy work [49].

Quality Performance and Improvement Planning for Early Lung Cancer Detection Programs

The ever-emerging science and evolving healthcare landscape require programs to constantly adapt and adjust to maintain a competitive position at the forefront of the field and succeed at delivering high-quality care. To do so, program leads and staff must maintain accurate and timely awareness of program performance metrics, act on frequent evaluations, and perform routine literature reviews to identify needed changes. Such changes may include exploring the adoption of emerging technology, newly integrated diagnostics and imaging tools, clinical care guidelines, shifts in care delivery workflows, attention to patient characteristics and care delivery and uptake patterns, and observed health outcomes within the program. Continuous evaluation and quality improvement initiatives ensure that programs operate at the highest level and deliver the safest care.

Establishing a quality dashboard and collecting data for analysis and routine evaluation of clinical program performance is crucial to ensuring high-quality outcomes. When designed to include critical information, quality dashboards also ensure that high-risk populations are represented and appropriately benefiting from the ELCD services. Measurable information assists programs in understanding how close they are to achieving their programmatic goals, including those around health equity. National benchmarks often inform programmatic goals.

Adherence as a Quality Measure Critical to Quality Outcomes

Select quality metrics are critical to determining ELCD programs' effectiveness, with annual adherence rates being one of the most important factors in saving lives from lung cancer. Annual follow-up adherence rates after initial screening for LCS are known to be as low as 35% [53], with adherence to important annual repeat LDCT or recommended routine follow-up decreasing each subsequent year [54]. Similarly, IPN follow-up adherence rates are as low as 40% [55]. There is a positive and direct correlation between adherence to routine repeat follow-up scan rates and the benefit of earlier stage lung cancer detection [54]. The extent to which routine and effective follow-up responsibility resides with the patient and ELCD programs is ill-defined. ELCD programs must proactively recall patients with every attempt to ensure they follow through on required imaging, benefit from LCS and IPN follow-up, and receive the value ELCD programs offer.

Healthcare Effectiveness Data and Information Set (HEDIS) Measures

The National Committee for Quality Assurance (NCQA) focuses on improving healthcare quality through several mechanisms, including Healthcare Effectiveness Data and Information Set (HEDIS) measures. The NCQA will release a HEDIS measure for LCS soon, which health systems should be preparing to respond to now. At any given time, more than 90 HEDIS measures are active and directed to measuring preventive services, treatment outcomes, and patient satisfaction across the care continuum in different disease areas where improvement is needed to improve related morbidity and mortality. Health plans use HEDIS elements to measure specific aspects of healthcare and associated services, monitoring, and evaluating health system performance. This monitoring and outcomes measurement improves health outcomes and addresses health disparities and inequities for at-risk and vulnerable populations [56, 57].

Growth and Sustainability of Early Lung Cancer Detection Programs

A growth mindset is crucial to the expansion and sustainability of ELCD programs. Program sustainability is multifaceted and hinges on the ability to collaborate. Partnerships and communication with local providers, hospitals, community-based organizations, and other groups enhance feedback and referral networks to ensure patients can access comprehensive care programs. Ultimately, healthcare is a service industry that depends on programs to effectively communicate and offer services and healthcare experiences that referring clinicians and patients expect and deserve.

Conclusion

Developing effective ELCD programs that are high-performing and effective at improving lung cancer outcomes requires careful attention to implementing current evidence, best practice standards, clinical guidelines, and agency (CMS) requirements. Multidisciplinary and cross-collaborative teams positively contribute to meeting the complex needs of people who need support and care through ELCD programs. Addressing health disparities and ensuring equitable access to screening and care, as well as continuous quality improvement, program evaluation, adaptation, and the effective utilization of technology, are all paramount to achieving long-term success in the fight against lung cancer.

Key Takeaways

- Organizational/system and community stakeholder engagement and support are a priority when building and growing the ELCD program
- Program success begins with establishing a governance structure
- Investment in multidisciplinary and collaborative relationships is broadly beneficial
- Leveraging technology to power and enhance ELCD programs is crucial to optimization and quality performance
- Prioritizing comprehensive services that promote the highest level of adherence is critical to early-stage lung cancer detection
- Integration of smoking cessation services in the context of ELCD programs improves abstinence and lung cancer survival rates

Key Readings and Resources

- United States Preventive Services Task Force Final Recommendation for Lung Cancer Screening [10]
- CMS National Coverage Determination [11]
- Lung-RADS 2022 [28]
- Fleischner Guidelines 2017 [29]
- GO2 for Lung Cancer Thoracic Oncology Business Model [45]
- GO2 for Lung Cancer Lung Cancer Screening Models [41]

Conflict of Interest Joelle Thirsk Fathi—No conflicts of interest
- Jonathan T. Hontzas—Reports receiving financial remuneration for speaking on behalf of Biodesix
- Sarah A. Weston—No conflicts of interest

References

1. Bray F, Laversanne M, Sung H, Ferlay J, Siegel RL, Soerjomataram I, et al. Global cancer statistics 2022: GLOBOCAN estimates of incidence and mortality worldwide for 36 cancers in 185 countries. CA Cancer J Clin. 2024;74(3):229–63.
2. National Cancer Institute. 61-Year Trends in U.S. Cancer Death Rates. National Cancer Institute; 2010. Available from: https://seer.cancer.gov/archive/csr/1975_2010/results_merged/topic_historical_mort_trends.pdf.
3. Wingo PA, Cardinez CJ, Landis SH, Greenlee RT, Ries LA, Anderson RN, et al. Long-term trends in cancer mortality in the United States, 1930–1998. Cancer. 2003;97(12 Suppl):3133–275.
4. Barta JA, Powell CA, Wisnivesky JP. Global epidemiology of lung cancer. Ann Glob Health. 2019;85(1)
5. Thandra KC, Barsouk A, Saginala K, Aluru JS, Barsouk A. Epidemiology of lung cancer. Contemp Oncol (Pozn). 2021;25(1):45–52.
6. American Lung Association. State of Lung Cancer 2024; 2024. Available from: https://www.lung.org/getmedia/12020193-7fb3-46b8-8d78-0e5d9cd8f93c/SOLC-2024.pdf.
7. Henschke CI, McCauley DI, Yankelevitz DF, Naidich DP, McGuinness G, Miettinen OS, et al. Early lung cancer action project: overall design and findings from baseline screening. Lancet. 1999;354(9173):99–105.
8. Aberle DR, Adams AM, Berg CD, Black WC, Clapp JD, Fagerstrom RM, et al. Reduced lung-cancer mortality with low-dose computed tomographic screening. N Engl J Med. 2011;365(5):395–409.
9. de Koning HJ, van der Aalst CM, de Jong PA, Scholten ET, Nackaerts K, Heuvelmans MA, et al. Reduced lung-cancer mortality with volume CT screening in a randomized trial. N Engl J Med. 2020;382(6):503–13.
10. U. S. Preventive Services Task Force, Krist AH, Davidson KW, Mangione CM, Barry MJ, Cabana M, et al. Screening for lung cancer: US preventive services task force recommendation statement. JAMA. 2021;325(10):962–70.
11. Centers for Medicare & Medicaid Services. Screening for Lung Cancer with Low Dose Computed Tomography (LDCT); 2022. Available from: https://www.cms.gov/medicare-coverage-database/view/ncacal-decision-memo.aspx?proposed=Y&ncaid=304&#:~:text=In%202021%2C%20the%20most%20recent,within%20the%20past%2015%20years.
12. American Lung Association. State of Lung Cancer; 2024. Available from: https://www.lung.org/research/state-of-lung-cancer/key-findings.
13. Farjah F, Monsell SE, Smith-Bindman R, Gould MK, Banegas MP, Ramaprasan A, et al. Fleischner society guideline recommendations for incidentally detected pulmonary nodules and the probability of lung cancer. J Am Coll Radiol. 2022;19(11):1226–35.
14. Vachani A, Zheng C, Amy Liu IL, Huang BZ, Osuji TA, Gould MK. The probability of lung cancer in patients with incidentally detected pulmonary nodules: clinical characteristics and accuracy of prediction models. Chest. 2022;161(2):562–71.
15. Burnett-Hartman A, Rendle K, Saia C, Greenlee R, Carroll N, Honda S, Hixon B, Kim R, Neslund-Dudas C, Oshiro C, Wain K, Rizwoller D, Vachani A. Lung cancer yield among those undergoing lung cancer screening in community-based healthcare systems. Cancer Epidemiol Biomarkers Prev [Internet]. 2025;32(6).:[863 p.]. Available from: https://aacrjournals.org/cebp/article/32/6/863/726584/Lung-Cancer-Yield-Among-Those-Undergoing-Lung.

16. Wolf AMD, Oeffinger KC, Shih TY, Walter LC, Church TR, Fontham ETH, et al. Screening for lung cancer: 2023 guideline update from the American Cancer Society. CA Cancer J Clin. 2024;74(1):50–81.
17. Gould MK, Tang T, Liu IL, Lee J, Zheng C, Danforth KN, et al. Recent trends in the identification of incidental pulmonary nodules. Am J Respir Crit Care Med. 2015;192(10):1208–14.
18. Mazzone PJ, White CS, Kazerooni EA, Smith RA, Thomson CC. Proposed quality metrics for lung cancer screening programs: a national lung cancer roundtable project. Chest. 2021;160:–368.
19. Luis A, Encinas JL, Leal N, Hernandez F, Gamez M, Murcia J, et al. Multidisciplinary approach in the management of intestinal failure. Cir Pediatr. 2007;20(2):71–4.
20. Eisenberg RL, Bankier AA, Boiselle PM. Compliance with Fleischner Society guidelines for management of small lung nodules: a survey of 834 radiologists. Radiology. 2010;255(1):218–24.
21. Esmaili A, Munden RF, Mohammed TL. Small pulmonary nodule management: a survey of the members of the society of thoracic radiology with comparison to the Fleischner society guidelines. J Thorac Imaging. 2011;26(1):27–31.
22. Tanner NT, Aggarwal J, Gould MK, Kearney P, Diette G, Vachani A, et al. Management of pulmonary nodules by community pulmonologists: a multicenter observational study. Chest. 2015;148(6):1405–14.
23. Mets OM, de Jong PA, Chung K, Lammers JJ, van Ginneken B, Schaefer-Prokop CM. Fleischner recommendations for the management of subsolid pulmonary nodules: high awareness but limited conformance – a survey study. Eur Radiol. 2016;26(11):3840–9.
24. Mankidy BJ, Mohammad G, Trinh K, Ayyappan AP, Huang Q, Bujarski S, et al. High risk lung nodule: a multidisciplinary approach to diagnosis and management. Respir Med. 2023;214:107277.
25. Stone CJL, Vaid HM, Selvam R, Ashworth A, Robinson A, Digby GC. Multidisciplinary clinics in lung cancer care: a systematic review. Clin Lung Cancer. 2018;19(4):323–30. e3.
26. Snoeckx A, Franck C, Silva M, Prokop M, Schaefer-Prokop C, Revel MP. The radiologist's role in lung cancer screening. Transl Lung Cancer Res. 2021;10(5):2356–67.
27. American College of Radiology. Adult Lung Cancer Screening: Technical Specifications – Adult Chest for Lung Cancer Screening; 2014. Available from: https://scottalexander.me/wp-content/uploads/2021/12/7dd83-acr-str-lung-cancer-screening-guidelines-2014.pdf.
28. Christensen J, Prosper AE, Wu CC, Chung J, Lee E, Elicker B, et al. ACR Lung-RADS v2022: assessment categories and management recommendations. J Am Coll Radiol. 2024;21(3):473–88.
29. MacMahon H, Naidich DP, Goo JM, Lee KS, Leung ANC, Mayo JR, et al. Guidelines for management of incidental pulmonary nodules detected on CT images: from the Fleischner society 2017. Radiology. 2017;284(1):228–43.
30. Maniaci MJ, Torres-Guzman RA, Avila FR, Maita K, Garcia JP, Forte AJ, et al. Development and evaluation of best practice advisory alert for patient eligibility in a hospital-at-home program: a multicenter retrospective study. J Hosp Med. 2024;19(3):165–74.
31. Basilio R, Carvalho AR, Rodrigues R, Conrado M, Accorsi S, Forghani R, et al. Natural language processing for the identification of incidental lung nodules in computed tomography reports: a quality control tool. JCO Glob Oncol. 2023;9:e2300191.
32. Parikh A, Gupta K, Wilson AC, Fields K, Cosgrove NM, Kostis JB. The effectiveness of outpatient appointment reminder systems in reducing no-show rates. Am J Med. 2010;123(6):542–8.
33. Prakashini K, Babu S, Rajgopal KV, Kokila KR. Role of Computer Aided Diagnosis (CAD) in the detection of pulmonary nodules on 64 row multi detector computed tomography. Lung India. 2016;33(4):391–7.
34. Aredo JV, Luo SJ, Gardner RM, Sanyal N, Choi E, Hickey TP, et al. Tobacco smoking and risk of second primary lung cancer. J Thorac Oncol. 2021;16(6):968–79.

35. Wang X, Romero-Gutierrez CW, Kothari J, Shafer A, Li Y, Christiani DC. Prediagnosis smoking cessation and overall survival among patients with non-small cell lung cancer. JAMA Netw Open. 2023;6(5):e2311966.
36. Caini S, Del Riccio M, Vettori V, Scotti V, Martinoli C, Raimondi S, et al. Quitting smoking at or around diagnosis improves the overall survival of lung cancer patients: a systematic review and meta-analysis. J Thorac Oncol. 2022;17(5):623–36.
37. Cinciripini PM, Kypriotakis G, Blalock JA, Karam-Hage M, Beneventi DM, Robinson JD, et al. Survival outcomes of an early intervention smoking cessation treatment after a cancer diagnosis. JAMA Oncol. 2024;10:1689–96.
38. Caini S, Gorini G, Del Riccio M, Saieva C, Carreras G, Bonomo P, et al. Upgrading your best chances: postdiagnosis smoking cessation boosts life expectancy of patients with cancer – a systematic review and meta-analysis. Tob Control. 2025.
39. National Institute of Health, National Cancer Institute Division of Cancer Control & Population Sciences. Smoking Cessation at Lung Examination: The SCALE Collaboration; 2025. Available from: https://cancercontrol.cancer.gov/brp/tcrb/scale-collaboration.
40. Joseph AM, Rothman AJ, Almirall D, Begnaud A, Chiles C, Cinciripini PM, et al. Lung cancer screening and smoking cessation clinical trials. SCALE (Smoking Cessation within the Context of Lung Cancer Screening) Collaboration. Am J Respir Crit Care Med. 2018;197(2):172–82.
41. GO2 for Lung Cancer. Lung Cancer Screening Clinical Workflow Models, 2025. https://hcp.go2.org/workflow-models/
42. Grover H, King W, Bhattarai N, Moloney E, Sharp L, Fuller L. Systematic review of the cost-effectiveness of screening for lung cancer with low dose computed tomography. Lung Cancer. 2022;170:20–33.
43. Behr CM, Oude Wolcherink MJ, IJzerman MJ, Vliegenthart R, Koffijberg H. Population-based screening using low-dose chest computed tomography: a systematic review of health economic evaluations. Pharmacoeconomics. 2023;41(4):395–411.
44. Gilbert CR, Ely R, Fathi JT, Louie BE, Wilshire CL, Modin H, et al. The economic impact of a nurse practitioner-directed lung cancer screening, incidental pulmonary nodule, and tobacco-cessation clinic. J Thorac Cardiovasc Surg. 2018;155(1):416–24.
45. GO2 for Lung Cancer. Thoracic Oncology Business Model; 2025. Available from: https://hcp.go2.org/business-model/.
46. Kratzer TB, Bandi P, Freedman ND, Smith RA, Travis WD, Jemal A, et al. Lung cancer statistics, 2023. Cancer. 2024;130(8):1330–48.
47. Das M, Raymond HF, Chu P, Nieves-Rivera I, Pandori M, Louie B, et al. Measuring the unknown: calculating community viral load among HIV-infected MSM unaware of their HIV status in San Francisco from National HIV Behavioral Surveillance, 2004–2011. J Acquir Immune Defic Syndr. 2013;63(2):e84–6.
48. Haddad DN, Sandler KL, Henderson LM, Rivera MP, Aldrich MC. Disparities in lung cancer screening: a review. Ann Am Thorac Soc. 2020;17(4):399–405.
49. Rivera MP, Katki HA, Tanner NT, Triplette M, Sakoda LC, Wiener RS, et al. Addressing disparities in lung cancer screening eligibility and healthcare access. Am J Respir Crit Care Med. 2020;202(7):e95–e112.
50. Lee K, Haramati LB, Ye K, Lin J, Mardakhaev E, Gohari A. Lung cancer screening penetration in an urban underserved county. Lung. 2023;201(2):243–9.
51. Simkin J, Khoo E, Darvishian M, Sam J, Bhatti P, Lam S, et al. Addressing inequity in spatial access to lung cancer screening. Curr Oncol. 2023;30(9):8078–91.
52. Pua BB, O'Neill BC, Ortiz AK, Wu A, D'Angelo D, Cahill M, et al. Results from lung cancer screening outreach utilizing a mobile CT scanner in an urban area. J Am Coll Radiol. 2024;21(5):778–88.
53. Gillespie C, Wiener RS, Clark JA. Patient experience of managing adherence to repeat lung cancer screening. J Patient Exp. 2022;9:23743735221126146.

54. Han SS, Erdogan SA, Toumazis I, Leung A, Plevritis SK. Evaluating the impact of varied compliance to lung cancer screening recommendations using a microsimulation model. Cancer Causes Control. 2017;28(9):947–58.
55. Wang Z, Mortani Barbosa EJ Jr. Socio-economic factors and clinical context can predict adherence to incidental pulmonary nodule follow-up via machine learning models. J Am Coll Radiol. 2024;21(10):1620–31.
56. Malik S. A quick guide to HEDIS measures and measurement-based care: Linear Health; 2024. Available from: https://linear.health/clinical-assessments/hedis-measures/.
57. National Committee for Quality Assurance. HEDIS Measures and Technical Resources: National Committee for Quality Assurance; 2025. Available from: https://www.ncqa.org/.

Open Access This chapter is licensed under the terms of the Creative Commons Attribution-NonCommercial 4.0 International License (http://creativecommons.org/licenses/by-nc/4.0/), which permits any noncommercial use, sharing, adaptation, distribution and reproduction in any medium or format, as long as you give appropriate credit to the original author(s) and the source, provide a link to the Creative Commons license and indicate if changes were made.

The images or other third party material in this chapter are included in the chapter's Creative Commons license, unless indicated otherwise in a credit line to the material. If material is not included in the chapter's Creative Commons license and your intended use is not permitted by statutory regulation or exceeds the permitted use, you will need to obtain permission directly from the copyright holder.

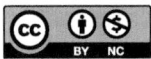

Imaging for Screening, Diagnosis, and Staging of Lung Cancer

8

Debra S. Dyer

Contents

Navigation Vignette.	92
Introduction.	92
Lung Cancer Screening.	92
Diagnosis of Lung Cancer.	97
Staging of Lung Cancer.	99
Conclusion.	102
Key Takeaways.	102
Key Readings and Resources.	102
References.	102

Abbreviations

CT	Computed tomography
CTDIvol	Computed tomography dose index volume
CXR	Chest radiograph
FDG	Fluorodeoxyglucose
FNA	Fine needle aspiration
IPN	Incidental pulmonary nodule
LDCT	Low-dose computed tomography
LCS	Lung cancer screening
Lungs-RADS	Lung imaging reporting and data system
mGy	Milligray
MIP	Maximum intensity projection

D. S. Dyer (✉)
Department of Radiology, National Jewish Health, Denver, CO, USA
e-mail: DyerD@NJHealth.org

© The Author(s) 2026
J. T. Fathi, M. F. Mortman (eds.), *Lung Cancer Navigation and Care*,
https://doi.org/10.1007/978-3-032-02200-4_8

MRI	Magnetic resonance imaging
MPR	Multiplanar reconstruction
PET-CT	Positron emission tomography-computed tomography
SUV	Standardized uptake value
TNM	Tumor, node, metastasis

Navigation Vignette

B.B. is a navigator at a rural facility who manages both the lung cancer screening (LCS) program and the incidental pulmonary nodule (IPN) program. Both programs are based within the radiology department. They have monthly multidisciplinary tumor board meetings where lung cancer screening (LCS) Lung-RADS 3–4 cases and patients with suspicious nodules (based on Fleischner Society guidelines) are discussed. B.B. reviews all LCS and IPN cases, discusses findings with her team, and prepares information for the monthly tumor board. She communicates the results of all scans and decisions made at the tumor board to the patients and the referring providers. She works closely with thoracic surgery, interventional pulmonology, medical oncology, and radiation oncology teams. She reports to the Director of Radiology; they meet weekly to review and discuss the programs. B.B. developed a quality dashboard to monitor both clinical programs. This dashboard facilitates their program activity reporting to the American College of Radiology Lung Cancer Screening Registry (ACR LCSR) to maintain their Lung Cancer Screening Designation and GO2 for Lung Cancer to maintain their Centers of Excellence for Lung Cancer Screening Designation. B.B. assists patients with scheduling and following up on their next steps if their scan is concerning for malignancy. Since the programs are so busy, B.B. works closely with her manager to establish and maintain clear job roles and responsibilities.

Introduction

This chapter provides an overview of the imaging procedures and reporting lexicons related to lung cancer screening, diagnosis, and staging.

Lung Cancer Screening

Lung cancer remains the number one cancer killer in men and women. Low-dose chest CT (LDCT) is the only test proven to reduce mortality from lung cancer in high-risk individuals [1, 2]. The goal of lung cancer screening CT is to identify lung cancer at an early stage when it can be treated and cured.

CT Technique

Use of appropriate low-dose CT technical parameters for performing LDCT is essential to achieve the lowest radiation dose while maintaining adequate exam quality. This is particularly important in LCS since patients are expected to undergo annual screening CTs, and some patients may need follow-up diagnostic chest CTs. A low-dose protocol should also be used for the diagnostic LCS follow-up CTs.

The protocol for an LDCT examination should include specific parameters [3]. Specific details of LDCT protocol include:

- Use of a multidetector CT scanner with at least 16 detectors
- Scan obtained at full inspiration during a single breath-hold
- Acquire axial images from the lung apices through the costophrenic sulci
- Obtain a slice thickness of 2.5 mm or less (1.0 mm slice thickness preferred)
- Creation of maximum intensity projection (MIP) reconstruction series to increase sensitivity for nodule detection
- Inclusion of multiplanar reconstruction (MPR) series showing coronal and sagittal reformats to better demonstrate the location of a nodule
- Perform without the use of intravenous contrast

The utilization of the appropriate low-dose protocol should yield a radiation exposure equivalent to a dose index volume (CTDIvol) of 3 mGy or less for a standard-sized patient. Automated dose modulating features on advanced scanners adjust the radiation exposure, reducing it for smaller-sized patients and increasing it for larger-sized patients. Sample LCS CT protocols for specific CT manufacturers and models are available through the American Association of Physicists in Medicine [4].

CT Interpretation and Reporting

A structured reporting system, such as Lung-RADS, should be utilized to promote consistent classification and management of the findings on LDCT [5]. The latest version of Lung-RADS, Lung-RADS 2022, is shown in Fig. 8.1.

This updated version not only addresses the management of lung nodules but also guides the classification and management of atypical pulmonary cysts, juxtapleural nodules, airway-centered nodules, and potentially infectious findings. In addition, it provides clarification for determining nodule growth and introduces stepped management for nodules that are stable or decreasing in size [6].

Utilization of Lung-RADS 2022 is nicely illustrated in Fig. 8.2. Figures 8.2a, 8.2c, and 8.2d demonstrate an atypical pulmonary cyst with irregular wall thickening in the right upper lobe.

The nodule is new since a prior chest CT performed 5 years earlier shows no evidence of the cystic nodule, as illustrated in Fig. 8.2b.

American College of Radiology — **Lung-RADS® v2022** Release Date: November 2022

Lung-RADS	Category Descriptor	Findings	Management
0	**Incomplete** Estimated Population Prevalence: ~1%	Prior chest CT examination being located for comparison (see note 9)	Comparison to prior chest CT;
		Part or all of lungs cannot be evaluated	Additional lung cancer screening CT imaging needed;
		Findings suggestive of an inflammatory or infectious process (see note 10)	1-3 month LDCT
1	**Negative** Estimated Population Prevalence: 39%	No lung nodules OR	12-month screening LDCT
		Nodule with benign features: • Complete, central, popcorn, or concentric ring calcifications OR • Fat-containing	
2	**Benign** - Based on imaging features or indolent behavior Estimated Population Prevalence: 45%	Juxtapleural nodule: • < 10 mm (524 mm³) mean diameter at baseline or new AND • Solid; smooth margins; and oval, lentiform, or triangular shape	12-month screening LDCT
		Solid nodule: • < 6 mm (< 113 mm³) at baseline OR • New < 4 mm (< 34 mm³)	
		Part solid nodule: • < 6 mm total mean diameter (< 113 mm³) at baseline	
		Non solid nodule (GGN): • < 30 mm (< 14,137 mm³) at baseline, new, or growing OR • ≥ 30 mm (≥ 14,137 mm³) stable or slowly growing (see note 7)	
		Airway nodule, subsegmental - at baseline, new, or stable (see note 11)	
		Category 3 lesion that is stable or decreased in size at 6-month follow-up CT OR Category 4B lesion proven to be benign in etiology following appropriate diagnostic workup	
3	**Probably Benign** - Based on imaging features or behavior Estimated Population Prevalence: 9%	Solid nodule: • ≥ 6 to < 8 mm (≥ 113 to < 268 mm³) at baseline OR • New 4 mm to < 6 mm (34 to < 113 mm³)	6-month LDCT
		Part solid nodule: • ≥ 6 mm total mean diameter (≥ 113 mm³) with solid component < 6 mm (< 113 mm³) at baseline OR • New < 6 mm total mean diameter (< 113 mm³)	
		Non solid nodule (GGN): • ≥ 30 mm (≥ 14,137 mm³) at baseline or new	
		Atypical pulmonary cyst: (see note 12) • Growing cystic component (mean diameter) of a thick-walled cyst	
		Category 4A lesion that is stable or decreased in size at 3-month follow-up CT (excluding airway nodules)	
4A	**Suspicious** Estimated Population Prevalence: 4%	Solid nodule: • ≥ 8 to < 15 mm (≥ 268 to < 1,767 mm³) at baseline OR • Growing < 8 mm (< 268 mm³) OR • New 6 to < 8 mm (113 to < 268 mm³)	3-month LDCT; PET/CT may be considered if there is a ≥ 8 mm (≥ 268 mm³) solid nodule or solid component
		Part solid nodule: • ≥ 6 mm total mean diameter (≥ 113 mm³) with solid component ≥ 6 mm to < 8 mm (≥ 113 to < 268 mm³) at baseline OR • New or growing < 4 mm (< 34 mm³) solid component	
		Airway nodule, segmental or more proximal - at baseline (see note 11)	
		Atypical pulmonary cyst: (see note 12) • Thick-walled cyst OR • Multilocular cyst at baseline OR • Thin- or thick-walled cyst that becomes multilocular	
4B	**Very Suspicious** Estimated Population Prevalence: 2%	Airway nodule, segmental or more proximal - stable or growing (see note 11)	Referral for further clinical evaluation
		Solid nodule: • ≥ 15 mm (≥ 1767 mm³) at baseline OR • New or growing ≥ 8 mm (≥ 268 mm³)	Diagnostic chest CT with or without contrast; PET/CT may be considered if there is a ≥ 8 mm (≥ 268 mm³) solid nodule or solid component; tissue sampling; and/or referral for further clinical evaluation Management depends on clinical evaluation, patient preference, and the probability of malignancy (see note 13)
		Part solid nodule: • Solid component ≥ 8 mm (≥ 268 mm³) at baseline OR • New or growing ≥ 4 mm (≥ 34 mm³) solid component	
		Atypical pulmonary cyst: (see note 12) • Thick-walled cyst with growing wall thickness/nodularity OR • Growing multilocular cyst (mean diameter) OR • Multilocular cyst with increased loculation or new/increased opacity (nodular, ground glass, or consolidation)	
		Slow growing solid or part solid nodule that demonstrates growth over multiple screening exams (see note 8)	
4X	Estimated Population Prevalence: <1%	Category 3 or 4 nodules with additional features or imaging findings that increase suspicion for lung cancer (see note 14)	
S	**Significant or Potentially Significant** Estimated Population Prevalence: 10%	Modifier: May add to category 0-4 for clinically significant or potentially clinically significant findings unrelated to lung cancer (see note 15)	As appropriate to the specific finding

© 2022 American College of Radiology® | All rights reserved

Fig. 8.1 Lung-RADS 2022

The patient is a 60-year-old female who currently smokes cigarettes and has a 50-pack-year history of cigarette smoking. The irregular wall thickening is suspicious for lung cancer, and the interpreting radiologist assigned the exam a Lung-RADS 4B with a recommendation for surgical referral consistent with Lung-RADS category 4B (Fig. 8.2e).

A multidisciplinary (nodule-review) committee review agreed there was not adequate soft tissue to be hypermetabolic on PET-CT (which would support an

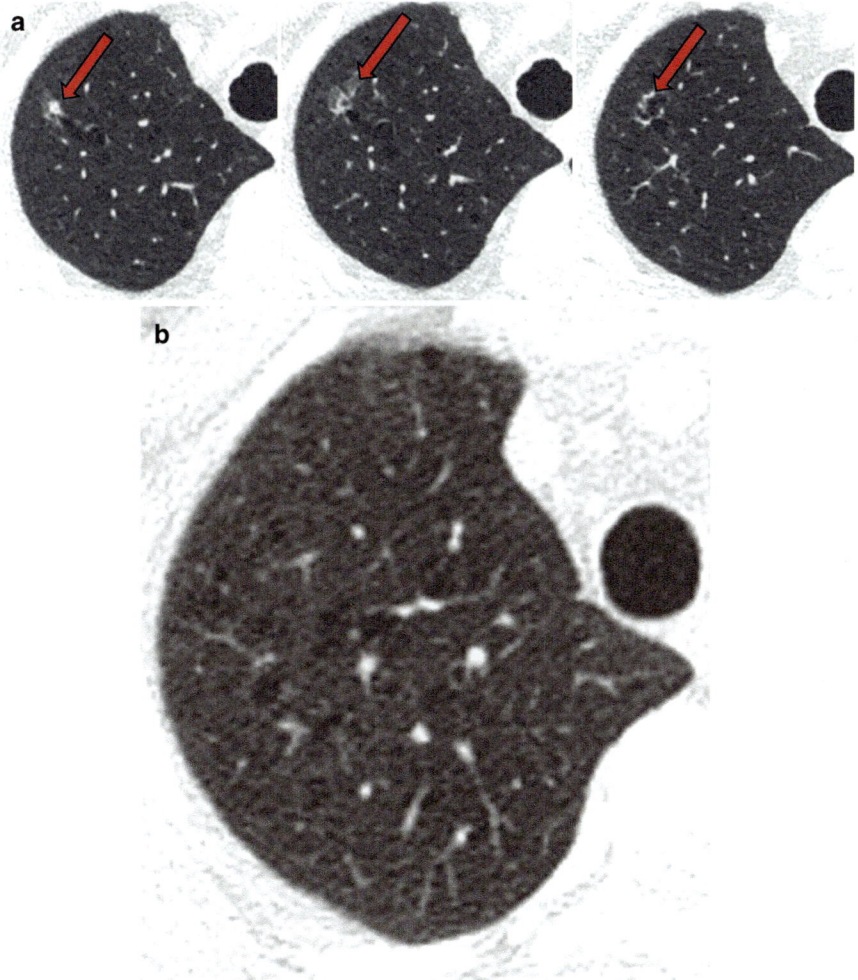

Fig. 8.2 (**a**) Axial images of cystic nodule in RUL (**b**) Comparison axial image of RUL showing no nodule in RUL (**c**) Coronal image with close up view of cystic nodule in RUL (**d**) Sagittal image of chest with close up view of cystic nodule in RUL (**e**) Illustrates section of Lung-RADS category 4B outlining management recommendation for Atypical pulmonary cyst

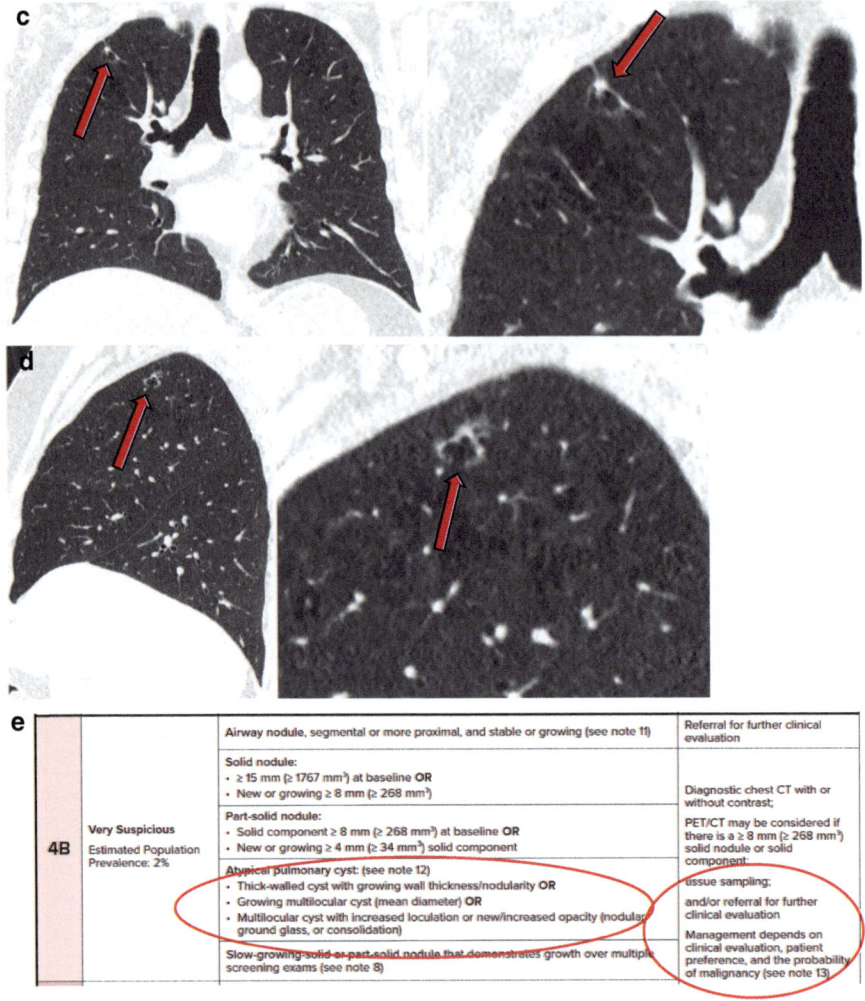

Fig. 8.2 (continued)

increased suspicion for cancer) or accessible (easily reached by interventional pulmonologist by bronchoscopy or by interventional radiologist by CT-guided biopsy for tissue sampling) so surgical resection was recommended. The patient had an uncomplicated wedge biopsy, which was positive for adenocarcinoma.

The radiologist should use appropriate "window" and "level" settings to enhance the visibility of specific tissues or structures when viewing the LDCT images. These settings allow the radiologist to adequately evaluate the lung parenchyma, mediastinal structures, bones, chest wall, lower neck, and upper abdomen. Lung nodules are assessed predominantly on lung windows; mediastinal windows help the radiologist look for fat or calcification within a nodule. The radiologist should describe the location of a nodule by including the lobe (or airway) where the nodule resides and the series/image number that best demonstrates the nodule. An adequate description of a nodule's characteristics and appearance should include size, attenuation (CT density), type of opacity (solid, part solid, ground glass), margins (smooth, lobulated, irregular, spiculated), and other important features such as cystic components. When available, a comparison with prior imaging is essential to determine any nodule size or appearance change.

The interpreting radiologist should recommend follow-up and a specific Lung-RADS category in the dictated report. Using a structured reporting system by the radiologist assists with data acquisition, tracking results, care management, and referral to a multidisciplinary conference when necessary.

Diagnosis of Lung Cancer

Potential lung cancer is identified by a radiologist on an imaging exam, usually a CXR or chest CT. Referring providers typically order a CXR first for patients with respiratory symptoms. The CXR may show an abnormality needing a diagnostic chest CT. A chest CT done for a variety of symptoms may show an incidental pulmonary nodule (meaning it was an unsuspected finding identified at the time of imaging done for another clinical indication or reason).

Further imaging is usually indicated if a suspicious pulmonary nodule is identified, whether on a diagnostic chest CT or a screening chest CT. Multidisciplinary committee or lung nodule board review can help determine the best next steps. Follow-up CT may be appropriate as outlined in the Fleischner Society guidelines for incidental nodules or Lung-RADS for nodules identified in the screening setting. If a nodule is highly suspicious, escalation of care involving a PET-CT and/or tissue sampling is typically needed.

PET-CT

PET (positron emission tomography) with integrated CT is a first-line tool for diagnosing lung cancer. PET-CT combines the functional data provided by PET with the anatomic and morphological information from CT. PET-CT helps assess the likelihood of malignancy within a suspicious nodule to help guide further work-up. It can demonstrate the extent of disease inside and outside the chest.

PET-CT uses a radiotracer, fluorodeoxyglucose (FDG), a glucose analog, to assess the cellular uptake of glucose in a target area. Cancer cells appear as bright "hot spots" since they use more glucose than normal healthy cells. The brightness is measured as the standard uptake value (SUV). An SUV of >2.5 has been used to differentiate benign from malignant nodules. However, SUV values can be lower in slowly growing cancers, carcinoids, and well-differentiated tumors.

PET is most effective and best used for solid nodules >8 mm in diameter or part solid nodules with a solid component >8 mm in diameter. Pure ground glass nodules are generally unsuitable for PET since they have no solid component. PET can be falsely positive in infection, inflammation, and sarcoidosis [7].

PET-CT is the preferred exam for identifying intrathoracic and extra-thoracic metastases. Since PET-CT includes imaging of the head through the level of the thighs, it can show the extent of disease in the body and is increasingly used for staging. It can detect intrathoracic lymph nodes, pleural disease, adrenal, liver, and bone metastases. It helps improve selection of patients appropriate for surgery or radiation therapy. It is particularly useful in identifying patients who are not surgical candidates but can be treated with radiation therapy. For example, a patient with a growing PET-positive nodule and no evidence of metastatic disease may be identified as having Clinical Stage 1 disease and referred for radiation therapy.

PET-CT is not useful for identifying metastatic disease in the brain since there is high glucose uptake (and therefore high FDG uptake) in normal brain tissue. Consequently, brain MRI is the exam of choice for diagnosing potential brain metastases.

Patients with evidence of hypermetabolic lesions with high FDG uptake on PET-CT are usually referred for tissue sampling. Nodules that are not hypermetabolic but have suspicious morphologic features are also appropriate for tissue sampling. Tissue is generally obtained via CT-guided biopsy or navigational bronchoscopy. However, if metastatic disease is present, PET-CT may show an alternate route for biopsy, such as sampling a supraclavicular lymph node to confirm diagnosis.

Tissue Sampling

If tissue sampling is needed, tissue can be obtained via percutaneous CT-guided lung biopsy (needle biopsy through the chest wall guided by imaging in radiology) or navigational bronchoscopy (through the airway performed by a pulmonologist).

CT-Guided Lung Biopsy

This procedure is typically appropriate if the nodule is in the periphery of the lung. Using real-time CT imaging for guidance, a needle is inserted through the chest wall and advanced into the nodule in the lung. A fine needle aspirate (FNA) and/or core biopsy is obtained for histologic analysis. CT-guided biopsy is a minimally invasive procedure with a high diagnostic yield. The most common complication is pneumothorax, occurring in 9–43% of cases, but only a minority of patients require a chest tube [8].

Navigational Bronchoscopy with Endobronchial Ultrasound

This procedure uses a bronchoscope to visually inspect the airways and obtain samples of the nodule and adjacent lymph nodes. Bronchoscopy is particularly useful for more centrally located nodules. Many institutions now have robotic-assisted bronchoscopy, which can improve diagnostic accuracy. The complication rate is lower than that of CT-guided biopsy, but the diagnostic yield is often lower [9].

Staging of Lung Cancer

Following a diagnosis of lung cancer, the disease should be staged to guide optimal treatment. Staging involves assessment of tumor size, location, nodal involvement (extent of lymph node invasion), and presence of metastases (tumor spread beyond the primary site). The staging process requires a combination of imaging modalities and, often, tissue sampling.

The TNM Staging System

The TNM staging system for lung cancer is used worldwide. The ninth edition was released in January 2025 [10, 11, 12]. The system assesses the anatomic extent of the primary tumor (T), lymph node involvement (N), and the extent and location of metastases (M). Stage classification is the cornerstone to optimize patient stratification and predict survival. By stratifying patients into similar groups, stage classification provides a consistent description of the anatomic extent of the tumor. Clear and concise communication, especially in multidisciplinary discussions, is vital for selecting appropriate treatment.

The TNM staging system applies to both clinical and pathological staging. The clinical stage, designated by the prefix "c" (c-stage or cTNM), involves information gathered before the initiation of treatment. Clinical staging relies heavily on imaging. Pathological staging, designated by the prefix "p" (p-stage or pTNM), includes information available from a surgical resection [13].

The T descriptor delineates tumor size and extent of local invasion. Increased size of the primary tumor correlates with progressive T status. For example, a nodule ≤ 1 cm is a T1a, while a nodule >1 cm to ≤ 2 cm is a T1b. Accurate measurements are essential. Tumor measurements should be done on lung windows and thin sections, preferably 1 mm or less. The largest diameter is recorded on the axial, coronal, or sagittal plane. For part-solid nodules, the longest diameter of the solid component is measured.

The N descriptor indicates the presence or absence of nodal disease, an important factor in determining treatment decisions. The anatomic location of lymph nodes is assessed using the IASLC lymph node map. There are 14 different nodal stations. Nodal stations are reported rather than descriptions of individual lymph nodes [10].

The N classification includes the N0, N1, N2, and N3 categories. N0 indicates no lymph node involvement. The N1 category includes ipsilateral peribronchial, hilar, and intrapulmonary lymph nodes. The N3 category includes contralateral mediastinal, contralateral hilar, scalene, and supraclavicular lymph nodes. The N2 category includes ipsilateral mediastinal and subcarinal lymph nodes. The ninth edition of the TNM Staging subdivides the N2 category into single station (N2a) and multiple station (N2b) involvement. Separating the N2 category better quantifies the disease burden since single-station disease has a better prognosis than multiple-station disease [13].

The M descriptor includes the M0 and M1 categories. M0 indicates no distant metastases. The M1 category is divided into subtypes. The M1a category includes one or more contralateral lesions and includes pleural and pericardial metastases. The M1b involves a single extra-thoracic metastatic lesion in a single organ system. The M1c involves multiple extra-thoracic metastatic lesions. In the ninth edition of the TNM staging, the M1c is split into two subcategories: The M1c1 subcategory indicates multiple metastases in a single organ system; the M1c2 subcategory indicates multiple metastases in multiple organ systems. Single-organ system metastatic disease has a better prognosis than multiple-organ system metastatic disease.

Some of the changes in the TNM category classification have resulted in changes in stage. For example, with the ninth edition, a patient with T1N2a disease is considered to have stage IIB disease, while previously, the patient would have been considered to have Stage IIIA disease [12].

Use of CT and PET-CT imaging for lung cancer staging is well demonstrated in Figs. 8.3a, b, and c. The patient is a 73-year-old male with a significant history of smoking cigarettes. Figure 8.3a shows a lung window on the chest CT with a new 2.6 × 1.1 cm pleural-based nodule in the left upper lobe (LUL). Figure 8.3b shows a mediastinal window on the chest CT and demonstrates station 7 mediastinal lymph node and left-sided pleural deposits. Figure 8.3c of a PET-CT image shows the LUL pleural-based nodule is hypermetabolic (SUV of 18.1) and hypermetabolic mediastinal and hilar lymph nodes and hypermetabolic pleural disease. This information indicates the TNM classification is T1cN2bM1c1, compatible with clinical stage IVB.

Imaging is a key contributor to the accurate staging of lung cancer and significantly impacts treatment decisions for optimal patient care.

Fig. 8.3 (**a**) Lung windows show 2.6 × 1.1 cm pleural based nodule in left upper lobe (**b**) Mediastinal windows show mildly enlarged precarinal lymph node (station 7) and nodular left sided pleural thickening (**c**) PET-CT demonstrates hypermetabolic pleural based nodule in the LUL (white arrowhead) with SUV 18.1, hypermetabolic station 7 mediastinal lymph node with SUV 11.2 and hypermetabolic left hilar station 10L lymph node with SUV 5.1. Metastatic left pleural disease (white arrow) is noted with hypermetabolic pleural deposit with SUV 9.9

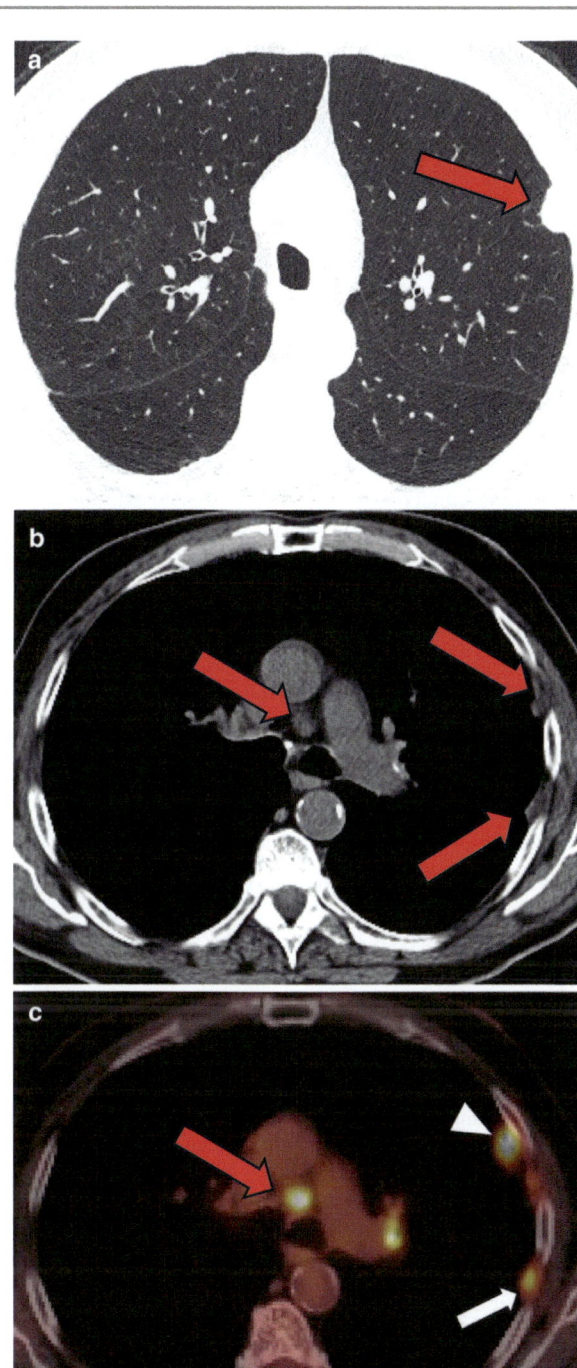

Conclusion

Appropriate imaging techniques and adherence to recognized reporting systems are essential in lung cancer screening and the diagnosis and staging of lung cancer.

Key Takeaways

- Annual lung cancer screening CT using a low-dose technique and structured reporting can identify lung cancer at an early stage and save lives.
- A multidisciplinary Nodule Review Board helps determine the best next steps for suspicious nodules identified through screening or as incidental lung nodules.
- Patients with suspicious nodules may need care escalation with PET-CT and/or tissue sampling to further assess the nodule.
- If lung cancer is identified, the cancer should be appropriately staged using the latest TNM taging System to help guide optimal treatment.

Key Readings and Resources

- Reduced lung cancer mortality with low-dose computed tomographic screening [1]
- American College of Radiology. Lung-RADS v2022 [6]
- Staging Cards in Thoracic Oncology ninth edition 2024 [10]

Conflict of Interest GO2 for Lung Cancer Global Advisory Council

References

1. National Lung Screening Trial Research Team, Aberle DR, Adams AM, et al. Reduced lung-cancer mortality with low-dose computed tomographic screening. N Engl J Med. 2011;365:395–409.
2. de Koning HJ, van der Aalst CM, de Jong PA, et al. Reduced lung-cancer mortality with volume CT screening in a randomized trial. N Engl J Med. 2020;382:503–13.
3. American College of Radiology (ACR) - Society of Thoracic Radiology (STR) Practice Parameters for the Performance and Reporting of Lung Cancer Screening Thoracic Computed Tomography (CT). Revised 2024. Available at: https://gravitas.acr.org. Accessed 4.22.25.
4. Lung Cancer Screening CT Protocols Version 6.0 Released November 2023. Available at AAPM.org. Accessed 4.22.25.
5. American College of Radiology. Lung-RADS v2022. Available at: https://www.acr.org/-/media/ACR/Files/RADS/Lung-RADS-2022.pdf. Accessed 4.22.25.
6. Christensen J, Prosper AE, Wu CC, Chung J, et al. ACR lung-RADS v2022: assessment categories and management recommendations. J Am Coll Radiol. 2024;21:473–88. https://doi.org/10.1016/j.jacr.2023.09.009.

7. Volpi S, Ali MA, Tasker A, Peryt A, et al. The role of positron emission tomography in the diagnosis, staging and response assessment of non-small cell lung cancer. Ann Transl Med. 2018;6(5):95. https://doi.org/10.21037/atm.2018.01.25.
8. Nakamura K, Matsumoto K, Inujii Soue C, Matsusue E, Fujii S. Computed tomography-guided lung biopsy: a review of techniques for reducing the incidence of complications. Intervent Radiol. 2021;6:83–92.
9. Chaudry FA, Thivierge-Southidara M, Molina JC, Farooqui SM, et al. CT-guided vs. navigational bronchoscopic biopsies for solitary pulmonary nodules: a single-institution retrospective comparison. Cancer. 2023;14:5258. https://doi.org/10.3390/cancers15215258.
10. Staging Cards in Thoracic Oncology 9th edition 2024.pdf. Available from the International Association for the Study of Lung Cancer at: https://www.education.iaslc.org. Accessed 4.22.25.
11. Detterbach FC, Woodard GA, Bader AS, Dacic S, et al. The proposed ninth TNM classification of lung cancer. Chest. 2024;166(4):882–95. https://doi.org/10.1016/j.chest.2024.05.026.
12. Rami-Porta R, Nishimura KK, Giroux DJ, Detterbach F, et al. International Association for the Study of Lung Cancer Lung Cancer Staging Project: proposals for revision of the TNM stage groups in the forthcoming (ninth) edition of the TNM classification of lung cancer. J Thorac Oncology. 2024;19(7):1007–27. https://doi.org/10.1016/j.jtho.2024.02.011.
13. Klug M, Kirshenboim Z, Truong MT, Sorin V, et al. Proposed ninth edition TNM staging system for lung cancer: guide for radiologists. Radiographics. 2024;44(12):e240057. https://doi.org/10.1148/rg.240057.

Open Access This chapter is licensed under the terms of the Creative Commons Attribution-NonCommercial 4.0 International License (http://creativecommons.org/licenses/by-nc/4.0/), which permits any noncommercial use, sharing, adaptation, distribution and reproduction in any medium or format, as long as you give appropriate credit to the original author(s) and the source, provide a link to the Creative Commons license and indicate if changes were made.

The images or other third party material in this chapter are included in the chapter's Creative Commons license, unless indicated otherwise in a credit line to the material. If material is not included in the chapter's Creative Commons license and your intended use is not permitted by statutory regulation or exceeds the permitted use, you will need to obtain permission directly from the copyright holder.

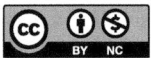

Lung Cancer Screening and Early Detection

9

Mary Pasquinelli and Linda Dowling

Contents

Navigation Vignette.	106
Lung Cancer Screening: History, Advances, Guidelines, and Implementation.	106
Race and Sex Disparities in USPSTF and CMS Guidelines.	108
Racial Disparities and the Need for Inclusive Criteria.	109
Risk-Based Screening and the PLCOm2012 Model.	109
Updated NCCN and ACS Screening Guidelines.	110
Current Screening and Implementation.	111
Integration of Smoking Cessation into LDCT Programs.	113
Opportunity for Early Detection Through Incidentally Detected Pulmonary Nodules (IPNs).	113
Artificial Intelligence and the Future of Lung Cancer Screening.	114
Key Takeaways.	115
Key Readings and Resources.	116
References.	116

Abbreviations

ACS	American Cancer Society
AI	Artificial intelligence
BMI	Body mass index
CMS	Centers for Medicare and Medicaid Services
COPD	Chronic obstructive pulmonary disease
EHR	Electronic health record
ELCAP	Early Lung Cancer Action Project
IPN	Incidental pulmonary nodule
LDCT	Low-dose computed tomography

M. Pasquinelli (✉) · L. Dowling
University of Illinois Chicago, Chicago, IL, USA
e-mail: mpasqu3@uic.edu

© The Author(s) 2026
J. T. Fathi, M. F. Mortman (eds.), *Lung Cancer Navigation and Care*,
https://doi.org/10.1007/978-3-032-02200-4_9

Lungs-RADS	Lung imaging reporting and data system
NCCN	National Comprehensive Cancer Network
NELSON	Nederlands-Leuvens Longkanker Screenings Onderzoek
NLST	National Lung Screening Trial
PLCO	Prostate, Lung, Colorectal, Ovarian
SDM	Shared decision-making
USPSTF	United States Preventive Services Task Force

Navigation Vignette

Mr. S., a 58-year-old retired construction worker with a history of tobacco use, presented to his primary care physician for a routine check-up. He formerly smoked one pack per day for 25 years and quit 12 years ago. Additionally, he has a family history of lung cancer—his father passed away from the disease—and a diagnosis of chronic obstructive pulmonary disease (COPD). As a Black individual with a high school education, his demographic and clinical profile further highlighted his elevated risk. These factors prompted his physician to consult a lung cancer screening (LCS) navigator for a comprehensive assessment.

The LCS navigator evaluated Mr. S's eligibility under the USPSTF guidelines, noting that he narrowly met the criteria based on his smoking history and cessation timeline. To refine the risk assessment, the navigator utilized the PLCOm2012 risk prediction model, which incorporates variables such as age, smoking history, race, COPD, BMI, family history of lung cancer, personal history of cancer, and educational attainment. The model estimated his 6-year risk of lung cancer at 3.4%, far exceeding the high-risk threshold ($\geq 1.5\%$).

The navigator initiated shared decision-making (SDM), explaining the benefits and limitations of low-dose computed tomography (LDCT). Mr. S. consented to screening, and his baseline scan revealed a 7-mm pulmonary nodule classified as Lung-RADS 3. His primary care physician discussed the LDCT results with him, and the navigator coordinated a follow-up LDCT in 6 months and counseled him on remaining smoke-free.

This case illustrates how lung cancer screening navigation ensures guideline-based care and early detection for high-risk individuals.

Lung Cancer Screening: History, Advances, Guidelines, and Implementation

Lung cancer screening has evolved significantly due to technological advancements, clinical research, and shifting epidemiological trends. Early screening efforts, such as chest X-rays and sputum cytology, aimed to detect lung cancer at an earlier, more treatable stage but lacked sufficient sensitivity for early-stage detection.

The Mayo Lung Project (1971–1983) is one of the earliest notable trials in this domain. The study—a randomized, controlled clinical trial—assessed the effectiveness of regular chest X-rays and sputum cytology in reducing lung cancer mortality. It included 9211 male participants aged 45 or older with significant tobacco exposure (≥ 1 pack per day) and no prior history of lung cancer. Participants were randomized into two groups: one undergoing chest X-rays and sputum cytology every 4 months, and the other advised to undergo annual chest X-rays and sputum cytology. Although the intervention group had higher detection rates and more early-stage diagnoses, the trial found no significant reduction in mortality between the groups [1]. These findings highlighted the need for more effective screening methods.

Subsequent advancements, such as the Early Lung Cancer Action Project (ELCAP), demonstrated the potential of LDCT in early lung cancer detection. ELCAP's work set a new benchmark in oncology by showcasing LDCT's superior sensitivity for identifying early-stage lung cancer, ultimately influencing clinical practices and policy worldwide [2, 3].

The National Lung Screening Trial (NLST), conducted from 2002 to 2010, marked a watershed moment in lung cancer screening. This randomized controlled trial involved 53,454 high-risk participants, including those with a current or former heavy smoking history of 30 pack-years, and compared LDCT with standard chest X-rays. Results revealed a 20% reduction in lung cancer mortality among those screened with LDCT, firmly establishing it as the preferred screening modality for high-risk populations [4]. Following the NLST findings, organizations like the US Preventive Services Task Force (USPSTF) revised guidelines to recommend annual LDCT for individuals aged 55–80 with a 30-pack-year smoking history (current or quit within the past 15 years) [5]. These recommendations significantly influenced public health policies, including insurance coverage for LDCT under the Affordable Care Act. The Centers for Medicare & Medicaid Services (CMS) adopted lung screening in 2015 for individuals aged 55–77 with a 30-pack-year smoking history (current or quit within the past 15 years) after a shared decision-making visit [6].

The NELSON Trial (Nederlands-Leuvens Longkanker Screenings Onderzoek) is another landmark study that demonstrated the efficacy of LDCT in reducing lung cancer mortality. Conducted in the Netherlands and Belgium with over 15,000 participants aged 50–74, the trial included current and former tobacco users with a smoking history of at least 10 cigarettes per day for 30 years or 15 cigarettes per day for 25 years. It utilized volumetric nodule assessment for follow-up, a more precise approach than diameter-based methods. Results showed a 24% reduction in lung cancer mortality among men and up to 33% among women, underscoring the importance of sex-specific analyses in screening [7]. By minimizing unnecessary follow-ups and interventions, the trial set new standards for LDCT implementation. Its findings have influenced global guidelines, including the USPSTF, emphasizing earlier detection, personalized care, and improved outcomes, particularly for women and high-risk populations. See Table 9.1 for a summary of pivotal lung screening trials.

Table 9.1 Pivotal lung screening trials: eligibility, screening interventions, and outcomes

Trial	Eligibility	Screening intervention	Outcomes
Mayo Lung Project [25]	Males, age 45–80; smoked ≥1 pack/day; no known lung cancer; life expectancy >5 years	Chest X-ray and sputum cytology every 4 months (intervention) vs. annual recommendation (control)	No reduction in lung cancer mortality in the intervention group compared to the control
National Lung Screening Trial (NLST) [4]	Age 55–74; ≥30 pack-years smoking history; current or quit ≤15 years ago	Low-dose CT (LDCT) annually for 3 years vs. chest X-ray	20% reduction in lung cancer mortality with LDCT; 6.7% all-cause mortality reduction
Danish lung cancer screening trial (DLCST) [26]	Smoking history, current or former, aged 50–70; ≥20 pack-years	LDCT annually for 5 years	No significant reduction in lung cancer mortality
NELSON (Dutch-Belgian trial) [7]	Men and women aged 50–74; with a current or former smoking history (quit <10 years); ≥15 cigarettes/day for 25 years or ≥ 10 cigarettes/day for 30 years	LDCT at 0, 1, 3, and 5.5 years	24% reduction in lung cancer mortality (33% in women)
LUSI (German lung cancer screening intervention trial) [27]	Smoking history—Current or formerly smoked, aged 50–69; ≥25 pack-years	LDCT annually for 5 years	Suggested reduction in lung cancer mortality (not statistically significant)
ELCAP (early lung cancer action project) [3]	Adults aged ≥60; smoking history or other risk factors	Baseline LDCT screening followed by annual scans	Detection of lung cancer at earlier stages with higher surgical cure rates
Multicentric Italian lung detection (mild trial) [28]	Adults aged 49–75, ≥ 20 pack-years, current or former smoking history (quit <10 years)	Randomized to LDCT every 12 months or every 24 months vs. control arm without intervention for a period of 6 years	58% reduction in lung cancer mortality at 5 years and 39% at 10 years in the LDCT arm

Race and Sex Disparities in USPSTF and CMS Guidelines

While the NLST provided a foundation for USPSTF and CMS recommendations, earlier guidelines unintentionally excluded large segments of the population at high risk for lung cancer, particularly Black individuals and women. The 2013 USPSTF guidelines, based on NLST data, restricted screening to individuals aged 55–80 with a smoking history of at least 30 pack-years, including those who had quit within the past 15 years. Similarly, the CMS guidelines 2015 mirrored this eligibility framework, limiting access to Medicare beneficiaries meeting these strict criteria [5, 6]. Research has demonstrated that these guidelines disproportionately excluded high-risk populations who did not meet the rigid age or smoking history thresholds. For instance, Black individuals often develop lung cancer with fewer pack-years of smoking compared to White individuals, and women are more likely to develop lung cancer with lower cumulative tobacco exposure [8, 9].

Racial Disparities and the Need for Inclusive Criteria

Black individuals were underrepresented in the NLST, comprising only 4.5% of the study cohort. The Aldrich et al. study highlighted significant racial disparities in lung cancer risk and screening eligibility, particularly for Black individuals [10]. It found that Black individuals with a smoking history were at higher risk of developing lung cancer at younger ages and with lower cumulative smoking exposure compared to White individuals. For example, Black individuals with a 20-pack-year smoking history had a comparable risk to White individuals with a 30-pack-year history. The study also revealed that the 2013 USPSTF guidelines disproportionately excluded high-risk Black individuals due to the 30-pack-year threshold and starting age of 55, which failed to account for their younger age of onset and higher risk at lower smoking intensities. These findings emphasized the need for more inclusive screening criteria, such as lowering the pack-year threshold and starting age, changes that were incorporated in the updated 2021 USPSTF guidelines. Aldrich et al. underscored the importance of addressing these disparities to improve access to early detection and reduce lung cancer mortality among Black individuals.

Risk-Based Screening and the PLCOm2012 Model

Pasquinelli et al.'s research advanced lung cancer screening by highlighting the value of the PLCOm2012 risk prediction model in addressing disparities and improving risk stratification. Unlike traditional guidelines, such as those issued by the USPSTF, which relied primarily on age, smoking history, and time since quitting, the PLCOm2012 model incorporates a broader range of variables, including age, race, smoking intensity and duration, time since quitting, personal and family history of cancer, chronic obstructive pulmonary disease (COPD), body mass index (BMI), and highest level of education. This personalized approach calculates a 6-year lung cancer risk, with a threshold of $\geq 1.5\%$, to determine screening eligibility. Pasquinelli's studies demonstrated that this model reduces disparities by better identifying high-risk populations, such as Black individuals and women, who often develop lung cancer at lower smoking intensities. Her 2020 and 2022 research showed that adopting the PLCOm2012 model could expand eligibility to historically excluded groups while improving predictive accuracy [11–13]. Some lung screening programs, such as those in Ontario and British Columbia, have adopted the PLCOm2012 model, and the NCCN now endorses its optional use for identifying high-risk individuals outside traditional pack-year thresholds. Pasquinelli's work underscores how risk-based models like PLCOm2012 improve lung cancer screening programs' precision, equity, and efficiency. These inequities highlighted the need for more nuanced screening approaches, including tools like the PLCOm2012 model, which incorporates demographic and clinical variables beyond traditional criteria. By identifying a broader at-risk population, the model has demonstrated its potential to reduce disparities in lung cancer detection, particularly among women and Black individuals, who were often excluded under previous guidelines [14, 15]

Eligibility criteria for lung screening have been refined over time to enhance inclusivity while maintaining clinical effectiveness. The US Preventive Services Task Force (USPSTF) guidelines, updated in 2021, specify eligibility for individuals aged 50–80, who are asymptomatic for lung cancer, have a 20-pack-year smoking history, and are either current tobacco users or have quit within the last 15 years. The guidelines also recommend discontinuing LDCT for individuals with life-limiting comorbidities or those unable to undergo curative treatment [16].

Similarly, the CMS guidelines, updated in 2021, align closely but specify eligibility for individuals aged 50–77, with the same smoking history and cessation criteria. Additionally, CMS requires a shared decision-making (SDM) visit before the initial LDCT screening. During this visit, a healthcare provider must engage the patient in a discussion about the benefits and risks of LDCT screening, assess eligibility, address tobacco cessation if applicable, and ensure the patient understands the importance of adherence to annual screenings. These SDM requirements emphasize patient-centered care and aim to support informed decision-making [6].

Updated NCCN and ACS Screening Guidelines

The American Cancer Society (ACS) has revised its LCS guidelines to expand eligibility and improve accessibility. The ACS now recommends annual low-dose computed tomography (LDCT) screening for individuals aged 50–80 with at least a 20-pack-year smoking history, including those who currently smoke or quit more than 15 years ago. By eliminating the quit smoking requirement to having quit within the past 15 years, the ACS guideline captures a larger group of individuals with a former smoking history who remain at significant risk for lung cancer. This adjustment reflects a commitment to inclusivity and equity, aiming to reduce lung cancer mortality by identifying at-risk populations who may have previously been overlooked [17].

Similarly, the National Comprehensive Cancer Network (NCCN) updated its (LCS) guidelines in 2024 to recommend screening for individuals with a 20-year history of smoking, regardless of the number of pack-years. This criterion captures individuals with long-term smoking habits who may have been excluded under previous guidelines that relied strictly on pack-year thresholds. By focusing on smoking duration rather than intensity, the NCCN's approach broadens access to screening for high-risk populations who would otherwise remain ineligible [18, 19].

Current Screening and Implementation

Eligibility criteria for low-dose computed tomography (LDCT) have been refined to balance inclusivity with clinical effectiveness. CMS guidelines, updated in 2021, specify eligibility for individuals aged 50–77 who are asymptomatic for lung cancer, have a 20-pack-year smoking history, and either currently smoke or have quit within the last 15 years (CMS 2021). The USPSTF guidelines, which extend the screening endpoint to age 80, recommend discontinuing LDCT for individuals with life-limiting comorbidities or those unable to undergo curative treatment [16].

Billing and reimbursement are critical for ensuring accessibility to LDCT screenings. The Affordable Care Act mandates coverage without cost-sharing, provided the screening meets established criteria. Accurate billing includes shared decision-making (CPT: G0296), the LDCT procedure (CPT: 71271), and, when applicable, tobacco cessation counseling (CPT: 99406 or 99,407) (CMS 2021). Patients undergoing interval diagnostic CTs are billed differently, often with CPT code 71250.

Structured reporting is an essential component of LDCT screening programs, providing a standardized method for documenting findings. The American College of Radiology's Lung-RADS® (Lung Imaging Reporting and Data System) is a widely used system that categorizes LDCT findings based on the likelihood of malignancy. Lung-RADS assigns a category ranging from 1 (negative) to 4 (suspicious for cancer), with subcategories (e.g., 4A, 4B) to provide even more precise guidance for follow-up. See Fig. 9.1: ACR Lung-Rads Categories [20].

For example:

- Lung-RADS 1 or 2: Represents benign findings requiring annual LDCT follow-up.
- Lung-RADS 3: Indicates findings with a low likelihood of malignancy, requiring follow-up in 6 months.
- Lung-RADS 4A/4B/4X: Suggests a higher likelihood of malignancy, requiring short-term or immediate diagnostic evaluation, such as biopsy or PET-CT.

This standardized approach improves communication between radiologists and referring clinicians, ensures appropriate follow-up, and reduces variability in management recommendations. Additionally, Lung-RADS can integrate with electronic health records (EHRs) and data registries, facilitating quality assurance, program analytics, and performance tracking.

Nodule tracking software enhances Lung-RADS utilization by ensuring patients are navigated appropriately across the continuum of care. This software automates

Lung-RADS	Category Descriptor	Findings	Management
0	**Incomplete** Estimated Population Prevalence: ~1%	Prior chest CT examination being located for comparison (see note 9)	Comparison to prior chest CT; Additional lung cancer screening CT imaging needed; 1-3 month LDCT
		Part or all of lungs cannot be evaluated	
		Findings suggestive of an inflammatory or infectious process (see note 10)	
1	**Negative** Estimated Population Prevalence: 39%	No lung nodules **OR**	12-month screening LDCT
		Nodule with benign features: • Complete, central, popcorn, or concentric ring calcifications **OR** • Fat-containing	
2	**Benign** - Based on imaging features or indolent behavior Estimated Population Prevalence: 45%	Juxtapleural nodule: • < 10 mm (524 mm³) mean diameter at baseline or new **AND** • Solid; smooth margins; and oval, lentiform, or triangular shape	12-month screening LDCT
		Solid nodule: • < 6 mm (< 113 mm³) at baseline **OR** • New < 4 mm (< 34 mm³)	
		Part solid nodule: • < 6 mm total mean diameter (< 113 mm³) at baseline	
		Non solid nodule (GGN): • < 30 mm (< 14,137 mm³) at baseline, new, or growing **OR** • ≥ 30 mm (≥ 14,137 mm³) stable or slowly growing (see note 7)	
		Airway nodule, subsegmental - at baseline, new, or stable (see note 11)	
		Category 3 lesion that is stable or decreased in size at 6-month follow-up CT **OR** Category 4B lesion proven to be benign in etiology following appropriate diagnostic workup	
3	**Probably Benign** - Based on imaging features or behavior Estimated Population Prevalence: 9%	Solid nodule: • ≥ 6 to < 8 mm (≥ 113 to < 268 mm³) at baseline **OR** • New 4 mm to < 6 mm (34 to < 113 mm³)	6-month LDCT
		Part solid nodule: • ≥ 6 mm total mean diameter (≥ 113 mm³) with solid component < 6 mm (< 113 mm³) at baseline **OR** • New < 6 mm total mean diameter (< 113 mm³)	
		Non solid nodule (GGN): • ≥ 30 mm (≥ 14,137 mm³) at baseline or new	
		Atypical pulmonary cyst: (see note 12) • Growing cystic component (mean diameter) of a thick-walled cyst	
		Category 4A lesion that is stable or decreased in size at 3-month follow-up CT (excluding airway nodules)	
4A	**Suspicious** Estimated Population Prevalence: 4%	Solid nodule: • ≥ 8 to < 15 mm (≥ 268 to < 1,767 mm³) at baseline **OR** • Growing < 8 mm (< 268 mm³) **OR** • New 6 to < 8 mm (113 to < 268 mm³)	3-month LDCT; PET/CT may be considered if there is a ≥ 8 mm (≥ 268 mm³) solid nodule or solid component
		Part solid nodule: • ≥ 6 mm total mean diameter (≥ 113 mm³) with solid component ≥ 6 mm to < 8 mm (≥ 113 to < 268 mm³) at baseline **OR** • New or growing < 4 mm (< 34 mm³) solid component	
		Airway nodule, segmental or more proximal - at baseline (see note 11)	
		Atypical pulmonary cyst: (see note 12) • Thick-walled cyst **OR** • Multilocular cyst at baseline **OR** • Thin- or thick-walled cyst that becomes multilocular	
4B	**Very Suspicious** Estimated Population Prevalence: 2%	Airway nodule, segmental or more proximal - stable or growing (see note 11)	Referral for further clinical evaluation
		Solid nodule: • ≥ 15 mm (≥ 1767 mm³) at baseline **OR** • New or growing ≥ 8 mm (≥ 268 mm³)	Diagnostic chest CT with or without contrast; PET/CT may be considered if there is a ≥ 8 mm (≥ 268 mm³) solid nodule or solid component; tissue sampling; and/or referral for further clinical evaluation Management depends on clinical evaluation, patient preference, and the probability of malignancy (see note 13)
		Part solid nodule: • Solid component ≥ 8 mm (≥ 268 mm³) at baseline **OR** • New or growing ≥ 4 mm (≥ 34 mm³) solid component	
		Atypical pulmonary cyst: (see note 12) • Thick-walled cyst with growing wall thickness/nodularity **OR** • Growing multilocular cyst (mean diameter) **OR** • Multilocular cyst with increased loculation or new/increased opacity (nodular, ground glass, or consolidation)	
		Slow growing solid or part solid nodule that demonstrates growth over multiple screening exams (see note 8)	
4X	Estimated Population Prevalence: < 1%	Category 3 or 4 nodules with additional features or imaging findings that increase suspicion for lung cancer (see note 14)	
S	**Significant or Potentially Significant** Estimated Population Prevalence: 10%	Modifier: May add to category 0-4 for clinically significant or potentially clinically significant findings unrelated to lung cancer (see note 15)	As appropriate to the specific finding

© 2022 American College of Radiology® | All rights reserved

Fig. 9.1 Lung-RADS® v2022 [20]. (Published in https://www.acr.org/Clinical-Resources/Clinical-Tools-and-Reference/Reporting-and-Data-Systems/Lung-RADS, under Reprinted with permission CC BY-ND 4.0 license)

follow-up scheduling, tracks changes in nodule size or density, and integrates artificial intelligence tools to streamline radiologist workflows. These advancements improve patient outcomes and reduce the risk of missed malignancies.

Integration of Smoking Cessation into LDCT Programs

Smoking cessation remains a cornerstone of lung cancer prevention, and its integration into LDCT screening programs underscores a comprehensive approach to lung health. Smoking is the leading cause of lung cancer, and evidence suggests that quitting smoking at any stage significantly reduces an individual's lung cancer risk. LDCT programs provide a critical opportunity to engage patients in tobacco cessation counseling, which not only complements the benefits of screening but also addresses the root cause of the disease.

Tobacco cessation counseling during LDCT visits is reimbursable under CMS guidelines and can be tailored to the patient's readiness to quit. Counseling includes discussing the benefits of quitting, addressing barriers, and providing pharmacologic and behavioral support. Billing codes such as CPT 99406 (3–10 min of counseling) or CPT 99407 (over 10 min) enable programs to formalize cessation efforts.

The shared decision-making (SDM) visit mandated by CMS provides an ideal framework for initiating tobacco cessation discussions. During SDM, healthcare providers educate patients about LDCT screening's benefits and limitations and incorporate smoking cessation guidance as part of the conversation. Recent updates to CMS guidelines now allow trained non-physician practitioners, including registered nurses, to deliver SDM, increasing accessibility and scalability of these services.

Smoking cessation programs integrated into LDCT screenings provide significant benefits, including improved long-term survival and quality of life. Comprehensive programs that offer cessation resources—such as referrals to smoking cessation Quitlines, access to FDA-approved pharmacologic support (e.g., nicotine replacement therapies and varenicline), and follow-up counseling—maximize the impact of LDCT by addressing smoking, the primary modifiable risk factor for lung cancer. Studies have demonstrated that combining LDCT screening with effective smoking cessation interventions not only reduces lung cancer incidence but also decreases all-cause mortality, underscoring the importance of a multifaceted approach to lung health [21, 22].

Opportunity for Early Detection Through Incidentally Detected Pulmonary Nodules (IPNs)

Incidentally detected pulmonary nodules (IPNs), commonly identified during imaging performed for reasons unrelated to lung cancer screening, represent a critical opportunity for early lung cancer detection. These nodules are frequently found on chest imaging ordered for evaluation of conditions such as infection, cardiac symptoms, or trauma. Given the widespread use of chest CT scans across clinical settings, the number of individuals with IPNs is substantial and continues to grow.

A national cohort study by Vachani et al. analyzed 23,780 individuals with incidentally detected pulmonary nodules measuring greater than 8 mm and found that nearly 10% (9.9%) were diagnosed with lung cancer within 27 months of nodule identification [23]. The likelihood of cancer varied significantly by tobacco exposure history: lung cancer was diagnosed in 5.4% of individuals with no history of tobacco use, 12.2% of individuals with a former history of tobacco use, and 17.7% of individuals with current tobacco exposure. Cancer risk also increased with nodule size: 5.7% of individuals with nodules measuring 9–15 mm, 12.1% of those with nodules greater than 15–20 mm, and 18.4% of those with nodules greater than 20–30 mm were diagnosed with lung cancer. These findings underscore the considerable malignancy risk associated with larger nodules and reinforce the importance of systematic surveillance.

Despite this elevated risk, many individuals with IPNs do not receive appropriate follow-up or timely diagnostic evaluation. Barriers include fragmented communication, unclear responsibility for nodule management, and lack of standardized tracking protocols. These gaps result in missed opportunities for diagnosing lung cancer at earlier, more treatable stages.

Integrating structured IPN follow-up programs within health systems—such as nurse navigator-led initiatives, centralized nodule tracking systems, or incorporation into a combined lung screening/IPN program—can significantly enhance the timeliness of diagnosis and improve clinical outcomes. In settings where lung cancer screening uptake is suboptimal or where eligibility criteria restrict access, systematic IPN tracking provides a complementary and impactful pathway for early detection, especially for individuals who may not qualify for traditional screening but remain at elevated risk.

Artificial Intelligence and the Future of Lung Cancer Screening

Integrating artificial intelligence (AI) into LCS is transforming the detection and management of the disease, with innovative machine learning models like Sybil leading the way. Developed by researchers at the Massachusetts Institute of Technology (MIT) and Massachusetts General Hospital (MGH), Sybil is a deep-learning model designed to predict lung cancer risk directly from low-dose computed tomography (LDCT) scans [24]. Unlike traditional methods that rely heavily on nodule detection, Sybil evaluates the entire lung and surrounding tissues, providing risk predictions for up to 6 years with remarkable accuracy. This approach allows for the identification of patients at high risk of developing lung cancer, even in the absence of visible nodules, making it a valuable tool for early detection and personalized care.

One of Sybil's most groundbreaking features is its ability to operate on a single LDCT scan without requiring additional clinical data or prior imaging for comparison. This innovation addresses a significant limitation in traditional screening models, enabling Sybil to deliver accurate risk predictions for patients with limited medical history or inconsistent access to care. In clinical studies, Sybil demonstrated high accuracy in predicting lung cancer risk across diverse datasets, including those from the National Lung Screening Trial (NLST) and international cohorts. Its ability to generalize across diverse populations further supports its potential to reduce disparities in lung cancer screening.

The application of Sybil and similar AI-driven models holds promise for enhancing lung cancer screening workflows. By integrating Sybil into LDCT programs, healthcare providers can improve screening precision, prioritize high-risk patients for follow-up, and reduce false positives, often leading to unnecessary procedures. Additionally, Sybil's ability to analyze volumetric and textural lung changes over time aligns with structured reporting systems like Lung-RADS®, enabling more accurate monitoring of indeterminate nodules.

Moreover, AI models like Sybil could complement traditional risk prediction tools by incorporating non-imaging data, such as demographic, genetic, and environmental factors, to further refine screening eligibility criteria. For example, Sybil could work alongside models like PLCOm2012 to address gaps in capturing high-risk individuals who do not meet traditional pack-year thresholds or those from historically underrepresented populations.

Despite its potential, adopting Sybil and similar AI technologies requires validation in diverse populations and addressing challenges such as integration with existing clinical workflows. Additionally, regulatory approval and clinician training will be essential for widespread implementation. Nevertheless, Sybil represents a significant step forward in leveraging machine learning to improve lung cancer screening outcomes.

Key Takeaways

- *Advancements in Screening*: Low-dose computed tomography (LDCT) has demonstrated its ability to significantly reduce lung cancer mortality in high-risk populations, solidifying its role as the gold standard in screening.
- *Addressing Disparities*: Updated guidelines, such as the USPSTF 2021, CMS 2021 criteria, and the PLCOm2012 risk prediction model, aim to reduce racial and sex-based disparities by broadening eligibility and improving inclusivity.
- *Comprehensive Care*: Structural reporting systems like Lung-RADS and integrating smoking cessation counseling into LDCT programs enhance diagnostic precision and promote better lung health outcomes.
- *AI Integration*: Advanced AI technologies, like Sybil, are revolutionizing lung cancer screening by improving risk assessment, streamlining workflows, and addressing screening inequities across diverse populations.
- *Global Impact*: Landmark studies, including NLST and NELSON, have shaped international screening guidelines, emphasizing early detection, personalized care, and equity in lung cancer prevention.

Key Readings and Resources

- ATS/ACCP Policy Statement: Guidance for implementing LDCT screening programs in clinical practice [29].
- 10 Pillars of Lung Cancer Screening: Rationale and logistics for building effective screening programs [30].
- Lung Cancer Screening Implementation Toolkit: Practical resources for initiating and scaling lung screening programs [31].
- GO2 for Lung Cancer: Thoracic Oncology Business Model [32].
- Best Practice Guide: Comprehensive guidance for building early detection programs [33].
- GO2 for Lung Cancer Global Knowledge Center: Free education for all healthcare professionals, repository of best practices and resources for LDCT programs [34].
- Patient Navigator Roadmap: Toolkit for lung cancer screening navigation [35].

Conflict of Interest Mary Pasquinelli reports no conflicts of Interest.

Disclosures
- Grant funding: Coleman Foundation, American Lung Association, LPOP
- Consulting: VA Cares, Center for Business Models in Healthcare, Jazz
- Grant Reviewer: Prevent Cancer Foundation

Linda Dowling No conflicts of interest.

References

1. Fontana RS, Sanderson DR, Woolner LB, Taylor WF, Miller WE, Muhm JR. Lung cancer screening: the Mayo program. J Occup Med. 1986;28(8):746–50.
2. Henschke CI, McCauley DI, Yankelevitz DF, Naidich DP, McGuinness G, Miettinen OS, et al. Early lung cancer action project: overall design and findings from baseline screening. Lancet. 1999;354(9173):99–105.
3. International Early Lung Cancer Action Program I, Henschke CI, Yankelevitz DF, Libby DM, Pasmantier MW, Smith JP, et al. Survival of patients with stage I lung cancer detected on CT screening. N Engl J Med. 2006;355(17):1763–71.
4. National Lung Screening Trial Research T, Aberle DR, Adams AM, Berg CD, Black WC, Clapp JD, et al. Reduced lung-cancer mortality with low-dose computed tomographic screening. N Engl J Med. 2011;365(5):395–409.
5. Moyer VA, Force USPST. Screening for lung cancer: U.S. Preventive Services Task Force recommendation statement. Ann Intern Med. 2014;160(5):330–8.
6. Centers for Medicare & Medicaid Services. Decision memo: screening for lung cancer with low dose computed tomography (LDCT); 2022.
7. de Koning HJ, van der Aalst CM, de Jong PA, Scholten ET, Nackaerts K, Heuvelmans MA, et al. Reduced lung-cancer mortality with volume CT screening in a randomized trial. N Engl J Med. 2020;382(6):503–13.
8. Haiman CA, Stram DO, Wilkens LR, Pike MC, Kolonel LN, Henderson BE, et al. Ethnic and racial differences in the smoking-related risk of lung cancer. N Engl J Med. 2006;354(4):333–42.

9. Jemal A, Miller KD, Ma J, Siegel RL, Fedewa SA, Islami F, et al. Higher lung cancer incidence in young women than young men in the United States. N Engl J Med. 2018;378(21):1999–2009.
10. Aldrich MC, Mercaldo SF, Sandler KL, Blot WJ, Grogan EL, Blume JD. Evaluation of USPSTF lung cancer screening guidelines among African American adult smokers. JAMA Oncol. 2019;5(9):1318–24.
11. Pasquinelli MM, Tammemagi MC, Kovitz KL, Durham ML, Deliu Z, Rygalski K, et al. Risk prediction model versus United States Preventive Services Task Force lung cancer screening eligibility criteria: reducing race disparities. J Thorac Oncol. 2020;15(11):1738–47.
12. Pasquinelli MM, Tammemagi MC, Kovitz KL, Durham ML, Deliu Z, Rygalski K, et al. Brief report: risk prediction model versus United States Preventive Services Task Force 2020 draft lung cancer screening eligibility criteria-reducing race disparities. JTO Clin Res Rep. 2021;2(3):100137.
13. Pasquinelli MM, Tammemagi MC, Kovitz KL, Durham ML, Deliu Z, Guzman A, et al. Addressing sex disparities in lung cancer screening eligibility: USPSTF vs PLCOm2012 criteria. Chest. 2021;161:248.
14. Tammemagi MC, Katki HA, Hocking WG, Church TR, Caporaso N, Kvale PA, et al. Selection criteria for lung-cancer screening. N Engl J Med. 2013;368(8):728–36.
15. Tammemagi MC, Church TR, Hocking WG, Silvestri GA, Kvale PA, Riley TL, et al. Evaluation of the lung cancer risks at which to screen ever- and never-smokers: screening rules applied to the PLCO and NLST cohorts. PLoS Med. 2014;11(12):e1001764.
16. U. S. Preventive Services Task Force, Krist AH, Davidson KW, Mangione CM, Barry MJ, Cabana M, et al. Screening for lung cancer: US Preventive Services Task Force recommendation statement. JAMA. 2021;325(10):962–70.
17. Wolf AMD, Oeffinger KC, Shih TY, Walter LC, Church TR, Fontham ETH, et al. Screening for lung cancer: 2023 guideline update from the American Cancer Society. CA Cancer J Clin. 2024;74(1):50–81.
18. Potter AL, Xu NN, Senthil P, Srinivasan D, Lee H, Gazelle GS, et al. Pack-year smoking history: an inadequate and biased measure to determine lung cancer screening eligibility. J Clin Oncol. 2024;42(17):2026–37.
19. Network NCC. Lung Cancer Screening (Version 1.2025); 2025. Available from: https://www.nccn.org/professionals/physician_gls/pdf/lung_screening.pdf.
20. Christensen J, Prosper AE, Wu CC, Chung J, Lee E, Elicker B, et al. ACR lung-RADS v2022: assessment categories and management recommendations. Chest. 2024;165(3):738–53.
21. Iaccarino JM, Duran C, Slatore CG, Wiener RS, Kathuria H. Combining smoking cessation interventions with LDCT lung cancer screening: a systematic review. Prev Med. 2019;121:24–32.
22. Minnix JA, Karam-Hage M, Blalock JA, Cinciripini PM. The importance of incorporating smoking cessation into lung cancer screening. Transl Lung Cancer Res. 2018;7(3):272–80.
23. Vachani A, Zheng C, Amy Liu IL, Huang BZ, Osuji TA, Gould MK. The probability of lung cancer in patients with incidentally detected pulmonary nodules: clinical characteristics and accuracy of prediction models. Chest. 2022;161(2):562–71.
24. Mikhael PG, Wohlwend J, Yala A, Karstens L, Xiang J, Takigami AK, et al. Sybil: a validated deep learning model to predict future lung cancer risk from a single low-dose chest computed tomography. J Clin Oncol. 2023;41(12):2191–200.
25. Marcus PM, Bergstralh EJ, Fagerstrom RM, Williams DE, Fontana R, Taylor WF, et al. Lung cancer mortality in the Mayo lung project: impact of extended follow-up. J Natl Cancer Inst. 2000;92(16):1308–16.
26. Wille MM, Dirksen A, Ashraf H, Saghir Z, Bach KS, Brodersen J, et al. Results of the randomized Danish lung cancer screening trial with focus on high-risk profiling. Am J Respir Crit Care Med. 2016;193(5):542–51.
27. Becker N, Motsch E, Trotter A, Heussel CP, Dienemann H, Schnabel PA, et al. Lung cancer mortality reduction by LDCT screening-results from the randomized German LUSI trial. Int J Cancer. 2020;146(6):1503–13.

28. Pastorino U, Silva M, Sestini S, Sabia F, Boeri M, Cantarutti A, et al. Prolonged lung cancer screening reduced 10-year mortality in the MILD trial: new confirmation of lung cancer screening efficacy. Ann Oncol. 2019;30(10):1672.
29. Wiener RS, Gould MK, Arenberg DA, Au DH, Fennig K, Lamb CR, et al. An official American Thoracic Society/American College of Chest Physicians policy statement: implementation of low-dose computed tomography lung cancer screening programs in clinical practice. Am J Respir Crit Care Med. 2015;192(7):881–91.
30. Fintelmann FJ, Bernheim A, Digumarthy SR, Lennes IT, Kalra MK, Gilman MD, et al. The 10 pillars of lung cancer screening: rationale and logistics of a lung cancer screening program. Radiographics. 2015;35(7):1893–908.
31. Lung Cancer Policy Network. Screening for lung cancer. Available from: https://www.lungcancerpolicynetwork.com/work/screening-for-lung-cancer/.
32. GO2 for Lung Cancer. Thoracic oncology business model. https://hcp.go2.org/business-model/.
33. National Lung Cancer Roundtable. Best Practice Guide for Building Lung Cancer Early Detection Programs. Available from: https://nlcrt.org/wp-content/uploads/NLCRT-Early-Detection-Playbook-Final.pdf.
34. GO2 for Lung Cancer. The Global Knowledge Center (GKC) for Lung Cancer. Available from: https://gkc.go2.org/.
35. Patient Navigation & Community Health Worker Training. Lung cancer screening: patient navigator roadmap. Available from: https://patientnavigatortraining.org/lung-cancer-screening-toolkit/.

Open Access This chapter is licensed under the terms of the Creative Commons Attribution-NonCommercial 4.0 International License (http://creativecommons.org/licenses/by-nc/4.0/), which permits any noncommercial use, sharing, adaptation, distribution and reproduction in any medium or format, as long as you give appropriate credit to the original author(s) and the source, provide a link to the Creative Commons license and indicate if changes were made.

The images or other third party material in this chapter are included in the chapter's Creative Commons license, unless indicated otherwise in a credit line to the material. If material is not included in the chapter's Creative Commons license and your intended use is not permitted by statutory regulation or exceeds the permitted use, you will need to obtain permission directly from the copyright holder.

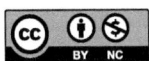

Tobacco Dependence Treatment and Lung Cancer Control

10

Chris Kotsen and Lisa Carter-Bawa

Contents

Navigator Vignette.	120
Introduction.	121
Tobacco Dependence Treatment for Cancer Control and Improved Health Outcomes.	121
Counseling.	121
Pharmacotherapy.	122
Effective Integration of Tobacco Treatment Services in Lung Cancer Screening.	122
Patient Barriers and Facilitators.	123
Clinician Barriers and Facilitators.	124
Systems Barriers and Facilitators.	125
Effective Integration of Tobacco Treatment within Lung Cancer Care.	126
Conclusion.	127
Key Takeaways.	127
Key Readings and Resources.	128
References.	129

C. Kotsen (✉)
Department of Psychiatry and Behavioral Sciences, Memorial Sloan Kettering Cancer Center, New York, NY, USA

Georgetown Lombardi Comprehensive Cancer Center, Washington, DC, USA
e-mail: kotsenc@mskcc.org

L. Carter-Bawa
Cancer Prevention Precision Control Institute, Center for Discovery & Innovation @ Hackensack Meridian Health, Nutley, NJ, USA
e-mail: lisa.carterbawa@hmh-cdi.org

© The Author(s) 2026
J. T. Fathi, M. F. Mortman (eds.), *Lung Cancer Navigation and Care*,
https://doi.org/10.1007/978-3-032-02200-4_10

Abbreviations

APN	Advanced practice nurse
BPA	Best practice advisory
CBT	Cognitive behavioral therapy
EHR	Electronic health record
FDA	Food and Drug Administration
LDCT	Low-dose computed tomography
MI	Motivational interviewing
NRT	Nicotine replacement therapy
PCP	Primary care physician
SDM	Shared decision-making
SEM	Socio-ecological model
TTS	Tobacco treatment specialist
U.S.	United States

Navigator Vignette

Mrs. R., a 58-year-old Latina with bipolar disorder and a 31-pack-year history of menthol cigarette use is referred by her primary care physician (PCP) to a centralized opt-out [1, 2] integrated low-dose computed tomography (LDCT)/tobacco treatment program. Presenting concerns include chronic pulmonary symptoms and coughing.

Despite moderate motivation to quit and low confidence, she completes six cognitive behavioral therapy (CBT) sessions with a psychologist/tobacco treatment specialist (TTS) for comprehensive biopsychosocial treatment. During the shared decision-making (SDM) visit, an advanced practice nurse (APN) navigator/TTS prescribes varenicline, addressing an initial barrier when insurance denies coverage by quickly securing prior authorization. Carbon monoxide testing at baseline is 29 ppm, reduced to 15 ppm by her third visit, encouraging her progress, then consistently under 6 ppm with quitting.

Treatment focuses on enhancing motivation, resolving ambivalence, proper use of varenicline, and implementing coping strategies, initially practicing stimulus control such as moving cigarettes out of reach and then deep breathing and delays for craving management. Psychologist/TTS reminds patient of proper use of varenicline and assists in monitoring for common side effects and craving reduction response. Both clinicians also work with the multidisciplinary care/tumor board/pulmonary nodule clinic, coordinating team care and a discussion of the LDCT Lung-RADs 3 and above findings. Cognitive restructuring helps replace old addictive self-talk with newer adaptive self-talk strategies, supporting her commitment to quit. At 6 months, she remains tobacco-free and is referred to a local therapist for ongoing support with pre-existing behavioral health challenges. This case demonstrates the importance of multidisciplinary collaboration and tailored interventions in addressing tobacco dependence within lung cancer care, emphasizing the critical role of navigators in bridging care gaps and overcoming barriers. This case also highlights the collaborative role of navigators and allied health professionals in tobacco treatment within a lung cancer screening program.

Introduction

Cigarette smoking is the leading lung cancer cause and a modifiable risk factor, as discussed. Lung cancer screening offers a critical "teachable moment" to address tobacco use [3, 4]. Tobacco companies have deliberately engineered cigarettes to optimize their addictive potential [5], with most individuals who smoke starting to experiment in their adolescence. Tobacco dependence can then quickly develop and become a chronic relapsing condition driven by addiction to nicotine [5–8]. People who smoke cigarettes may make at least 20–30 quit attempts before permanently quitting [9, 10]. However, evidence-based tobacco treatments can accelerate long-term quit rates [5, 9, 11]. Moreover, evidence demonstrates that 79% of lung cancer screening-eligible individuals who smoke attempt to quit smoking compared to the general population (50%), and lung cancer screening participation can promote interest and motivation in smoking cessation [12–14].

Tobacco Dependence Treatment for Cancer Control and Improved Health Outcomes

The gold standard for tobacco treatment involves motivational interviewing (MI) counseling [15] and CBT [16] for behavior change, coupled with first-line FDA-approved pharmacotherapy [5, 11]. The most recent version of the United States Preventive Services Task Force guideline continues to highlight that effective counseling can be combined with evidenced-based FDA-approved pharmacotherapy for the best quitting results [17].

Counseling

Many navigators and allied health professionals receive extensive training in interpersonal relationship skills, which is essential for effectively working with populations affected by addiction. The philosophy of MI is a patient-centered approach to counseling, which focuses on helping patients develop intrinsic motivation for behavior change. This counseling approach is also consistent with the shared decision-making (SDM) visit philosophy employed by clinical navigators and allied health professionals, as these clinicians jointly help patients explore a menu of screening and treatment options across the lung cancer care continuum within a framework of patient-centered empathic assessment, while assisting patients in healthcare decision-making.

A range of tobacco treatments can be effective and practical for the primary care setting and include the use of brief 5 A (Ask, Advise, Assess, Assist, and Arrange) interventions [11]. Clinicians can ask about tobacco use, advise to quit in a personalized manner taking into consideration tobacco-related symptoms, assess willingness to quit, advise on quitting strategies, and assist in ongoing counseling or refer to moderate intensity (i.e., Quitline) or intensive, comprehensive biopsychosocial treatments which are most effective [5, 18, 19].

Pharmacotherapy

There are five nicotine replacement therapies (NRTs) and two non-nicotine pill medications in the United States that treat nicotine withdrawal symptoms and tobacco cravings. Effective medications include an NRT patch, gum, lozenge, inhaler, or nasal spray. In the United States, the patch, lozenge, and gum are over the counter and covered by prescription with most insurances. Nicotine inhaler or nicotine nasal spray are prescription only and often covered. Varenicline and bupropion are non-nicotine pills and is often covered with a prescription by most US insurance payors. Current NCCN guidelines [18] recommend either varenicline or a combination long-acting (patch), with short-acting NRT (i.e., lozenge, gum, nasal spray, inhaler) as the preferred pharmacotherapy regimen. Finally, cytisine has shown strong efficacy, with recent approval in Canada, the United Kingdom, and the European Union [20–22].

All tobacco treatments, but particularly intensive tobacco treatments, lead to improved health outcomes beyond lung cancer risk reduction, such as cardiac, pulmonary, and for at least 11 other tobacco-caused cancer conditions [23, 24]. Additionally, most patients with a lung cancer diagnosis and patients attending LDCT screening programs, by definition, have a long-standing history of tobacco use (i.e., at least 20 pack-years), most with at least moderate-high levels of tobacco dependency [1, 25], so this review will highlight available evidence surrounding more intensive tobacco treatments (i.e., in-person, phone, video telehealth), which deliver the strongest treatment dose.

Effective Integration of Tobacco Treatment Services in Lung Cancer Screening

The socio-ecological model (SEM) (see Fig. 10.1) takes a multi-level perspective and focuses on patient-, clinician-, and systems barriers and facilitators, which can affect patient's health [26–28]. Recently, the National Cancer Institute published Monograph 23, *Treating Smoking in Cancer Patients: An Essential Component of Cancer Care* [29], which simplifies these components within the SEM model (see Fig. 10.2). These frameworks can help busy navigators and allied health clinicians in identifying effective clinical workflows to overcome barriers. Later, we will address tobacco treatments with patients already diagnosed with lung cancer.

Fig. 10.1 The socio-ecological model (SEM). (Reprinted with permission from Yesiltepe et al. [27])

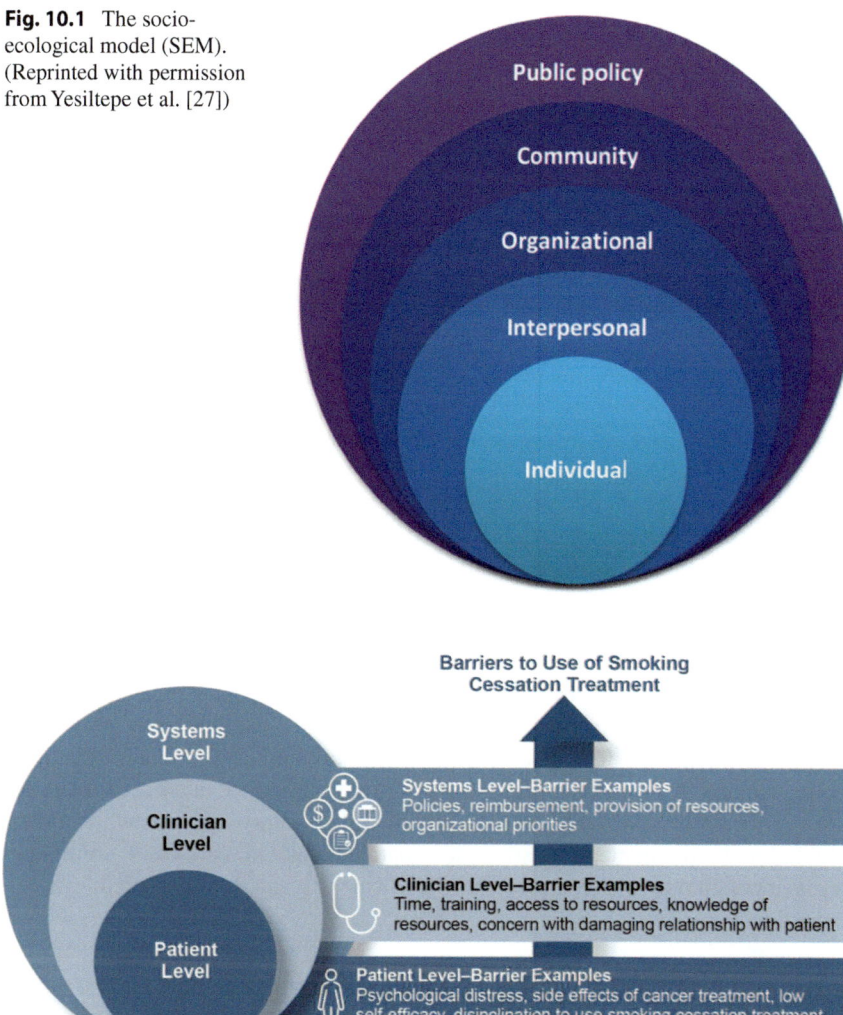

Fig. 10.2 Patient-, clinician-, and systems-level barriers to the use of smoking cessation treatment in cancer care settings. (Reprinted with permission from National Cancer Institute, 2023. Barriers to Use of Smoking Cessation Treatment. [Fig. 10.2]. Monograph 23. Treating Smoking in Cancer Patients Social Media Toolkit)

Patient Barriers and Facilitators

As discussed, teachable moments for tobacco treatment can arise during lung cancer screening. However, many patients experience significant tobacco-related stigma, which can serve as a major barrier to seeking care. In addition, patients may face compounded stigmas, such as those related to smoking, lung cancer, and co-occurring conditions, such as behavioral health issues or additional addictions. These overlapping stigmas may contribute to the avoidance of tobacco treatment and are reflected in lower lung cancer screening rates compared to other common cancer screenings with higher adherence rates. For example, stigma associated with smoking may lead to feelings of shame, embarrassment, or fear of judgment, deterring patients from disclosing smoking histories or seeking help [29].

In fact, patient factors often intersect with clinician or system-level barriers. Many clinicians are constrained by time, limiting their ability to obtain an accurate smoking history [29]. Additionally, limited training on how to empathetically assess smoking behavior and its stigma-related nuances can result in missed opportunities for effective tobacco treatment during the lung cancer screening referral [29]. According to recent reports, some healthcare systems have begun implementing solutions to these barriers by improving clinician support through electronic health records (EHR) and other systems-level interventions [30, 31]. However, it is common for patients, out of embarrassment or fear of stigma, to underreport their smoking history, necessitating more thorough and empathetic clinician-patient interactions to ensure accurate history-taking and proper referral for lung cancer screening and tobacco dependence treatment [29].

The influence of medical mistrust, particularly among African American/Black patients and other historically marginalized groups, adds another layer of complexity [32, 33]. This mistrust stems from a long history of unethical medical practices, which continues to affect perceptions of care today. While Hamman provides an in-depth discussion of stigma (in Chap. 1), it is important to acknowledge that intersecting stigmas and mistrust are major barriers to engagement in tobacco treatment. The healthcare system must prioritize trust-building interventions, such as culturally tailored communication strategies, patient-centered care, and community engagement initiatives, to overcome these barriers and foster equitable access to care.

Clinician Barriers and Facilitators

Lack of time and lack of clinician training remain major barriers leading to low delivery of evidence-based tobacco treatment [29]. Research has shown that busy primary care clinicians, oncologists, and clinicians in lung cancer screening programs often do an excellent job implementing the first 3 A's (Ask, Advise, Assist). Still, there is a significant drop-off in delivering treatment and providing ongoing follow-up visits [5, 34–36]. This is understandable, considering these clinicians are evaluating, managing, and treating multiple patient comorbidities beyond tobacco use.

Significant advancements have been made in delivering tobacco treatment services at the organizational, community, and societal levels. One key development is the growing role of TTSs, clinicians with advanced training in tobacco use assessment and treatment [37]. An emerging workforce of these specialists is now taking shape, supported by 28 specialized accredited training programs that equip clinicians with tobacco treatment skills and strategies for effectively collaborating within busy healthcare environments [19]. Many TTSs, particularly those in allied health roles, are highly motivated to assist people who use tobacco users who may be eligible for lung cancer screening and view patient navigation as an integral part of their responsibilities [38].

Research supports that TTSs provide the highest quit rates [19]. This may be due to the specialized training, full-time or majority-time of clinical focus on tobacco treatment, ongoing clinical supervision, and having the dedicated time to deliver more intensive treatments. While many clinicians work in community settings, primary care, or behavioral health, TTSs are increasingly working in cancer centers, specifically lung cancer screening programs [29].

While it is beyond the scope of this chapter to review all clinical studies involving tobacco treatment within lung cancer screening, a few important summaries are noted. First, Leone et al. (2013) provided guideline recommendations for the American College of CHEST Physicians for lung cancer-eligible patients or those diagnosed with lung cancer: all benefit from combined behavioral and pharmacotherapy tobacco treatment [7]. Later, while discussing that more research is needed, Fucito et al. (2016) compiled a similar list of key guidelines integrating evidence-based tobacco treatments into visits within lung cancer screening centers [1]. Leone et al. (2020) subsequently developed pharmacotherapy clinical practice guidelines as part of the American Thoracic Society [39]. Finally, three important recent reviews examined smoking cessation efforts within lung cancer screening programs [3, 40, 41]. While reviews indicated some mixed results and limitations in study designs [3, 40, 41], each concluded that intensive multimodal tobacco treatment involving behavioral therapy and pharmacotherapy yielded the highest quit rates.

Systems Barriers and Facilitators

As previously noted, screening and accurately assessing tobacco use is often challenging due to patient-related stigma and complexities in documenting this information within EHRs. However, at the healthcare systems level, improvements in clinician decision-making support through EHR enhancements—such as automated calculations of patients' smoking pack-year history—have been shown to increase the rates of LDCT orders for eligible patients [31]. Furthermore, at the community and organizational levels, Presant et al. [30] demonstrated that EHR improvements, including best practice alerts (BPAs) for lung cancer screening referrals and tobacco treatment, combined with other quality improvement initiatives, resulted in significant increases in tobacco treatment engagement and screening referrals, particularly among minority populations.

At the community level, Volk et al. [2] discussed systems tradeoffs—pluses and minuses of decentralized referral pathways for LDCT referral, PCPs who have a larger reach, and, alternatively, centralized facilities (e.g., radiology centers or LDCTs in cancer centers), which have fewer staff, so their staff can be trained more easily with standardized SDM workflows. In either setting, navigators and allied health professionals are well suited to assist busy clinicians in assessing, documenting in EHR, and conversing with patients about tobacco use and the risk of lung cancer.

At the institutional level and community level, LDCT-screened eligible patients who also smoke can be connected with tobacco treatment services using an opt-out referral [29, 30, 42]. Again, healthcare systems can take advantage of these macro barriers by bringing in navigators, allied health clinicians, and TTSs to fill in gaps in the healthcare system, assist with clinical workflows, and deliver treatments.

At the public policy level, another major issue is insurance-related barriers, including perceived or actual low coverage for follow-up procedures, which may deter patients from pursuing lung cancer screening [43]. Uninsured or underinsured patients often face significant social determinants of health challenges, exacerbating their risk of delayed or foregone care. For example, financial toxicity—a well-known consequence of cancer treatment—creates additional barriers for patients who may already be concerned about the cost of care [43]. Healthcare systems must be prepared to offer financial navigation services and other support to ensure equitable access to screening and treatment.

Addressing these barriers is essential to achieving health equity in lung cancer screening and tobacco treatment. In this context, health equity means ensuring that all patients—regardless of race/ethnicity, income, or insurance status—have access to timely, high-quality tobacco treatment and screening services. Solutions at the systems level should include expanded insurance coverage for lung cancer screening and related follow-up care, improved patient education about coverage, and efforts to streamline referral and treatment pathways to minimize delays in care [44]. Furthermore, training for navigators and clinicians on mitigating stigma and addressing medical mistrust is critical. These strategies will support patients in overcoming both personal and structural barriers, ensuring that the benefits of lung cancer screening and tobacco treatment reach the populations most in need.

Finally, new macro national and local public health policies impacting the delivery of care access are improving. For instance, recent updates to Medicare guidelines have modified the requirements for SDM visits between patients and clinicians [45]. This new policy allows lung cancer screening to expand by allowing allied health providers—such as health educators, social workers, and other clinicians—to conduct the SDM visits "incident to" physicians. Additionally, a significant advancement is the option to deliver SDM visits via telehealth [2, 45], which has already been shown to increase patient access and engagement, as demonstrated by higher show rates for tobacco treatment services compared to in-person [46, 47].

Effective Integration of Tobacco Treatment within Lung Cancer Care

All tobacco treatments can be integrated into care with populations who are diagnosed with lung cancer [29], across all cancer stages [48]. Like screening for LDCT, the diagnosis of lung cancer itself may be a teachable moment. Navigators and allied health clinicians can listen to patient expressions such as "cancer is a wake-up call for me about the importance of my health." These patients are processing the shock of a lung cancer diagnosis, and clinicians can often use MI skills to validate losses/fears, use reflective listening to bolster interest in behavior change, build quitting motivation, and often resolve ambivalence about taking action around reduction of tobacco use. Clinicians can additionally treat cancer-related distress concurrently, including addressing any pre-existing psychiatric comorbidities that may be present, at the same time as delivering tobacco dependence treatment [29]. While there are few studies that specifically only focus on lung cancer alone, consistently high quit rates have been published with all cancer patients involving CBT coupled with best practices pharmacotherapy [18, 49, 50] and with lung cancer patients undergoing all cancer treatments [7]. A recent prospective cohort study showed that referral to a specialized and structured intensive tobacco treatment program for all cancer patients who smoke (including 20% of patients with lung cancer) led to significant survival benefits across all cancer types [48]. Moreover, effective training of oncology providers to deliver tobacco treatment who work in oncology settings now exists [51].

Conclusion

While there is no one-size-fits-all approach to tobacco treatment within lung cancer screening programs [41, 52]—given variations in geographic settings, healthcare system capacity, and staffing resources—a multimodal approach, combining first-line FDA-approved pharmacotherapy with intensive CBT, continues to show the highest efficacy. Scaling and sustaining tobacco treatment services within multidisciplinary lung cancer screening workflows is critical for long-term success. Embedding TTSs, patient navigators, and allied health clinicians who can deliver tobacco treatment within these programs has emerged as a best practice [1]. The NCI-funded SCALE studies [53] and other research initiatives will provide valuable insights into overcoming implementation challenges and refining scalable models for diverse healthcare settings. By addressing these key components, lung cancer screening programs can effectively integrate and sustain tobacco treatment services, leading to improved patient outcomes and broader public health impact. Finally, for all lung cancer survivors, there is a clear benefit in living longer with stopping tobacco use, and effective tobacco treatments can be delivered by navigators and allied health professionals across the continuum of cancer care.

Key Takeaways

1. *Cigarette Smoking and Lung Cancer*
    - Cigarette smoking remains the leading cause of lung cancer and is a modifiable risk factor. Lung cancer screening and/or a lung cancer diagnosis presents a powerful "teachable moment" to address tobacco use effectively.

2. *Role of Navigators and Allied Health Professionals*
   - Navigators and allied health professionals are vital contributors to tobacco treatment efforts with their strong interpersonal and communication skills. Within multidisciplinary care teams, they support shared decision-making and connect patients to cessation resources. In some cases, allied health professionals such as nurse practitioners may also be positioned to prescribe pharmacotherapies, enabling a more streamlined, inclusive approach to delivering comprehensive care and enhancing the likelihood of successful quitting.

3. *Barriers to Tobacco Treatment Integration*
   - *Patient-Level Barriers*: Tobacco-related stigma, often compounded by medical mistrust and adverse social determinants of health, can deter patients from engaging in treatment.
   - *Clinician-Level Barriers*: Time constraints and limited training in empathic communication hinder effective tobacco treatment delivery.
   - *Systems-Level Barriers*: Challenges in EHR documentation and insurance coverage gaps impact screening and treatment engagement.

4. *Facilitators for Successful Tobacco Treatment*
   - *Multilevel Frameworks*: The socio-ecological model provides a useful lens to identify and address barriers at patient, clinician, and systems levels.
   - *Emerging Workforce*: Tobacco treatment specialists deliver the highest quit rates, supported by specialized training and integration into cancer centers.
   - *Technology Integration*: EHR enhancements, such as automated pack-year history calculations, best practice advisories, and opt-out referrals, streamline care pathways for lung cancer screening referrals and tobacco treatment delivery.

5. *Best Practices in Tobacco Treatment*
   - Intensive multimodal interventions—combining CBT with FDA-approved pharmacotherapy medications—accelerate long-term quit rates, particularly in lung cancer screening programs.

6. *Addressing Stigma and Health Equity*
   - Tailored communication strategies and trust-building interventions are critical to overcoming stigma and medical mistrust, particularly among historically marginalized populations.
   - Expanding insurance coverage and offering financial navigation support are essential to ensure equitable access to lung cancer screening and tobacco treatment services.

Key Readings and Resources

Tobacco Dependence Treatment Guidelines
- Tobacco Use and Dependence Guideline Panel. Treating Tobacco Use and Dependence: 2008 Update [11].

- U.S. Department of Health and Human Services: Public Health Service. Smoking Cessation: A Report of the Surgeon General Rockville, MD 2020 [5].
- Initiating Pharmacologic Treatment in Tobacco-Dependent Adults. An Official American Thoracic Society Clinical Practice Guideline [39].
- Treating Smoking in Cancer Patients: An Essential Component of Cancer Care. National Cancer Institute Tobacco Control Monograph 23 [29].
- Quit Smoking: NCCN Clinical Practice Guidelines in Oncology (NCCN Guidelines®) for Smoking Cessation [18].

National Coverage Determination and Oncology Guidelines for Smoking Cessation at Time of Lung Cancer Screening
- Screening for Lung Cancer with Low Dose Computed Tomography (LDCT) Centers for Medicare & Medicaid Services (CMS). Medicare coverage database: Screening for Lung Cancer with Low Dose Computed Tomography (LDCT) [45].
- Lung Cancer Screening: Clinical Practice Guidelines in Oncology (NCCN Guidelines®) [24].

Tobacco Treatment at Time of Lung Cancer Screening Guideline
- Pairing Smoking Cessation Services with Lung Cancer Screening: A Clinical Guideline from the Association for the Treatment of Tobacco Use and Dependence and Society for Research on Nicotine and Tobacco [1].

Acknowledgments We appreciate the support of Christopher S. Webster, Vanessa Brooks, and Francis Valenzona for assistance in preparing this manuscript.

Conflict of Interest The authors have no conflicts of interest to declare relevant to this chapter's content.

References

1. Fucito LM, Czabafy S, Hendricks PS, Kotsen C, Richardson D, Toll BA. Pairing smoking-cessation services with lung cancer screening: a clinical guideline from the Association for the Treatment of Tobacco Use and Dependence and the Society for Research on Nicotine and Tobacco. Cancer. 2016;122(8):1150–9.
2. Volk RJ, Myers RE, Arenberg D, Caverly TJ, Hoffman RM, Katki HA, et al. The American Cancer Society National Lung Cancer Roundtable strategic plan: current challenges and future directions for shared decision making for lung cancer screening. Cancer. 2024;130(23):3996–4011.
3. Williams PJ, Philip KE, Alghamdi SM, Perkins AM, Buttery SC, Polkey MI, et al. Strategies to deliver smoking cessation interventions during targeted lung health screening – a systematic review and meta-analysis. Chron Respir Dis. 2023;20:14799731231183446.
4. Williams RM, Cordon M, Eyestone E, Smith L, Luta G, McKee BJ, et al. Improved motivation and readiness to quit shortly after lung cancer screening: evidence for a teachable moment. Cancer. 2022;128(10):1976–86.

5. U.S. Department of Health and Human Services. Smoking Cessation. A Report of the Surgeon General. Atlanta, GA: U.S. Department of Health and Human Services, Centers for Disease Control and Prevention, National Center for Chronic Disease Prevention and Health Promotion, Office on Smoking and Health, 2020. 2020 [cited 2025 April 14]. Available from: https://www.hhs.gov/sites/default/files/2020-cessation-sgr-full-report.pdf.
6. Bernstein SL, Toll BA. Ask about smoking, not quitting: a chronic disease approach to assessing and treating tobacco use. Addict Sci Clin Pract. 2019;14(1):29.
7. Leone FT, Evers-Casey S, Toll BA, Vachani A. Treatment of tobacco use in lung cancer: diagnosis and management of lung cancer, 3rd ed: American College of Chest Physicians evidence-based clinical practice guidelines. Chest. 2013;143(5 Suppl):e61S–77S.
8. Steinberg MB, Schmelzer AC, Richardson DL, Foulds J. The case for treating tobacco dependence as a chronic disease. Ann Intern Med. 2008;148(7):554–6.
9. Borland R, Partos TR, Cummings KM. Systematic biases in cross-sectional community studies may underestimate the effectiveness of stop-smoking medications. Nicotine Tob Res. 2012;14(12):1483–7.
10. Chaiton M, Diemert L, Cohen JE, Bondy SJ, Selby P, Philipneri A, Schwartz R. Estimating the number of quit attempts it takes to quit smoking successfully in a longitudinal cohort of smokers. BMJ Open. 2016;6(6):e011045.
11. U.S. Department of Health and Human Services, Fiore MC, Jaén CR, Baker TB, Bailey WC, Benowitz NL, et al. Tobacco use and dependence guideline panel. Treating tobacco use and dependence: 2008 Update. Rockville; 2008 [cited 2025 April 10]. Available from: https://www.ncbi.nlm.nih.gov/books/NBK63952/ & https://www.ncbi.nlm.nih.gov/books/NBK63950/.
12. American Cancer Society. The American Cancer Society's principles of oncology: prevention to survivorship. In: Glynn TJ, Hurt RD, Lee Westmaas J, editors. Section 1 | Cancer causes, prevention, and early detection 1 (tobacco; chapter 6). Hoboken: Wiley Black; 2018. p. xv, 456 pages (58–71).
13. Ostroff JS, Buckshee N, Mancuso CA, Yankelevitz DF, Henschke CI. Smoking cessation following CT screening for early detection of lung cancer. Prev Med. 2001;33(6):613–21.
14. Piñeiro B, Simmons VN, Palmer AM, Correa JB, Brandon TH. Smoking cessation interventions within the context of low-dose computed tomography lung cancer screening: a systematic review. Lung Cancer. 2016;98:91–8.
15. Miller WR, Rollnick S. Motivational interviewing: helping people change and grow. 4th ed. New York: The Guilford Press; 2023. p. xiv, 338 pages p.
16. Abrams DB, Niaura R, Brown RA, Emmons KM, Goldstein MG, Monti PM. The tobacco dependence treatment handbook: a guide to best practices. New York: Guilford Press; 2003. p. xviii, 365 p.
17. United States Preventive Services Task Force, Krist AH, Davidson KW, Mangione CM, Barry MJ, Cabana M, et al. Screening for lung cancer: U.S. Preventive Services Task Force recommendation statement. JAMA. 2021;325(10):962–70.
18. National Comprehensive Cancer Network®. Quit smoking: NCCN clinical practice guidelines in oncology (NCCN Guidelines®) for smoking cessation, Version 1.2024 – April 30, 2024, Plymouth Meeting, Pennsylvania [cited 2025 April 10]. Available from: https://www.nccn.org/patients/guidelines/content/PDF/quitting-smoking-patient.pdf & https://www.nccn.org/patientresources/patient-resources/guidelines-for-patients.
19. Sheffer CE, Al-Zalabani A, Aubrey A, Bader R, Beltrez C, Bennett S, et al. The emerging global tobacco treatment workforce: characteristics of tobacco treatment specialists trained in council-accredited training programs from 2017 to 2019. Int J Environ Res Public Health. 2021;18(5)
20. Fathi, JT, Evison, M. Cytisine: a new opportunity in the UK for the Treatment of Tobacco Dependency. IASLC-The International Association for the Study of Lung Cancer: Tobacco Control & Smoking Cessation [Internet] 2024 April 10, 2025. Available from: https://www.ilcn.org/cytisine-a-new-opportunity-in-the-uk-for-the-treatment-of-tobacco-dependency/.

21. Rigotti NA, Benowitz NL, Prochaska J, Leischow S, Nides M, Blumenstein B, et al. Cytisinicline for smoking cessation: a randomized clinical trial. JAMA. 2023;330(2):152–60.
22. Dixit SM. Cytisine: a new smoking cessation treatment in spain. MEDICOS Next [Internet]. 2025 April 10. Available from: https://medicosnext.com/?p=3984.
23. U.S Department of Health & Human Services, Personal Author(s):, Lushniak BD, Samet JM, Pechacek TF, Norman LA, et al. The Health consequences of smoking—50 years of progress: a report of the Surgeon General, Published Date: 2014, [cited 2025 April 14]. Available from: https://stacks.cdc.gov/view/cdc/21569 & https://stacks.cdc.gov/view/cdc/21569_cdc_21569_DS1.pdf.
24. National Comprehensive Cancer Network®. Lung Cancer Screening: Clinical Practice Guidelines in Oncology (NCCN Guidelines®) Guidelines Version 2.2024, Plymouth Meeting, Pennsylvania [cited 2025 April 14]. Available from: https://www.nccn.org/patientresources/patient-resources/guidelines-for-patients/lung-cancer-resources.
25. Shoenbill KA, Goldstein AO. Better together: advancing tobacco use treatment and lung cancer screening. J Thorac Oncol. 2024;19(4):531–3.
26. Sallis JF, Owen N, Fisher EB. Ecological models of health behavior. Health behavior and health education: theory, research, and practice. 4th ed. San Francisco: Jossey-Bass; 2008. p. 465–85.
27. Yesiltepe D, Pepping R, Ling FCM, Tempest G, Mauw S, Janssen M, Hettinga F. A tale of two cities: understanding children's cycling behavior from the socio-ecological perspective. Front Public Health. 2022;10:864883. https://doi.org/10.3389/fpubh.2022.864883.
28. Bronfenbrenner U. The ecology of human development: experiments by nature and design. Harvard University Press; 1979.
29. U.S. National Cancer Institute. Treating Smoking in Cancer Patients: An Essential Component of Cancer Care. National Cancer Institute Tobacco Control Monograph 23. Bethesda, MD: U.S. Department of Health and Human Services, National Institutes of Health, National Cancer Institute; 2022. [cited 2025 April 10]. Available from: https://cancercontrol.cancer.gov/sites/default/files/2023-01/Monograph_23-ALL-PageNumbered-011223.pdf.
30. Presant CA, Ashing K, Raz D, Yeung S, Gascon B, Stewart A, et al. Overcoming barriers to tobacco cessation and lung cancer screening among racial and ethnic minority groups and underserved patients in academic centers and community network sites: the City of Hope experience. J Clin Med. 2023;12(4)
31. Steinberg MB, Young WJ, Miller Lo EJ, Bover-Manderski MT, Jordan HM, Hafiz Z, et al. Electronic health record prompt to improve lung cancer screening in primary care. Am J Prev Med. 2023;65(5):892–5.
32. Carter-Bawa L. Shifting the lens on lung cancer screening inequities. JAMA Netw Open. 2024;7(5):e2412782.
33. Richmond J, Fernandez JR, Bonnet K, Sellers A, Schlundt DG, Forde AT, et al. Patient lung cancer screening decisions and environmental and psychosocial factors. JAMA Netw Open. 2024;7(5):e2412880.
34. Park ER, Gareen IF, Japuntich S, Lennes I, Hyland K, DeMello S, et al. Primary care provider-delivered smoking cessation interventions and smoking cessation among participants in the National Lung Screening Trial. JAMA Intern Med. 2015;175(9):1509–16.
35. Ostroff JS, Reilly EM, Burris JL, Warren GW, Shelton RC, Mullett TW. Current practices, perceived barriers, and promising implementation strategies for improving quality of smoking cessation support in accredited cancer programs of the American College of Surgeons. JCO Oncol Pract. 2024;20(2):212–9.
36. Warren GW, Marshall JR, Cummings KM, Toll BA, Gritz ER, Hutson A, et al. Addressing tobacco use in patients with cancer: a survey of American Society of Clinical Oncology members. J Oncol Pract. 2013;9(5):258–62.
37. Sheffer CE, Payne T, Ostroff JS, Jolicoeur D, Steinberg M, Czabafy S, et al. Increasing the quality and availability of evidence-based treatment for tobacco dependence through unified certification of tobacco treatment specialists. J Smok Cessat. 2016;11(4):229–35.

38. Carter-Bawa L, Kotsen C, Schofield E, Fathi J, Frederico V, Walsh LE, et al. Tobacco treatment specialists' knowledge, attitudes and beliefs about lung cancer screening: potential piece of the puzzle for increasing lung cancer screening awareness. Patient Educ Couns. 2023;115:107871.
39. Leone FT, Zhang Y, Evers-Casey S, Evins AE, Eakin MN, Fathi J, et al. Initiating pharmacologic treatment in tobacco-dependent adults. An official American Thoracic Society clinical practice guideline. Am J Respir Crit Care Med. 2020;202(2):e5–e31.
40. Iaccarino JM, Duran C, Slatore CG, Wiener RS, Kathuria H. Combining smoking cessation interventions with LDCT lung cancer screening: a systematic review. Prev Med. 2019;121:24–32.
41. Moldovanu D, de Koning HJ, van der Aalst CM. Lung cancer screening and smoking cessation efforts. Transl Lung Cancer Res. 2021;10(2):1099–109.
42. Evans WK, Tammemägi MC, Walker MJ, Cameron E, Leung YW, Ashton S, et al. Integrating smoking cessation into low-dose computed tomography lung cancer screening: results of the Ontario. Can Pilot J Thorac Oncol. 2023;18(10):1323–33.
43. Kota KJ, Ji S, Bover-Manderski MT, Delnevo CD, Steinberg MB. Lung cancer screening knowledge and perceived barriers among physicians in the United States. JTO Clin Res Rep. 2022;3(7):100331.
44. Copeland J, Neal E, Phillips W, Hofferberth S, Lathan C, Donington J, Colson Y. Restructuring lung cancer care to accelerate diagnosis and treatment in patients vulnerable to healthcare disparities using an innovative care model. MethodsX. 2023;11:102338.
45. Centers for Medicare & Medicaid Services (CMS): Medicare Coverage Database. Screening for Lung Cancer with Low Dose Computed Tomography (LDCT), [cited 2025 May 1]. Available from: https://www.cms.gov/medicare-coverage-database/view/ncacal-decision-memo.aspx?proposed=N&NCAId=304.
46. Kotsen C, Dilip D, Carter-Harris L, O'Brien M, Whitlock CW, de Leon-Sanchez S, Ostroff JS. Rapid scaling up of telehealth treatment for tobacco-dependent cancer patients during the COVID-19 outbreak in new York City. Telemed J E Health. 2021;27(1):20–9.
47. Cancer Center Cessation Initiative Telehealth Working Group. Telehealth delivery of tobacco cessation treatment in cancer care: an ongoing innovation accelerated by the COVID-19 pandemic. J Natl Compr Cancer Netw. 2021;19(Suppl_1):S21-s4
48. Cinciripini PM, Kypriotakis G, Blalock JA, Karam-Hage M, Beneventi DM, Robinson JD, et al. Survival outcomes of an early intervention smoking cessation treatment after a cancer diagnosis. JAMA Oncol. 2024;10(12):1689–96.
49. Cinciripini PM, Karam-Hage M, Kypriotakis G, Robinson JD, Rabius V, Beneventi D, et al. Association of a Comprehensive Smoking Cessation Program with Smoking Abstinence among Patients with Cancer. JAMA Netw Open. 2019;2(9):e1912251.
50. Park ER, Perez GK, Regan S, Muzikansky A, Levy DE, Temel JS, et al. Effect of sustained smoking cessation counseling and provision of medication vs shorter-term counseling and medication advice on smoking abstinence in patients recently diagnosed with cancer: a randomized clinical trial. JAMA. 2020;324(14):1406–18.
51. Ostroff JS, Bolutayo Gaffney KL, O'Brien M, deLeon-Sanchez ST, Whitlock CW, Kotsen CS, et al. Training oncology care providers in the assessment and treatment of tobacco use and dependence. Cancer. 2021;127(16):3010–8.
52. Roughgarden KL, Toll BA, Tanner NT, Frazier CC, Silvestri GA, Rojewski AM. Tobacco treatment specialist training for lung cancer screening providers. Am J Prev Med. 2021;61(5):765–8.
53. Joseph AM, Rothman AJ, Almirall D, Begnaud A, Chiles C, Cinciripini PM, et al. Lung cancer screening and smoking cessation clinical trials. SCALE (smoking cessation within the context of lung cancer screening) collaboration. Am J Respir Crit Care Med. 2018;197(2):172–82.

Open Access This chapter is licensed under the terms of the Creative Commons Attribution-NonCommercial 4.0 International License (http://creativecommons.org/licenses/by-nc/4.0/), which permits any noncommercial use, sharing, adaptation, distribution and reproduction in any medium or format, as long as you give appropriate credit to the original author(s) and the source, provide a link to the Creative Commons license and indicate if changes were made.

The images or other third party material in this chapter are included in the chapter's Creative Commons license, unless indicated otherwise in a credit line to the material. If material is not included in the chapter's Creative Commons license and your intended use is not permitted by statutory regulation or exceeds the permitted use, you will need to obtain permission directly from the copyright holder.

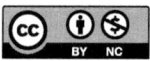

Clinical Manifestations and Presentations of Lung Cancer

11

Martina Block

Contents

Navigation Vignette	136
Introduction	137
Intrathoracic Presentations	137
Extrathoracic Presentations	140
Paraneoplastic	142
Conclusion	144
Key Takeaways	144
Key Readings and Resources	145
References	145

Abbreviations

ADH	Anti-diuretic hormone
CAT	Cancer-associated thrombosis
CNS	Central nervous system
COPD	Chronic obstructive pulmonary disease
CT	Computed tomography
DPOA	Medical Durable Power of Attorney
FMLA	Family Medical Leave Act
G-CSF	Granulocyte colony stimulating factor

M. Block (✉)
Department of Medical Oncology, Providence Regional Cancer Partnership, Everett, WA, USA

Department of Biobehavioral Nursing and Health Informatics, School of Nursing, University of Washington, Seattle, WA, USA
e-mail: marpgor@uw.edu

© The Author(s) 2026
J. T. Fathi, M. F. Mortman (eds.), *Lung Cancer Navigation and Care*,
https://doi.org/10.1007/978-3-032-02200-4_11

MRI	Magnetic resonance imaging
NSCLC	Non-small cell lung cancer
PET	Positron emission tomography
PNS	Paraneoplastic syndromes
SCC	Squamous cell cancer
SCLC	Small cell lung cancer
SIADH	Syndrome of inappropriate anti-diuretic hormone
SVC	Superior vena cava
TMA	Thrombotic microangiopathy
VEGF	Vascular endothelial growth factor

Navigation Vignette

A 73-year-old female presents with unexplained failure to thrive, mild confusion, and a persistent wet cough. Imaging identifies a hilar mass with adenopathy, as well as lytic lesions to the pelvis and right rib. PET scan confirms metastatic disease, consistent with stage IV small cell lung cancer. While MRI of the brain is unremarkable, lab findings reveal hyponatremia and hypercalcemia, consistent with syndrome of inappropriate antidiuretic hormone and hypercalcemia (both commonly occurring clinical presentations of advanced small cell lung cancer) likely contributing to her confusion and fatigue. She experiences severe low back pain and significant weakness, though she remains able to get out of bed. A biopsy of the lymph node confirms the diagnosis, and the oncology team begins planning for systemic chemotherapy.

Due to her confusion, the patient cannot fully comprehend her diagnosis or participate in treatment discussions. Her daughter, designated as her durable power of attorney (DPOA), is overwhelmed by the rapid progression of her mother's illness and concerned about her ability to manage care at home. She expresses anxiety over her mother's frailty and pain and uncertainty about how to balance her full-time job with caregiving needs, especially without financial resources to hire help. Despite these challenges, she is committed to ensuring her mother receives the best possible care and seeks guidance on what to expect.

The lung cancer nurse navigator provides clarity, support, and coordination at this critical juncture. Recognizing the urgency of addressing pain and metabolic imbalances, the navigator advocates for early palliative care consultation. This allows immediate pain management interventions, including appropriate pharmacologic treatment and the potential initiation of bone-modifying agents to help stabilize skeletal lesions and reduce fracture risk. Correcting hyponatremia and hypercalcemia will also help improve the patient's cognitive status and quality of life before and during initial treatment.

To support the patient and caregiver, the navigator connects the daughter with a hospital social worker to explore home health services, including visiting nurse support and physical therapy, which may be covered by insurance. Additionally, the navigator helps facilitate a family meeting with the oncology and palliative teams to set realistic expectations and goals of care while also discussing options for short-term skilled nursing or hospice evaluation if needed.

Understanding the caregiver strain, the navigator links the daughter to caregiver support groups and provides information on community-based respite services. Together, they review workplace resources such as the Family and Medical Leave Act (FMLA) and employee assistance programs, empowering the daughter to advocate for flexible support from her employer.

With the navigator's guidance, the family begins to feel less isolated and more informed. Treatment is initiated with a focus on improving symptoms, stabilizing function, and preserving dignity. While the prognosis remains serious, the coordinated, supportive care led by the navigator helps optimize the patient's quality of life and reduces the caregiver's emotional and logistical burden—ensuring that both mother and daughter feel supported through every step of the journey.

Introduction

Lung cancer histopathology is divided into small cell (SCLC) and non-small cell lung cancer (NSCLC) subtypes. SCLC makes up 15–20% of new lung cancer diagnoses and has distinctly neuroendocrine pathology [1]. It is typically more advanced at presentation than NSCLC, with extrathoracic metastasis in greater than 50% of cases [22]. SCLC often arises from the lobar bronchi as a hilar or perihilar mass visible by computed tomography (CT) [23]. Non-small cell carcinomas, comprised primarily of squamous cell (SCC), adenocarcinoma, and large cell carcinoma, arise from either the bronchial epithelium (SCC) or submucosal glands (adenocarcinoma). Definitive diagnosis requires tissue acquisition for histopathologic confirmation. Clinical manifestations of all lung cancers can be most easily classified into (1) intrathoracic, (2) extrathoracic, or (3) paraneoplastic.

Intrathoracic Presentations

Physical Exam Findings

Intrathoracic manifestations of lung cancer typically present with non-specific physical exam findings of intrathoracic disease (see Table 11.1). An astute clinician might note dull or absent lung sounds, dull percussion, tactile fremitus (palpable vibrations felt over the chest used to assess densities in the chest), positive whispered pectoriloquy (a sign of consolidation in the lung), pain or reduced expansion with deep breathing, hypoxia/tachypnea, tachycardia, fingernail clubbing, or lymphadenopathy. Exam findings associated with peripherally located tumors include diminished lung sounds in specific lung fields, localized dullness to percussion, or pleural rub. Conversely, exam findings of centrally located tumors include generalized rales, wheezing, hoarseness, or tachypnea.

Table 11.1 Common presenting symptoms of lung cancer and etiology by subtype [1, 4, 8, 9, 19, 25–28, 32, 39–41, 46]

Common presenting symptoms of lung cancer and etiology by subtype			
	Small cell lung cancer	Non-small cell lung cancer	
		Squamous cell carcinoma	Adenocarcinoma
Origin and behavior	Neuroendocrine Most aggressive	Bronchial epithelium	Submucosal glands Least aggressive
Radiographic appearance	Hilar Spiculated nodules Necrosis	Central Large Cavitary appearance	Peripheral nodules Size variable
Chest pain causes	Bulky adenopathy	Chest wall invasion Malignant effusion	Chest wall invasion
Dyspnea and causes	Central obstruction SVC syndrome Bulky adenopathy	Central compression	Airway compression Pleural effusion
Superior vena cava syndrome	Most common	Less common	Least common
Pancoast syndrome Horner's syndrome	Rare	Most common	Most common
Paraneoplastic	SIADH PNS	Hypercalcemia CAT	Hypercalcemia Leukocytosis Thrombocytosis CAT

Radiologic Presentation

The presence of other pathologic processes in the chest, such as infection or COPD, may confound radiographic evidence of lung cancer [24]. Signs of lung cancer by radiography include hilar or perihilar mass, lymphadenopathy, wide mediastinum, and pleural or pericardial effusion [25]. Any presumed pulmonary infection or effusion not responsive to first-line management or with atypical appearance should warrant early CT imaging and involvement of pulmonary specialists to discern the underlying pathology. If malignancy is strongly suspected, full-body CT or PET-CT should be obtained to capture the presence of the primary tumor and any body metastasis [25]. Central nervous system (CNS) metastasis is also a prime concern in suspected lung cancer, and neurologic abnormalities in this setting should prompt urgent CNS imaging [29].

By CT, SCLC typically presents as a hilar mass or spiculated nodules, often accompanied by bulky mediastinal adenopathy that variably represents true nodal metastasis [25]. Malignant nodes by CT are enlarged and frequently have heterogeneous enhancement with central necrosis and/or irregular borders. In SCLC, necrosis and hemorrhagic changes are common due to its rapid growth and aggressive biochemical resource allocation. Regarding NSCLC subtypes, SCC masses often appear larger and are more centrally located with cavitation or subsegmental collapse [25]. Presentation of adenocarcinoma by CT is frequently parenchymal nodularity, with nodules less than 3 centimeters [25].

Intrathoracic Symptoms

Cough is reported by 30–70% of patients at the time of lung cancer diagnosis (see Table 11.1) [2–4]. It is often not responsive to traditional treatment modalities. Cough is more prevalent in advanced stages of disease, and a nationwide registry study reported a slightly higher prevalence in SCLC [4]. Many patients have baseline cough due to smoking, COPD, or underlying respiratory infection; therefore, it is critical to obtain a detailed history of these symptoms to determine if the severity or character of the cough has changed from baseline.

Chest pain is prevalent in 20–40% of new diagnoses and is more common in younger patients [4]. Notably, the lung parenchyma is not sensitive to pain; dull, aching pain may be due to central tumor progression into the chest wall, large vessels, bronchi (parabronchial nerves), or mediastinum [4, 26]. Pleuritic pain can occur in the setting of pleural involvement but may also occur in cases of concurrent tumor-associated pulmonary embolism or obstructive pneumonitis [26, 27]. Shoulder pain in lung cancer may be due to phrenic nerve irritation caused by Pancoast tumor or mediastinal invasion. Radiation of pain down the arm is concerning for tumor involvement of the brachial plexus, and pain of this nature is correlated with advanced disease and inoperability [27].

Approximately 20% of new hemoptysis is reported to be in the setting of a lung malignancy, and hemoptysis occurs in around 10% of new lung cancer diagnoses [4, 5, 29, 47]. When present in any patient, hemoptysis indicates bronchial involvement of a pathogenic process and should be investigated promptly with dedicated CT imaging and pulmonology specialty consultation for consideration of further evaluation by bronchoscopy. Non-oncologic differentials for hemoptysis include infection, infarction, bronchiectasis, adenoma, or benign erosion.

Dyspnea occurs in 25–60% of new lung cancer diagnoses [4]. Dyspnea in lung cancer can arise from numerous etiologies, including obstruction of the airway, obstructive pneumonitis, anemia, cachexia, lymphangitic spread, pulmonary emboli, pathogenic pneumothorax, and pleural effusion. Cardiac compromise may also occur due to tumor compression or malignant pericardial effusion. Diaphragmatic tumor invasion resulting in phrenic nerve paralysis may also result in dyspnea [28]. A detailed medical history of this symptom can be key to differentiating between malignant etiology and other conditions such as asthma, infection, or cardiac etiology.

Unexplained wheezing, particularly if unilateral, should prompt concern for lung cancer [6]. Stridor may be noted with tracheal invasion or local compression and is managed with steroids, radiation, or stenting. Both wheezing and stridor, particularly when gradually occurring, should raise clinical suspicion for tumor invasion of the airway and prompt pulmonology referral for bronchoscopy. Lung cancer-associated hoarseness may occur on presentation in up to 10% of cases and is due to tumor involvement/compression of the laryngeal nerve, resulting in vocal cord paralysis. Lung cancer-associated dysphagia may occur due to nodal pressure on the esophagus, CNS, or local nerve involvement [4, 49].

Pleural involvement of lung cancer is a frequent cause of pain. Resultant effusions can be either malignant or benign. Pleural involvement may appear on imaging as pleural thickening or nodularity, with or without effusion. Malignant effusions preclude resection with curative intent, so differentiating malignant from non-malignant effusions is relevant for staging in many cases. If the effusion is not amenable to sampling, PET-CT is typically needed to differentiate malignant from benign findings [30]. Sampling of the pleural fluid for cytology is common and straightforward, though cytology has variable diagnostic yield. Fluid in malignant effusion is typically exudative and may be serous to grossly sanguineous with atypical cells present on cell count.

Intrathoracic Syndromes

Superior vena cava syndrome (SVC syndrome) occurs when SVC compression prevents blood return to the heart from the upper limbs, head, and neck, resulting in a medical emergency due to venous distention and impaired cardiac return. Lung cancer is one of the most frequent causes of these clinical stigmata [31]. Symptoms include dyspnea, cough, face/neck/arm swelling, venous distention of the neck, facial plethora, and cyanosis. Treatment is often accomplished by stenting, surgery, or radiation [31]. Any characteristic symptoms should prompt urgent CT imaging. If SVC syndrome appears in the setting of suspected malignancy, staging imaging and tissue acquisition for treatment should be conducted urgently. SVC syndrome is more commonly noted at diagnosis of SCLC than other histologic types and also in tumors arising from the right side of the chest due to vessel proximity [32]. Management prior to cancer treatment often includes steroids, diuretics to optimize volume status, and radiation/stenting.

Pancoast syndrome represents a constellation of symptoms seen in tumors of the superior sulcus of the lung, resulting in damage near the thoracic inlet. It may be caused by any expansile lesion in this region [8, 50]. Hallmark symptoms include severe, radiating shoulder pain, weakness/atrophy of thenar hand muscles on the affected side, and oculosympathetic paresis (Horner's syndrome). Horner's syndrome is a triad of symptoms, including unilateral ptosis (drooping eyelid), miosis (pupillary constriction), and anhidrosis on the side of the tumor. It is important to note that patients often do not present with all three triad elements. It can additionally present with enophthalmos, conjunctival changes, or color changes to the impacted side of the face [33]. The majority of tumors associated with Pancoast syndrome are NSCLC, most frequently adenocarcinoma. Only a small percentage of tumors of the superior sulcus have an underlying etiology of SCLC [8, 9, 50].

Extrathoracic Presentations

Extrathoracic signs and symptoms of lung cancer are typically due to metastatic disease. Bone metastases are present in 20–50% of patients at diagnosis [10–13]. Typical presentations include pain, commonly to the hip and back, hypercalcemia, and elevated alkaline phosphatase. Imaging may reveal lytic lesions or pathologic fractures [10–13]. These can result in skeletal instability or spinal cord compression. A French study reported that up to 80% of patients presenting with bony metastasis have multiple sites of metastatic bony disease [14]. Common sites of bony involvement include the spine (40–53%), ribs (62%), and pelvis (17–22%) [7, 10–14]. X-ray is poorly sensitive to detect these lesions. Bone scintigraphy has higher sensitivity than X-ray; however, MRI or PET-CT are considered best practices for complete staging [17, 18, 51]. Spinal cord compression as a result of pathologic fracture or expansile bony lesions should be managed emergently. Even if the patient is relatively asymptomatic, cord compression requires hospitalization for radiation or surgical intervention. Hypercalcemia of malignancy is common in the setting of bony metastasis and may be life-threatening [19]. Standard medical management of hypercalcemia with intravenous fluid and calcitonin may be needed until treatment is initiated. Additionally, bisphosphonate therapy not only corrects hypercalcemia definitively but these agents have been shown to reduce skeletal complications in patients with known bony metastatic disease [15, 16].

Adrenal metastases are equally common among all histologic types of lung cancer. They are less commonly noted at time of diagnosis than other metastatic sites [20]. Their presence is correlated with higher disease stage at diagnosis and with progressive/refractory disease [20, 21]. Patients with large or invasive adrenal metastasis may present with symptoms of back, chest, or abdominal pain or with renal failure. Symptoms may also include failure to thrive that is poorly explained, manifesting as poor appetite, weight loss, nausea, weakness, or electrolyte imbalance. Adrenal masses are often incidental findings, and it is difficult to differentiate benign from metastatic etiology without PET-CT or tissue acquisition [21].

CNS metastases are present in 10–30% of patients with newly diagnosed lung cancer [48]. Manifestations of intracranial disease depend on location of the tumor within the brain. They may include headaches—often severe and more prominent in the morning—vomiting, vision changes, hemiparesis, or seizures [34]. Specialist neurosurgery, radiation oncology, and medical oncology expertise are required for the co-management of lung cancer with CNS metastasis.

The liver is a common site of metastatic disease for both patients with SCLC and NSCLC, though it is more common among patients with SCLC [35]. Metastatic liver disease often presents initially with isolated elevated liver enzymes. Only after sufficient progression of liver disease does the patient begin to develop hyperbilirubinemia and loss of function [36]. Exam and lab findings may include hepatomegaly, abdominal pain, ascites, jaundice, bleeding, or coagulopathy.

Lymphadenopathy may represent either true metastasis or reactivity to underlying inflammation. Common sites of nodal metastasis in lung cancer include hilar, clavicular, and cervical nodes. A 2021 study noted that non-calcified mediastinal adenopathy on screening CT was associated with increased lung cancer diagnosis, earlier diagnosis, and increased mortality [37]. By exam, metastatic nodes are frequently large, hard, and fixed. They are often not painful; however, when pathologically enlarged, they may cause local compression, resulting in pain.

Constitutional symptoms of lung malignancy include weight loss, anorexia, low-grade fever, and progressive fatigue [4]. Generalized weakness and functional decline are common, particularly in geriatric patients. These symptoms are highly variable from patient to patient, but malignancy should be strongly suspected in their collective presence [4, 49]. In patients with lung cancer, these symptoms may also occur secondary to infection, progressive dyspnea (energy expenditure), dysphagia or local compression of nerves, vasculature or GI organs. Enlarged fingertips and curved nail appearance, known as "clubbing," are thought to occur in lung cancer due to tumor secretion of VEGF and prostaglandins, as well as hypoxia. This occurs in about 30% of lung cancer patients and is more common in NSCLC than SCLC [38].

Paraneoplastic

Endocrine Syndromes

Paraneoplastic endocrine syndromes are defined by abnormal endocrine function without evidence of physiologic feedback regulation. These characteristically worsen with advancing disease and improve with treatment. In many cases, there is evidence of tumor hormone synthesis driving this process [39].

Hypercalcemia of malignancy occurs in about 10% of lung cancer patients and is more common in NSCLC. It occurs in advanced disease and is associated with poor overall prognosis [19, 39, 40]. In lung cancer patients, it occurs most frequently due to tumor secretion of parathyroid hormone-related protein but may also be secondary to extensive bony metastasis or primary hyperparathyroidism [39]. Initial symptoms often include anorexia, nausea, vomiting, constipation, lethargy, polyuria/polydipsia, and dehydration. Confusion and coma are late signs and should be immediately managed with hydration, calcitonin, and/or dialysis [52]. Cancer treatment is the only definitive solution, though the above therapeutic modalities can be used to stabilize patients temporarily.

Syndrome of inappropriate antidiuretic hormone (SIADH) occurs at lung cancer diagnosis due to tumor secretion of antidiuretic hormone (ADH) and is most common in SCLC, occurring in about 15% of new diagnoses [39, 40]. Patients may be mildly or profoundly hyponatremic. Symptoms include fatigue, headache, anorexia, nausea/vomiting, restlessness, or irritability. Untreated, there is a concern for cerebral edema manifesting as seizure and eventually progressing to coma or death. Management includes typical SIADH strategies such as hypertonic fluids, urea or vasopressin, and fluid restriction. SIADH typically resolves within several weeks of SCLC treatment with combination chemotherapy [40].

Other less common endocrinopathies or clinical findings associated with lung cancer include Ectopic Cushing's syndrome, hypoglycemia, acromegaly, and gynecomastia [39].

Neurologic Syndromes

Paraneoplastic neurologic syndromes (PNS) are thought to be due to the presence of onconeural antibodies generated by T-lymphocytes in the presence of certain malignancies [41]. They may be associated with any lung cancer histologic type but are most common in SCLC, occurring in 3–5% of cases [39, 41]. Paraneoplastic neurologic syndromes may precede, follow, or present concurrently with the primary symptoms of malignancy. One study reported that in up to 80% of cases, PNS presented prior to any other clinical evidence of lung cancer [41]. Types of PNS are numerous and presentations variable. Symptoms may include muscle weakness, difficulty swallowing, balance changes, headache, vision changes, changes in behavior, or seizures [39–41]. If a patient presents with these symptoms, an MRI and spinal fluid evaluation should be completed to rule out metastatic disease, alternative etiologies, and to evaluate for the presence of paraneoplastic antibodies [39]. If PNS is suspected, dedicated neurology specialist evaluation should be conducted. Often, symptoms improve or resolve with cancer treatment initiation; however, at times, immunosuppressive therapies such as steroids, plasmapheresis, or intravenous immunoglobulin are utilized to stabilize patients until treatment is underway [39].

Hematologic Syndromes

Hematologic paraneoplastic conditions occurring in the setting of lung cancer are typically cytokine mediated. Granulocytosis, eosinophilia, and thrombocytosis are commonly associated with NSCLC due to granulocyte colony-stimulating factor (G-CSF) tumor secretion, which stimulates the myeloid lineage in the marrow [40]. These hematologic abnormalities are typically associated with poorer overall prognosis due to the role of G-CSF in fostering inflammatory-mediated tumor progression and promoting immune dysregulation [42]. Thrombocytosis at presentation is felt to be an independent predictor of overall survival regardless of histology or initial stage [43].

Thrombotic microangiopathy (TMA) of malignancy may occur due to tumor damage to the vascular endothelium, resulting in endothelial dysregulation leading to thrombosis of the microvasculature and shearing hemolysis. Lung cancer accounts for approximately 10% of malignancy-associated TMAs, and the only evidence-based management strategy is to treat the underlying malignancy [44]. Unlike other TMA syndrome subtypes, immunosuppression, plasmapheresis, or complement blockade do not typically provide benefit.

Cancer-associated thrombosis (CAT) is common in lung cancers, occurring in up to 15% of patients at the time of diagnosis, and is a frequent cause of pretreatment mortality [46]. CAT is an independent predictor of early lung cancer mortality [46]. It can occur as deep venous thrombosis, central sinus venous thrombosis, and even as non-bacterial thrombotic endocarditis. Pathogenesis of thrombosis in lung cancer is mediated by tissue factor secretion by the tumor [45]. Local compression by bulky tumors impacting blood flow may also result in thrombosis [45]. Most CAT occurs in NCLSC, specifically in patients with ROS1 or ALK fusion. EGFR and KRAS mutations are considered to be at a lower risk with respect to thrombotic events [46]. Patients with lung cancer who are hospitalized, undergoing surgery, or acutely ill should receive Deep Vein Thrombosis (DVT) prophylaxis. High-risk patients with lung cancer in the community may also benefit from DVT prophylaxis.

Conclusion

As the prevalence of lung cancer remains high in comparison with other malignancies, so too does the focus on identifying at-risk patients, improving screening guideline adherence, and educating clinicians to recognize hallmark signs and symptoms. In order to achieve a timely diagnosis, it is critical that all clinicians are not only able to recognize early manifestations of lung cancer but feel empowered and adequately resourced to pursue the evaluations needed. This chapter aims to support early recognition and increase lung cancer survival, ultimately providing patients with the best possible experience as they begin their cancer treatment journey.

Key Takeaways

- Both individuals who smoke and those who do not may develop lung cancer—screening all patients for common signs and symptoms is critical to obtain a timely diagnosis
- Any intrathoracic symptom (cough, dyspnea, pain, hemoptysis) that is recalcitrant or poorly explained should result in further diagnostic exploration and pulmonary evaluation
- Lung cancer frequently causes paraneoplastic syndromes—patients with any suspected malignancy should have a thorough screening assessment for paraneoplastic phenomena
- Thrombotic events are common at lung cancer diagnosis; all patients with lung cancer who are hospitalized or acutely ill should have adequate DVT prophylaxis
- For patients with skeletal metastasis, bisphosphonate therapy has been found to reduce skeletal complications, including pathologic fractures
- Multiple concurrent constitutional symptoms, such as weight loss, anorexia, low-grade fever, and progressive fatigue, should always heighten concern for underlying malignancy and prompt thorough exam and clinical evaluations

Key Readings and Resources

- Lung Cancer Symptoms at Diagnosis [4]
- Paraneoplastic Syndromes in Lung Cancers [41]
- A Patient Perspective: Identifying and Understanding the Barriers Associated with the Diagnostic Delay of Lung Cancer [53]
- Learn Oncology: Lung Cancer [54]

Conflict of Interest None.

References

1. Wang Q, Gümüş ZH, Colarossi C, Memeo L, Wang X, Kong CY, et al. SCLC: epidemiology, risk factors, genetic susceptibility, molecular pathology, screening, and early detection. J Thorac Oncol. 2023;18(1):31–46.
2. Kocher F, Hilbe W, Seeber A, Pircher A, Schmid T, Greil R, et al. Longitudinal analysis of 2293 NSCLC patients: a comprehensive study from the TYROL registry. Lung Cancer. 2015;87(2):193–200.
3. Harle A, Molassiotis A, Buffin O, Burnham J, Smith J, Yorke J, et al. A cross sectional study to determine the prevalence of cough and its impact in patients with lung cancer: a patient unmet need. BMC Cancer. 2020;20(1):9.
4. Ruano-Raviña A, Provencio M, Calvo De Juan V, Carcereny E, Moran T, Rodriguez-Abreu D, et al. Lung cancer symptoms at diagnosis: results of a nationwide registry study. ESMO Open. 2020;5(6):e001021. https://linkinghub.elsevier.com/retrieve/pii/S2059702920327563.
5. Singer ED, Faiz SA, Qdaisat A, Abdeldaem K, Dagher J, Chaftari P, et al. Hemoptysis in cancer patients. Cancers. 2023;15(19):4765.
6. Chernecky C, Sarna L, Waller JL, Becht ML. Assessing coughing and wheezing in lung cancer: a pilot study. Oncol Nurs Forum. 2004;31(6):1095–101.
7. Kuchuk M, Addison CL, Clemons M, Kuchuk I, Wheatley-Price P. Incidence and consequences of bone metastases in lung cancer patients. J Bone Oncol. 2013;2(1):22–9.
8. Zarogoulidis K, Porpodis K, Domvri K, Eleftheriadou E, Ioannidou D, Zarogoulidis P. Diagnosing and treating pancoast tumors. Expert Rev Respir Med. 2016;10(12):1255–8.
9. Tohme S, Parikh K, Lee PC. Pancoast tumors: current management and outcomes—a narrative review. Curr Chall Thorac Surg. 2024;6:34.
10. Roato I. Bone metastases: when and how lung cancer interacts with bone. WJCO. 2014;5(2):149.
11. Katakami N, Kunikane H, Takeda K, Takayama K, Sawa T, Saito H, et al. Prospective study on the incidence of bone metastasis (BM) and skeletal-related events (SREs) in patients (pts) with stage IIIB and IV lung cancer—CSP-HOR 13. J Thorac Oncol. 2014;9(2):231–8.
12. Nistor CE, Ciuche A, Cucu AP, Nitipir C, Slavu C, Serban B, et al. Management of lung cancer presenting with solitary bone metastasis. Medicina. 2022;58(10):1463.
13. Knapp BJ, Devarakonda S, Govindan R. Bone metastases in non-small cell lung cancer: a narrative review. J Thorac Dis. 2022;14(5):1696–712.
14. Wu S, Pan Y, Mao Y, Chen Y, He Y. Current progress and mechanisms of bone metastasis in lung cancer: a narrative review. Transl Lung Cancer Res. 2021;10(1):439–51.
15. Wei Z, Pan B, Jia D, Yu Y. Long-term safety and efficacy of bisphosphonate therapy in advanced lung cancer with bone metastasis. Future Oncol. 2022;18(18):2257–67.
16. El-Hajj Fuleihan G, Clines GA, Hu MI, Marcocci C, Murad MH, Piggott T, et al. Treatment of hypercalcemia of malignancy in adults: an Endocrine Society clinical practice guideline. J Clin Endocrinol Metab. 2023;108(3):507–28.

17. Ban J, Fock V, Aryee DNT, Kovar H. Mechanisms, diagnosis and treatment of bone metastases. Cells. 2021;10(11):2944.
18. Farsad M. FDG PET/CT in the staging of lung cancer. CRP. 2020;13(3):195–203.
19. Chan VWQ, Henry MT, Kennedy MP. Hyponatremia and hypercalcemia: a study of a large cohort of patients with lung cancer. Transl Cancer Res TCR. 2020;9(1):222–30.
20. Kocijančič I, Vidmar K, Zwitter M, Snoj M. The significance of adrenal metastases from lung carcinoma. Eur J Surg Oncol. 2003;29(1):87–8.
21. Spartalis E, Drikos I, Ioannidis A, Chrysikos D, Athanasiadis DI, Spartalis M, et al. Metastatic carcinomas of the adrenal glands: from diagnosis to treatment. Anticancer Res. 2019;39(6):2699–710.
22. Ko J, Winslow MM, Sage J. Mechanisms of small cell lung cancer metastasis. EMBO Mol Med. 2021;13(1):e13122.
23. Carter BW, Glisson BS, Truong MT, Erasmus JJ. Small cell lung carcinoma: staging, imaging, and treatment considerations. Radiographics. 2014;34(6):1707–21.
24. Bradley SH, Abraham S, Callister ME, Grice A, Hamilton WT, Lopez RR, et al. Sensitivity of chest X-ray for detecting lung cancer in people presenting with symptoms: a systematic review. Br J Gen Pract. 2019;69(689):e827–35.
25. Panunzio A, Sartori P. Lung cancer and radiological imaging. CRP. 2020;13(3):238–42.
26. Mercadante S, Vitrano V. Pain in patients with lung cancer: pathophysiology and treatment. Lung Cancer. 2010;68(1):10–5.
27. Cuadrado DG, Grogan EL. Management of superior sulcus tumors: posterior approach. Oper Tech Thorac Cardiovasc Surg. 2011;16(2):154–66.
28. Quint LE. Thoracic complications and emergencies in oncologic patients. Cancer Imaging. 2009;9(Special Issue A):S75–82.
29. Mpika GSM, Kechnaoui S, Tourane LOEI, Fikri O, Amro L. Hemoptysis: epidemiological, clinical and etiological aspects. SAS J Med. 2023;9(11):1139–43.
30. Bai JH, Hsieh MS, Liao HC, Lin MW, Chen JS. Prediction of pleural invasion using different imaging tools in non-small cell lung cancer. Ann Transl Med. 2019;7(2):33.
31. Azizi AH, Shafi I, Shah N, Rosenfield K, Schainfeld R, Sista A, et al. Superior Vena Cava Syndrome. J Am Coll Cardiol Intv. 2020;13(24):2896–910.
32. Lepper PM, Ott SR, Hoppe H, Schumann C, Stammberger U, Bugalho A, et al. Superior vena cava syndrome in thoracic malignancies. Respir Care. 2011;56(5):653–66.
33. Baik D, Alghanim F, Arvan W. Horner syndrome as a late manifestation of non-small cell lung cancer. Chest. 2023;164(4):A4466.
34. Myall NJ, Yu H, Soltys SG, Wakelee HA, Pollom E. Management of brain metastases in lung cancer: evolving roles for radiation and systemic treatment in the era of targeted and immune therapies. Neuro-oncology. Advances. 2021;3(Supplement_5):v52–62.
35. Ren Y, Dai C, Zheng H, Zhou F, She Y, Jiang G, et al. Prognostic effect of liver metastasis in lung cancer patients with distant metastasis. Oncotarget. 2016;7(33):53245–53.
36. Choi MG, Choi CM, Lee DH, Kim SW, Yoon S, Kim WS, et al. Different prognostic implications of hepatic metastasis according to front-line treatment in non-small cell lung cancer: a real-world retrospective study. Transl Lung Cancer Res. 2021;10(6):2551–61.
37. Chalian H, McAdams HP, Lee Y, Duan F, Wu Y, Khoshpouri P, et al. Mediastinal lymphadenopathy in the National Lung Screening Trial (NLST) is associated with interval lung cancer. Radiology. 2022;302(3):684–92.
38. Sridhar KS, Lobo CF, Altman RD. Digital clubbing and lung cancer. Chest. 1998;114(6):1535–7.
39. Soomro Z, Youssef M, Yust-Katz S, Jalali A, Patel AJ, Mandel J. Paraneoplastic syndromes in small cell lung cancer. J Thorac Dis. 2020;12(10):6253–63.
40. Iyer P, Ibrahim M, Siddiqui W, Dirweesh A. Syndrome of inappropriate secretion of antidiuretic hormone (SIADH) as an initial presenting sign of non small cell lung cancer-case report and literature review. Respir Med Case Rep. 2017;22:164–7.
41. Shamji FM, Beauchamp G, Maziak DE, Cooper J. Paraneoplastic syndromes in lung cancers. Thorac Surg Clin. 2021;31(4):519–37. https://www-clinicalkey-com.offcampus.lib.washington.edu/#!/content/playContent/1-s2.0-S1547412721000578?scrollTo=%23top

42. Kasuga I, Makino S, Kiyokawa H, Katoh H, Ebihara Y, Ohyashiki K. Tumor-related leukocytosis is linked with poor prognosis in patients with lung carcinoma. Cancer. 2001;92(9):2399–405.
43. Pedersen L, Milman N. Prognostic significance of thrombocytosis in patients with primary lung cancer. Eur Respir J. 1996;9(9):1826–30.
44. Babu KG, Bhat GR. Cancer-associated thrombotic microangiopathy. ecancer [Internet]. 2016 Jun 28 [cited 2025 Jan 6];10. Available from: http://www.ecancer.org/journal/10/full/649-cancer-associated-thrombotic-microangiopathy.php
45. Abdol Razak N, Jones G, Bhandari M, Berndt M, Metharom P. Cancer-associated thrombosis: an overview of mechanisms, risk factors, and treatment. Cancers. 2018;10(10):380.
46. Wei Xiong GX, Du H, Xu M, Zhao Y. Management of venous thromboembolism in patients with lung cancer: a state-of-the-art review. BMJ Open Resp Res. 2023;10(1):e001493.
47. Mondoni M, Carlucci P, Job S, Parazzini EM, Cipolla G, Pagani M, Tursi F, Negri L, Fois A, Canu S, Arcadu A, Pirina P, Bonifazi M, Gasparini S, Marani S, Comel AC, Ravenna F, Dore S, Alfano F, et al. Observational, multicentre study on the epidemiology of haemoptysis. Eur Respir J. 2018;51(1):1701813. https://doi.org/10.1183/13993003.01813-2017.
48. Newman SJ, Hansen HH. Frequency, diagnosis, and treatment of brain metastases in 247 consecutive patients with bronchogenic carcinoma. Cancer. 1974;33(2):492–6.
49. Key NS, Khorana AA, Kuderer NM, Bohlke K, Lee AYY, Arcelus JI, et al. Venous thromboembolism prophylaxis and treatment in patients with cancer: ASCO clinical practice guideline update. JCO. 2020;38(5):496–520.
50. Marulli G, Battistella L, Mammana M, Calabrese F, Rea F. Superior sulcus tumors (Pancoast tumors). Ann Transl Med. 2016;4(12):239.
51. National Comprehensive Cancer Network. Non-Small Cell Lung Cancer [Internet]. [cited 2025 Apr 5]. Available from: https://www.nccn.org/professionals/physician_gls/pdf/nscl.pdf.
52. Walker MD, Shane E. Hypercalcemia: a review. JAMA. 2022;328(16):1624.
53. Hill LLE, Collier G, Gemine RE. A patient perspective: identifying and understanding the barriers associated with the diagnostic delay of lung cancer. EMJ Respir. 2017;5:92–8. https://www.researchgate.net/publication/367047860_A_Patient_Perspective_Identifying_and_Understanding_the_Barriers_Associated_with_the_Diagnostic_Delay_of_Lung_Cancer
54. Ingledew, Paris. Learn Oncology: Lung Cancer [Internet]. Available from: https://www.learnoncology.ca/modules/lung-cancer

Open Access This chapter is licensed under the terms of the Creative Commons Attribution-NonCommercial 4.0 International License (http://creativecommons.org/licenses/by-nc/4.0/), which permits any noncommercial use, sharing, adaptation, distribution and reproduction in any medium or format, as long as you give appropriate credit to the original author(s) and the source, provide a link to the Creative Commons license and indicate if changes were made.

The images or other third party material in this chapter are included in the chapter's Creative Commons license, unless indicated otherwise in a credit line to the material. If material is not included in the chapter's Creative Commons license and your intended use is not permitted by statutory regulation or exceeds the permitted use, you will need to obtain permission directly from the copyright holder.

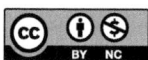

Classification and Staging of Lung Cancer

12

Nicholas C. Love and Arpan A. Patel

Contents

Navigation Vignette	150
Introduction	151
Cell Type of Origin and Histology	152
Diagnostic Evaluation	153
TNM Staging of Lung Cancer	154
Lymph Node Stations	157
VALG Staging of Small Cell Lung Cancer	160
Role of Molecular Diagnostic Studies	160
Key Takeaways	161
Key Readings and Resources	161
References	161

Abbreviations

AJCC	American Joint Committee on Cancer
ALK	Anaplastic lymphoma kinase
BRAF	V-Raf murine sarcoma viral oncogene homolog B
CT	Computed tomography
EGFR	Epidermal growth factor receptor
FDG	Fluorodeoxyglucose
FISH	Fluorescence in situ hybridization

N. C. Love (✉) · A. A. Patel
Wilmot Cancer Institute, University of Rochester Medical Center, Rochester, NY, USA
e-mail: NicholasC_Love@URMC.Rochester.edu; arpan_patel@urmc.rochester.edu

© The Author(s) 2026
J. T. Fathi, M. F. Mortman (eds.), *Lung Cancer Navigation and Care*,
https://doi.org/10.1007/978-3-032-02200-4_12

HER2	Human epidermal growth factor receptor 2
IASLC	International Association for the Study of Lung Cancer
KRAS	Kirsten rat sarcoma virus oncogene homolog
MRI	Magnetic resonance imaging
NGS	Next generation sequencing
NSCLC	Non-small cell lung cancer
NTRK	Neurotrophic tropomyosin receptor kinase
PD-L1	Programmed death-ligand 1
PET	Positron emission tomography
RET	Rearranged during transfection
ROS1	ROS proto-oncogene 1, receptor tyrosine kinase
SCLC	Small cell lung cancer
TNM	Tumor, nodal, and metastasis
TPS	Tumor proportion score
VALG	Veterans Administration Lung Cancer Study Group
WHO	World Health Organization

Navigation Vignette

Mr. J, a 64-year-old male with a 20-pack-year tobacco use history presents for initial oncology consultation for a left apical consolidation that was found on CXR during the workup of progressive non-productive cough with pleuritic chest discomfort and unintentional weight loss. Vital signs and laboratory testing are unremarkable. A comprehensive physical examination is notable for a patient with thin body habitus, normal cardiac and pulmonary examinations, normal abdominal examination without hepatosplenomegaly, and absent palpable lymphadenopathy.

Initial diagnostic evaluation includes a chest, abdomen, and pelvis CT with findings notable for a 4.5 × 2.5 cm left apical consolidation and a prominent 1.8 × 0.9 cm left pretracheal lymph node without other lymphadenopathy or evidence of distal metastatic disease. In this case, subsequent PET/CT should be considered to assess if this lymph node is fluorodeoxyglucose (FDG)-avid, which, if it is, would indicate hypermetabolic activity and suggest the presence of metastatic disease to regional lymph nodes.

Whole body PET/CT is obtained and shows a similarly sized left apical mass, the previously noted left pretracheal lymph node, which now measures 2.2 × 1.3 cm, and an additional subcarinal lymph node measuring 2.5 × 1.3 cm. All these findings are noted to be FDG-avid, and there are no additional FDG-avid foci.

Bronchoscopy sampled the areas of concern by needle biopsy. The left apical lesion, station 7 (subcarinal), and station 4 L (pretracheal) lymph nodes were all positive for adenocarcinoma. This is consistent with a diagnosis of NSCLC.

Based on the IASLC ninth edition of the tumor, node, metastasis (TNM) classification system, this patient is found to have *stage IIIa (cTNM cT2b, cN2a, cM0) lung cancer*.

- T2b designates tumors *>4 cm but ≤ 5 cm* in greatest dimension.
- N2 specifies metastasis in ipsilateral mediastinal and/or *subcarinal lymph nodes* and is further subdivided into *single N2 station involvement (N2a)* and multiple N2 station involvement (N2b).
- And there is no evidence of distant metastatic disease *(M0)* on whole-body PET/CT.

Note that the patient has two lymph nodes involved by his disease (4 L) and (7) at two different lymph node stations. The 4 L node, if this were the only lymph node involved, would qualify the patient as having N1 disease and is not an N2 station lymph node. However, the presence of a single N2-qualifying lymph node instead classifies the patient as having N2a disease, as only the highest N designation that would be suggested by the lymph node station is considered in the staging.

Given the locally advanced (stage IIIa) disease, an MRI of the brain was also performed and was negative for intracranial metastatic disease at the time of diagnosis.

Immunohistochemistry showed PD-L1 TPS (programmed death-ligand 1 tumor proportion score) <1% (indicating that PD-L1 is expressed on less than 1% of tumor cells), and a next-generation sequencing (NGS) panel revealed no actionable mutations (e.g., no EGFR, BRAF, or KRAS mutations, ALK, ROS1, or RET gene rearrangements).

At the time of discovery, a nurse navigator was introduced to the patient to guide the patient through the complex diagnostic and treatment planning process. The nurse navigator assisted in this process by explaining, scheduling, and coordinating the multitude of appointments and referrals (e.g., CT scan, PET/CT scan, and bronchoscopy/pulmonology consultation) required to accurately stage the patient's lung cancer. They also connected the patient with local support groups and resources to help them and their families come to terms with this new diagnosis. Additionally, when treatment modalities were discussed at a subsequent visit, they assisted in educating the patient regarding the potential side effects of chemotherapy and their treatment schedule.

Recognizing the emotional toll of a new cancer diagnosis, the navigator assessed the patient's psychosocial needs, connected the patient to support services, and addressed barriers to care such as transportation and insurance coverage. As part of the multidisciplinary tumor board discussions, the navigator ensured the patient's voice and preferences were represented and that follow-up was streamlined across providers.

Introduction

Lung cancer is a significant contributor to both global and nationwide cancer-related morbidity and mortality, with an estimated 234,580 new cases of lung cancer occurring in the United States in 2024. The incidence of lung cancer has declined in recent decades, from 65.2 per 100,000 persons in 1990 to 43.7 in 2021 [1], coinciding with a decrease in population trends in tobacco use. The implementation of widespread screening in high-risk patients has led to the earlier identification of lung cancer. This, combined with the advent of novel targeted and immunotherapies, has contributed to a similar decline in the death rate over this same period, from 58.9 per 100,000 persons in 1990 to 31.3 in 2021 [2]. Despite this, lung cancer remains the leading cause of cancer mortality in the United States, with 125,070 cancer deaths reported in 2024 (comprising 20.44% of all cancer deaths in the United States) [3].

Cell Type of Origin and Histology

Lung cancer is classified based on the cell type of origin and on histologic appearance and staining.

Bronchogenic carcinomas arise from the epithelial cells that line the lungs' airways. These are the most common of lung cancers and are typically broadly classified as small cell lung cancer (SCLC) or non-small cell lung cancer (NSCLC), with the distinction being made largely due to the comparatively poor prognosis of small cell compared with non-small cell lung cancer. NSCLC comprises approximately 80% and SCLC represents approximately 14% [3] of bronchogenic carcinomas.

The 2021 World Health Organization (WHO) Classification of Thoracic Tumors [4] further divides the bronchogenic carcinomas into numerous subtypes based on cell histology or microscopic appearance. A non-exhaustive list of the most clinically prevalent of these is (in descending order) adenocarcinoma, squamous cell carcinoma, and small cell carcinoma. Small cell carcinoma is synonymous with small cell lung cancer, and all of the other types of epithelial lung cancer are classified as non-small cell lung cancer (NSCLC).

Cancer can also arise from the mesenchymal tissues (e.g., mesothelioma) and hematolymphoid tissues (e.g., lymphoma). A more detailed discussion on lymphoma is outside of the scope of this review publication.

Mesothelioma is quite uncommon when compared with the bronchogenic carcinomas, with an incidence of 0.7 per 100,000 persons recorded in 2021 [5]. Malignant mesothelioma can arise from the mesothelial cells surrounding the lung (pleural, 81.4% of cases), abdomen (peritoneal, 10.5% of cases), or rarely the heart (pericardial, 0.2% of cases) [6]. Mesothelioma can arise from spindle cells (sarcomatoid), epithelial cells (epithelioid), or both cell types (biphasic). Epithelioid mesothelioma is the most common type of mesothelioma, comprising approximately 60% of cases at the time of diagnosis by WHO estimates [7] (although the estimated rate can vary from 50% to 70% depending on the source), and typically has a better prognosis than either sarcomatoid or biphasic mesothelioma. (See Chap. 17 for more information about mesothelioma.)

Diagnostic Evaluation

Initial Evaluation by Imaging

The initial evaluation of a patient with newly diagnosed lung cancer consists of imaging to assess the patient's disease burden and tissue sampling by biopsy in order to determine the pathology. Initial imaging typically consists of diagnostic contrast-enhanced or non-contrast CT scans of the chest, abdomen, and in some cases, the pelvis. This differs from the low-dose (so-named for the comparatively lower dose of radiation) spiral CT scans that are the recommended screening modality for patients at high risk for developing lung cancer [8]. Chest x-ray may be the initial diagnostic modality to suggest the presence of a potential lung cancer but is insufficient for staging purposes due to the inability to accurately assess the volume of disease burden.

Proper Imaging for Metastasis

PET/CT scans can either be used for initial staging (similar to a diagnostic CT scan), to subsequently evaluate for the presence of nodal metastatic disease, particularly in patients being evaluated for a curative-intent surgery, or to appraise indeterminate findings on traditional CT scan. Of note, PET/CT scans have a low sensitivity and specificity for lesions <1 cm and should not be used in these circumstances [9].

Brain MRI with contrast is recommended in addition to CT scans as part of the evaluation for all patients diagnosed with SCLC by biopsy and can be employed in patients with NSCLC in order to exclude intracranial metastatic disease (Stage II, Stage III, and Stage IV) prior to starting aggressive local or combined-modality treatments.

Tissue Biopsy of Cancer for Histologic Diagnosis

Tissue biopsy is essential to providing a histologic diagnosis. This can either be obtained from the primary lesion (the lung cancer itself) or the site of suspected metastatic disease in advanced lung cancer in order to minimize the amount of invasive testing that a patient undergoes. For example, a patient presenting with a 7-cm lung mass and a 4-cm liver lesion could be diagnosed with metastatic lung cancer by a single liver biopsy with histology that is consistent with adenocarcinoma derived from lung tissue. Biopsy can be obtained either by endoscopy/bronchoscopy, through interventional radiology, or concurrently at the time of surgical resection (typically after an initial tissue sampling via one of the other aforementioned modalities has already been obtained). Surgical approaches ideally include a lobectomy as opposed to a wedge resection [10, 11] or, less commonly, pneumonectomy, depending on the extent of disease.

Nodal Sampling to Assess Extent of Cancer

Pathologic mediastinal staging (either by mediastinoscopy, mediastinotomy, endobronchial ultrasound, or video-assisted thoracic surgery) to evaluate for nodal metastatic disease is typically performed prior to potentially curative surgery in NSCLC. It is used similarly to confirm limited rather than extensive stage (see the section on Veterans Administration Lung Cancer Study (VALG) staging below) in SCLC prior to proceeding with treatment.

Pleural Fluid Sampling to Assess Extent of Cancer

Thoracentesis or thoracoscopy (if thoracentesis is negative) can be used to analyze pleural fluid for suspected malignant effusion. Both thoracentesis and needle biopsy may be non-diagnostic in the evaluation of suspected malignant mesothelioma. In these cases, thoracoscopy can provide a more substantial tissue specimen that may assist in providing a diagnosis.

TNM Staging of Lung Cancer

The International Association for the Study of Lung Cancer (IASLC) has recently released its ninth edition of the Tumor, Node, Metastasis (TNM) classification system [12].

Tumor Component

The tumor (T) component of staging ranges from values of T0 to T4, with TX as a null value indicating that the primary tumor cannot be assessed. T0 indicates no evidence of a primary tumor. "Tis" corresponds to carcinoma in situ (when there is no evidence of tumor invasion into deeper tissue).

T1 tumors are surrounded by normal lung tissue or visceral pleura or are located in a lobar or more peripheral bronchus. T1 is further subdivided into:

- T1mi: Minimally invasive adenocarcinoma
- T1a: Tumors ≤1 cm in greatest dimension
- T1b: Tumors >1 cm but ≤2 cm in greatest dimension
- T1c: Tumors >2 cm but ≤3 cm in greatest dimension

T2 tumors are subdivided as follows:

- T2a: tumors >3 cm but ≤4 cm in greatest dimension, invasion of the visceral pleura or an adjacent lobe, involvement of the main bronchus (excluding the

carina), or associated atelectasis or obstructive pneumonitis extending to the hilar region
- T2b: tumors >4 cm but ≤5 cm in greatest dimension

T3 tumors include any of the following features: tumors >5 cm but ≤7 cm in greatest dimension, invasion of the parietal pleura, the chest wall, the pericardium, the phrenic nerve, the azygos vein, the thoracic nerve roots or stellate ganglion. The presence of separate tumor nodules in the same lobe as the primary tumor is also a qualifying feature for T3 classification.

T4 tumors are >7 cm in greatest dimension or are those that invade critical structures such as the mediastinum, thymus, trachea, carina, recurrent laryngeal nerve, vagus nerve, esophagus, diaphragm, heart, great vessels, supra-aortic arteries, brachiocephalic veins, subclavian vessels, vertebral bodies, lamina, spinal cord, cervical nerve roots, or brachial plexus. The presence of separate nodules in a different ipsilateral lobe than the primary tumor is also a qualifying feature for T4 classification.

Nodal Component

The nodal (N) component of staging ranges from values of N0–N3, with NX as a null value indicating that regional lymph nodes cannot be assessed.

- N0 signifies the absence of nodal metastatic disease.
- N1 classification denotes the presence of metastasis in ipsilateral peribronchial, hilar, and/or intrapulmonary lymph nodes.
- N2 specifies metastasis in ipsilateral mediastinal and/or subcarinal lymph nodes and is further subdivided into single N2 station involvement (N2a) and multiple N2 station involvement (N2b).
- N3 indicates metastasis in the contralateral mediastinal or hilar lymph nodes, the ipsilateral or contralateral scalene, or ipsilateral or contralateral supraclavicular lymph nodes. Direct extension of the primary tumor into lymph nodes is counted as lymph node involvement in this classification.

Metastasis Component

The metastasis (M) component of staging ranges from M0 to M1c. M0 indicates the absence, whereas M1 represents the presence of distant metastatic disease and is further subdivided as follows:

- M1a indicates a tumor with pleural or pericardial involvement, the presence of a malignant pleural or pericardial effusion, as well as the presence of separate tumor nodules in a contralateral lobe.

Table 12.1 TNM staging

9th Edition TNM Descriptors and Stages				N2		
T/M	Categories and Descriptors	N0	N1	N2a	N2b	N3
T1	T1a ≤1 cm	IA1	IIA	IIB	IIIA	IIIB
	T1b >1 to ≤2 cm	IA2	IIA	IIB	IIIA	IIIB
	T1c >2 to ≤3 cm	IA3	IIA	IIB	IIIA	IIIB
T2	T2a Visceral pleura / central invasion	IB	IIB	IIIA	IIIB	IIIB
	T2a >3 to ≤4 cm	IB	IIB	IIIA	IIIB	IIIB
	T2b >4 to ≤5 cm	IIA	IIB	IIIA	IIIB	IIIB
T3	T3 >5 to ≤7 cm	IIB	IIIA	IIIA	IIIB	IIIC
	T3 Invasion	IIB	IIIA	IIIA	IIIB	IIIC
	T3 Same lobe separate tumor nodules	IIB	IIIA	IIIA	IIIB	IIIC
T4	T4 >7 cm	IIIA	IIIA	IIIB	IIIB	IIIC
	T4 Invasion	IIIA	IIIA	IIIB	IIIB	IIIC
	T4 Ipsilateral separate tumor nodules	IIIA	IIIA	IIIB	IIIB	IIIC
M1	M1a Contralateral tumor nodules	IVA	IVA	IVA	IVA	IVA
	M1a Pleural / pericardial effusion, nodules	IVA	IVA	IVA	IVA	IVA
	M1b Single extrathoracic metastasis	IVA	IVA	IVA	IVA	IVA
	M1c1 Multiple metastases in 1 organ system	IVB	IVB	IVB	IVB	IVB
	M1c2 Multiple metastases in >1 organ systems	IVB	IVB	IVB	IVB	IVB

Reprinted courtesy of the International Association for the Study of Lung Cancer. Copyright ©2024
Adapted from the *Staging Manual in Thoracic Oncology*, 3rd Edition [12]
Reprinted courtesy of the International Association for the Study of Lung Cancer. Copyright ©2024

- M1b indicates a single extrathoracic metastasis occurring in a single organ system (including the involvement of a single non-regional lymph node).
- M1c indicates the presence of multiple extrathoracic metastases either isolated to a single organ system (M1c1) or occurring in multiple organ systems (M1c2).

These TNM parameters are then applied by both clinicians and pathologists in their staging process, as described below, and the patient is assigned the corresponding TNM stage (Table 12.1).

Clinical Staging

Clinical staging (cTNM) is often the first TMN stage assigned to a patient's disease and is determined by a clinician who is, in turn, informed by the results of a comprehensive physical examination, the aforementioned imaging modalities, and the result of biopsies.

Pathological Staging

Pathological staging (pTNM) is determined by a pathologist based on tissue sampling analysis, either from a biopsy sample or a surgical resection. Pathological staging based on a sample from a surgical resection can be discordant with clinical staging (either by upstaging or downstaging the patient's disease) if the pathology notes more or less extensive tissue invasion or nodal metastases than would be suggested by clinical examination or imaging. Therefore, pTNM is often considered the most accurate TNM stage, although both clinical and pathologic staging are used routinely in practice.

Lymph Node Stations

The IASLC lymph node classification system is the most widely used system to describe lymph node involvement by lung cancer and divides the regional lymph nodes of the thorax into seven zones and further into 14 lymph node "stations" (Fig. 12.1) which are described below [12]:

Supraclavicular Zone
- Station #1 (further classified as left/right relative to the midline of the trachea) includes the low cervical, supraclavicular, and sternal notch lymph nodes, which are bounded superiorly by the cricoid cartilage and inferiorly by the clavicles and manubrium.

Superior Mediastinal Nodes

Upper Zone
- Station #2 (further classified as left/right relative to the left lateral border of the trachea) includes the upper paratracheal nodes, which are bounded superiorly by the apex of lung, pleural space, and the manubrium, and bounded inferiorly on the right by the intersection of the innominate vein with the trachea, and on the left by the superior border of the aortic arch.
- Station #3 includes the prevascular and retrotracheal nodes. The prevascular nodes are bounded superiorly by the apex of the chest, inferiorly by the carina, anteriorly by the sternum, and posteriorly by the superior vena cava on the right and the left carotid artery on the left. The retrotracheal nodes are bounded superiorly by the apex of the chest and inferiorly by the carina.
- Station #4 (further classified as left/right relative to the left lateral border of the trachea) includes the lower paratracheal and pretracheal nodes. Those on the

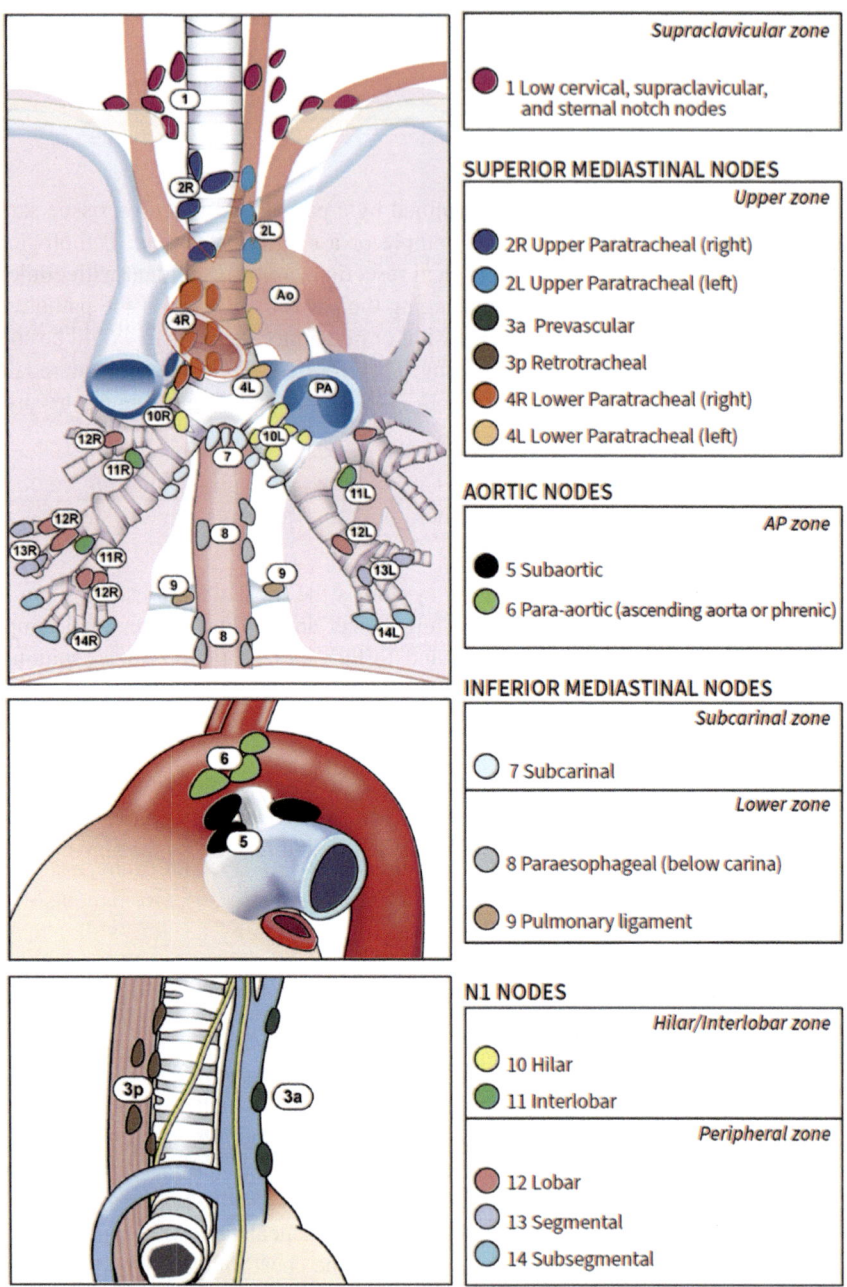

Fig. 12.1 Lymph node stations. (Adapted from the *Staging Manual in Thoracic Oncology*, 3rd Edition [12]. Reprinted courtesy of the International Association for the Study of Lung Cancer. Copyright ©2009 Memorial Sloan-Kettering Cancer Center)

right (4R) are bounded superiorly by the intersection of the innominate vein with the trachea and inferiorly by the lower border of the azygos vein. Those on the left (4 L) are bounded by the aortic arch and the left main pulmonary artery.

Aortic Nodes

Aorto-Pulmonary (AP) Zone
- Station #5 includes the subaortic (aorto-pulmonary window) lymph nodes, which are located lateral to the ligamentum arteriosum and between the aortic arch and the left main pulmonary artery.
- Station #6 includes the para-aortic nodes, which are located adjacent to the ascending aorta and aortic arch, extending from the upper to the lower borders of the aortic arch.

Inferior Mediastinal Nodes

Subcarinal Zone
- Station #7 includes the subcarinal nodes, extending from the carina to the upper border of the lower lobe bronchus on the left and the lower border of the bronchus intermedius on the right.

Lower Zone
- Station #8 (further classified as left/right) includes the para-esophageal nodes located inferior to the carina, which extend from the upper border of the lower lobe bronchus on the left and the lower border of the bronchus intermedius on the right down to the diaphragm.
- Station #9 (further classified as left/right) includes the pulmonary ligament nodes located between the inferior pulmonary vein and the diaphragm.

N1 Nodes

Hilar/Interlobar Zone
- Station #10 (further classified as left/right) includes the hilar nodes, which are located adjacent to the mainstem bronchus and hilar vessels and extends from the azygos vein on the right and pulmonary artery on the left to the origin of the lobar bronchi.
- Station #11 (further classified as left/right) includes the interlobar nodes that are located between the origin of the lobar bronchi, with additional optional subcategories ("11s" and "11i") that can be used to further classify right-sided nodes based on their location. Station #11s starts at the upper lobe bronchus and terminates at the bronchus intermedius, where station 11i starts, 11i and subsequently terminates at the lower lobe bronchus.

Peripheral Zone
- Stations #12–14 (further classified as left/right) include the lobar nodes (#12), the segmental nodes (#13), and the sub-segmental nodes (#14) that are so-named for their adjacency to their respective bronchi.

VALG Staging of Small Cell Lung Cancer

The Veterans Administration Lung Study Group (VALG) staging system is sometimes used in addition to the TNM classification system but is specific to SCLC and is not utilized in other lung cancer types. This system divides patients into those with limited-stage disease or extensive-stage disease and is traditionally defined as the ability to fit all of a patient's disease within a radiation field (limited-stage) or not (extensive-stage). More specifically, limited-stage disease consists of TNM stages I–III, any T (except for T3–4 due to the presence of multiple lung nodules that are either too extensive or too large to fit within a radiation field), any N, and M0. Conversely, extensive-stage disease consists of stage IV (any T, any N, M1 a/b/c) or T3–4 due to multiple lung nodules that are either too extensive or too large to fit within a radiation field.

Role of Molecular Diagnostic Studies

Molecular diagnostic studies are particularly important in the pretreatment evaluation of NSCLC, as detecting an ever-increasing number of mutations with available therapeutic targets significantly alters the therapy selection. Multiple modalities are available and can be performed on patient tissue samples obtained via biopsy, including panel-based next-generation sequencing (NGS) or other sequencing modalities, fluorescence in-situ hybridization (FISH) targeted to specific genetic rearrangements with available therapeutic targets (e.g., ALK), and immunohistochemistry (IHC) measurement of PD-L1 tumor proportion score (TPS). Additionally, so-called peripheral blood "liquid biopsy" (e.g., Guardant 360 testing) can be obtained to provide similar or additional information but does not eliminate the need for a tissue biopsy.

Some common examples of targetable gene mutations in NSCLC include epidermal growth factor receptor (EGFR, particularly exon 19 deletions and p.L858R point mutation in exon 21), ALK (anaplastic lymphoma kinase) gene rearrangements, and KRAS (KRAS proto-oncogene) point mutations. Some less commonly encountered but still clinically relevant mutations are ROS1 gene rearrangements, BRAF mutations (particularly V600E), HER2, and NTRK. (See Chap. 14 for more information on molecular testing and biomarkers.)

Key Takeaways

- Lung cancer is classified based on the cell type of origin and based on the histology of tissues.
- All lung cancer is staged based on the IASLC tumor, nodal, and metastasis (TNM) system, and small cell carcinoma is additionally referred to as either limited or extensive stage.
- The IASLC lymph node classification system describes lymph node involvement based on 14 standardized lymph node stations.
- Molecular diagnostic studies may highlight gene mutations with available therapeutic targets.

Key Readings and Resources

- Malignant Mesothelioma Treatment (PDQ®)–Health Professional Version [15]
- Non-Small Cell Lung Cancer Treatment (PDQ®)–Health Professional Version [13]
- Small Cell Lung Cancer Treatment (PDQ®)–Health Professional Version [14]
- *Staging Manual in Thoracic Oncology*, 3rd Edition [12]

Conflicts of Interest The authors report no relevant conflicts of interest to disclose.

References

1. SEER*Explorer: An interactive website for SEER cancer statistics [Internet]. Surveillance Research Program, National Cancer Institute; 2024 Apr 17. [updated: 2024 Nov 5; cited 2025 Jan 25]. Available from: https://seer.cancer.gov/statistics-network/explorer/. Data source(s): SEER Incidence Data, November 2023 Submission (1975–2021), SEER 8 registries.
2. SEER*Explorer: An interactive website for SEER cancer statistics [Internet]. Surveillance Research Program, National Cancer Institute; 2024 Apr 17. [updated: 2024 Nov 5; cited 2025 Jan 25]. Available from: https://seer.cancer.gov/statistics-network/explorer/. Data source(s): U.S. Mortality Data (1969-2022), National Center for Health Statistics, CDC.
3. American Cancer Society: Cancer Facts and Figures 2024. American Cancer Society; 2024. Available from: https://wwwcancerorg/content/dam/cancer-org/research/cancer-facts-and-statistics/annual-cancer-facts-and-figures/2024/2024-cancer-facts-and-figures-acspdf Cited 2025 Jan 25.
4. World Health Organization. Thoracic tumours. 5th ed. International Agency for Research on Cancer; 2021.
5. SEER*Explorer: An interactive website for SEER cancer statistics [Internet]. Surveillance Research Program, National Cancer Institute; 2024 Apr 17. [updated: 2024 Nov 5; cited 2025 Jan 25]. Available from: https://seer.cancer.gov/statistics-network/explorer/. Data source(s): SEER Incidence Data, November 2023 Submission (1975–2021), SEER 22 registries.
6. Centers for Disease Control and Prevention (CDC). United States cancer statistics: mesothelioma [Internet]. Atlanta: CDC; [updated 2024 Jan 26; cited 2025 Jan 25]. Available from: https://www.cdc.gov/united-states-cancer-statistics/publications/mesothelioma.html

7. Travis W, Brambilla E, Müller-Hermelink H, et al., editors. Pathology and genetics of tumours of the lung, pleura, and thymus. IARC Press/World Health Organization Classification of Tumours; 2004.
8. de Koning HJ, van der Aalst CM, de Jong PA, et al. Reduced lung-cancer mortality with volume CT screening in a randomized trial. N Engl J Med. 2020;382(6):503–13. https://doi.org/10.1056/NEJMoa1911793.
9. Vansteenkiste JF, Stroobants SS. PET scan in lung cancer: current recommendations and innovation. J Thorac Oncol. 2006;1(1):71–3.
10. Ginsberg RJ, Rubinstein LV. Randomized trial of lobectomy versus limited resection for T1 N0 non-small cell lung cancer. Lung Cancer Study Group. Ann Thorac Surg. 1995;60(3):615–23. https://doi.org/10.1016/0003-4975(95)00537-u.
11. Altorki N, Wang X, Kozono D, et al. Lobar or sublobar resection for peripheral stage IA non-small-cell lung cancer. N Engl J Med. 2023;388(6):489–98. https://doi.org/10.1056/NEJMoa2212083.
12. Asamura H, International Association for the Study of Lung Cancer. Staging manual in thoracic oncology. 3rd ed. Editorial Rx Press; 2024.
13. PDQ® Adult Treatment Editorial Board. PDQ Non-Small Cell Lung Cancer Treatment. Bethesda: National Cancer Institute. Updated 03/21/2025. Available at: https://www.cancer.gov/types/lung/hp/non-small-cell-lung-treatment-pdq. Accessed 14 Apr 2025. [PMID: 26389304]
14. PDQ® Adult Treatment Editorial Board. PDQ Small Cell Lung Cancer Treatment. Bethesda: National Cancer Institute. Updated 03/26/2025. Available at: https://www.cancer.gov/types/lung/hp/small-cell-lung-treatment-pdq. Accessed 14 Apr 2025. [PMID: 26389347]
15. PDQ® Adult Treatment Editorial Board. PDQ Malignant Mesothelioma Treatment. Bethesda: National Cancer Institute. Updated 04/24/2024. Available at: https://www.cancer.gov/types/mesothelioma/hp/mesothelioma-treatment-pdq. Accessed 14 Apr 2025. [PMID: 26389420]

Open Access This chapter is licensed under the terms of the Creative Commons Attribution-NonCommercial 4.0 International License (http://creativecommons.org/licenses/by-nc/4.0/), which permits any noncommercial use, sharing, adaptation, distribution and reproduction in any medium or format, as long as you give appropriate credit to the original author(s) and the source, provide a link to the Creative Commons license and indicate if changes were made.

The images or other third party material in this chapter are included in the chapter's Creative Commons license, unless indicated otherwise in a credit line to the material. If material is not included in the chapter's Creative Commons license and your intended use is not permitted by statutory regulation or exceeds the permitted use, you will need to obtain permission directly from the copyright holder.

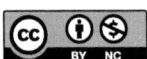

Surgical Interventions and Care for Lung Cancer Control

13

Keith D. Mortman and Bitana Saintilma

Contents

Navigation Vignette.	164
Introduction.	165
Surgical Management of Lung Cancer.	165
Determination of Resectability.	166
Functional Status/Appropriateness.	166
Preoperative Workup.	168
Types of Surgical Resection.	170
Postoperative Care.	171
Conclusion.	172
Key Takeaways.	172
Key Readings and Resources.	172
References.	173

Abbreviations

ACCP	American College of Chest Physicians
AJCC	American Joint Commission on Cancer
CPET	Cardiopulmonary exercise testing

K. D. Mortman (✉)
Thoracic Surgery, The George Washington University Hospital, Washington, DC, USA
e-mail: kmortman@mfa.gwu.edu

B. Saintilma
Transplant Surgery, MedStar Georgetown University Hospital, Washington, DC, USA
e-mail: bitana.saintilma@medstar.net

© The Author(s) 2026
J. T. Fathi, M. F. Mortman (eds.), *Lung Cancer Navigation and Care*,
https://doi.org/10.1007/978-3-032-02200-4_13

CT Scan	Computed tomography scan
DLCO	Diffusing capacity of the lung for carbon monoxide
EBUS	Endobronchial ultrasound
ERAS	Enhance recovery after surgery
FEV1	Forced expiratory volume in 1 second
LCSG	Lung Cancer Study Group
MRI	Magnetic resonance imaging
PAL	Prolonged air leak
PET	Positron emission tomography
PFT	Pulmonary function tests
ppoDLCO	Predicted postoperative diffusing capacity of the lung for carbon monoxide
TNM	Tumor node metastases
V/Q scan	Ventilation and perfusion scan
VAMLA	Video-assisted mediastinoscopic lymphadenectomy
VATS	Video-assisted thoracic surgery

Navigation Vignette

Mrs. M. is an 83-year-old diabetic female with a smoking history. She was referred to the thoracic surgeon by her oncologist due to an incidental finding of a right lung nodule on CT scan. The CT was then followed by a PET scan demonstrating hypermetabolic activity in the nodule. Mrs. M. denied any cardiopulmonary signs or symptoms. Upon first learning about the lung nodule, she was devastated. During her initial consultation with the thoracic surgeon, Mrs. M. met nurse navigator B.C.

Navigator B.C. had a lengthy discussion with Mrs. M. about the next steps, including all preparatory appointments needed for surgical clearance. Navigator B.C. helped Mrs. M. schedule all appointments, including a pulmonary function test and a visit with her primary care physician to ensure preoperative glycemic control. In addition to providing guidance, Navigator B. was present to alleviate anxiety by thoroughly explaining each step of the process. Throughout Mrs. M.'s postoperative recovery, Navigator B.C. remained a crucial contact point and was available for guidance. She provided verbal instructions and written resources on what to expect post-surgery, including recovery time and during the surveillance period. As part of her standard practice, Navigator B.C. called Mrs. M. two days post-operatively to check her pain control, bowel function, nutrition, and physical activity. These issues are common reasons patients are re-admitted to the hospital via the emergency department. Mrs. M. was grateful as she was experiencing pain and learned she was not taking her medication correctly.

Navigator B.C.'s role as a nurse navigator was instrumental in helping Mrs. M. navigate the complexities of lung cancer treatment and recovery. Mrs. M.'s work with Nurse Navigator B.C. motivated Mrs. M. to advocate for herself while gaining confidence and strength in moving forward with her care plan.

Introduction

Although the incidence of lung cancer in the United States has been decreasing in men since the 1980s and in women since the mid-2000s, it is still responsible for the most cancer deaths among both sexes [1]. Navigating through the complexities of a new lung cancer diagnosis can be a daunting task for a patient. Having a lung cancer navigator guide a patient through this process can make it less so. The inception of navigational services was created in the 1990s by Dr. Harold Freeman in Harlem, New York City [2]. He believed that if patients were provided with resources on how to steer through the complex world of cancer, their outcomes would improve. As time passed and the healthcare landscape became multifaceted, thoracic surgery navigation became what it is today. Navigational services support early diagnosis, appropriate staging, and aggressive treatment, which are associated with improved outcomes. Increasingly, lung cancer treatment has become a multimodal approach. Lung cancer navigators are instrumental in coordinating care among surgeons, medical oncologists, radiation oncologists, diagnostic and interventional radiologists, interventional pulmonologists, pathologists, and many other healthcare providers. This chapter will highlight the surgical management of lung cancer and the role of the navigator in that process.

Surgical Management of Lung Cancer

The approach to lung cancer surgery has evolved tremendously over the past 100 years. In 1929, Brunn described successful one-stage lobectomy (for bronchiectasis); in 1933, Graham performed the first successful one-stage pneumonectomy for lung cancer [3]. In 1947, Coleman published a case of long-term survival following en bloc excision of the chest wall with lung resection [4]. Sleeve lobectomy for a bronchial adenoma and for non-small cell lung cancer and the excision of superior sulcus tumors with neoadjuvant and adjuvant radiotherapy saw the increasing use of open thoracotomy to treat malignant pathology of the chest [5–8]. With significant advances in fiberoptic technology, the era of video-assisted thoracic surgery (VATS) began in the 1990s. As surgeons' experience and comfort level improved with VATS, more complex procedures were completed minimally invasively. The turn of the new millennium then bore witness to the introduction of robotic thoracic surgery. Regardless of the approach used, the principles of surgical management of lung cancer include determination of tumor resectability, determination of patient functional status, and complete tumor extirpation with negative margins and adequate lymph node sampling. In this process, the navigator reinforces patient and caregiver education, which helps reduce hospital readmissions and, in turn, promotes a continuum of quality and comprehensive care [9].

Determination of Resectability

Whereas operability refers to whether a patient can tolerate an operation (to be discussed in the next section), resectability refers to tumor-related factors that dictate whether the lung cancer can be completely removed with negative margins. The American Joint Commission on Cancer (AJCC) TNM staging system is most commonly used to guide the clinician when determining resectability. T4 cancers are generally considered unresectable when they invade the mediastinum, heart, great vessels, esophagus, or spine. Lung cancers may also be considered unresectable in the presence of advanced disease such as multistation or bulky N2 disease, N2 disease with extracapsular extension, N3 disease, or metastatic (M1) disease.

Another way to define the completeness of surgical resection is with the "R" status. The goal of any curative intent lung cancer surgery is an R0 resection. This means that the tumor margins are microscopically negative, systematic lymph node dissection is performed, extracapsular nodal extension is absent, the highest mediastinal lymph node is negative for cancer, and pleural or pericardial cytology is negative [10]. An R1 resection is one in which there is microscopic disease at the tumor resection margin. An R2 resection is one with macroscopic disease at the margin. The increasing use of neoadjuvant immunotherapy and chemotherapy adds complexity to the definition of resectability. Oftentimes, clinical and pathologic downstaging can occur in patients receiving induction regimens. A tumor that may not have been resectable at the time of initial lung cancer diagnosis may subsequently become resectable. Thus, surgical resection of lung cancer may now be offered to patients who were previously not candidates for this treatment.

Functional Status/Appropriateness

When thoracic surgery is planned, presurgical clearance (when required) must be completed promptly to expedite the patient's care. Aside from the physician, the navigator is the key source of information for the patient. In this role, navigator duties include describing the purpose of presurgical clearance and coordinating clearance appointments with providers such as cardiology, pulmonology, or primary care.

Before lung resection surgery, assessment of a patient's pulmonary reserve is mandatory. Thus, all patients seeking surgery for lung cancer will have pulmonary function tests (PFT). PFTs are a noninvasive way to measure how much air a patient can inhale and exhale, how quickly one can exhale, and how much air a patient's lungs can hold. Oftentimes, a room air arterial blood gas will be drawn with the PFTs to directly measure the amount of oxygen and carbon dioxide in a patient's blood along with the pH.

PFTs can indicate the severity of pulmonary dysfunction but do not provide a specific diagnosis. A patient's baseline PFTs are evaluated in light of the planned extent of surgical resection (wedge resection, lobectomy, or pneumonectomy) to determine if the patient can tolerate the procedure. Full PFTs are divided into 3

13 Surgical Interventions and Care for Lung Cancer Control

parts: spirometry, lung volumes, and diffusion capacity for carbon monoxide. Figure 13.1 shows an example of PFTs:

PFTs can be intimidating at first glance. To determine patient operability for lung surgery, two of the many PFT values have proven to be more important than the others. These are the forced expiratory volume in 1 second (FEV1) and the diffusion capacity for carbon monoxide (DLCO). FEV1 measures (in liters) the amount of air a patient can forcefully exhale in 1 second. DLCO measures how efficiently gas is exchanged at the level of the alveoli. PFTs are also normalized based on the patient's age, height, race, and sex. Therefore, FEV1 and DLCO can also be expressed as a percentage of predicted values. Although variability exists in acceptable preoperative measurements, Table 13.1 depicts minimum values for the planned extent of resection:

Sometimes, a patient's initial preoperative pulmonary assessment will fall into a "gray" area for operability. In these situations, additional tests can be performed to shed light on the suitability of surgery. Quantitative ventilation and perfusion scanning (V/Q scan) is one such test. V/Q scan is a nuclear imaging study that uses

	Pre-Bronch					Post-Bronch			
	Pred	Actual	%Pred	LLN	ULN	Actual	%Pred	%Chng
---- SPIROMETRY ----								
FVC (L)	2.39	2.49	104	1.76	3.04	2.49	104	+0
FEV1 (L)	1.87	1.61	85	1.35	2.38	1.71	91	+6
FEV1/FVC (%)	78.99	64.45	81	66.45	89.94	68.41	86	+6
FEF Max (L/sec)	5.19	4.33	83	3.58	6.80	2.84	54	-34
FEF 25-75% (L/sec)	1.63	0.81	49	0.74	2.93	1.09	66	+34
FEF 50% (L/sec)	3.28	1.08	32	1.47	5.10	1.75	53	+61
FIF 50% (L/sec)	3.08	3.15	102	1.65	4.52	4.14	134	+31
MVV (L/min)	81	73	90	63	98			
---- LUNG VOLUMES ----								
TGV (L)	2.71	2.75	101	1.85	3.57			
IC (L)	1.77	1.95	110					
TLC (Pleth) (L)	4.75	4.71	99	3.87	5.64			
SVC (L)	2.39	2.35	98	1.76	3.04			
RV (Pleth) (L)	2.13	2.36	111	1.50	2.76			
RV/TLC (Pleth) (%)	44.30	50.19	113	35.29	53.31			
ERV (L)	0.89	0.39	44					
sGaw (1/cmH2O*s)	0.20	0.13	61	0.14	0.26			
---- DIFFUSION ----								
DLCOunc (ml/min/mmHg)	18.11	10.67	58	13.79	23.39			
DLCOcor (ml/min/mmHg)	18.11			13.79	23.39			
VA (L)	4.32	4.19	97	3.47	5.26			
DL/VA (ml/min/mmHg/L)	4.19	2.55	60					
IVC (L)		2.27						

Fig. 13.1 PFTs demonstrating spirometry, lung volumes, and diffusion

Table 13.1 Minimum PFT values for surgical resection

	FEV1 (L)	DLCO (% predicted)
Wedge resection	0.8–1.0	>40%
Lobectomy	1.2	>60%
Pneumonectomy	2.0	>80%

aerosolized radiolabeled technetium or xenon to assess airflow and injectable radiolabeled technetium to assess blood flow in the lungs. The percentage of flow to one lung versus the other can be calculated, and the flow to each lung can be further divided into top, middle, and lower thirds. Although baseline (preoperative) PFTs provide crucial information about a patient's pulmonary function, it is even more important to gauge one's postoperative pulmonary reserve before surgery is performed. To that end, one can use the results of a quantitative V/Q scan and baseline PFTs to calculate predicted postoperative FEV1 (ppoFEV1) and ppoDLCO.

If the ppoFEV1 and ppoDLCO still fall within a gray zone after a quantitative V/Q scan, then cardiopulmonary exercise testing (CPET) can be performed. CPET is a specialized heart and lung stress test that uses a bicycle ergometer to measure exercise capability expressed as maximum oxygen consumption (VO2 max). Information about heart and lung physiology under stress helps the surgeon understand how a patient will recover and function post-surgery.

Formal cardiac risk assessment ("cardiac clearance") is reserved for patients with a history of coronary artery disease, cardiac valvular disease, coronary stent insertion, or cardiac surgery. Patients with multiple risk factors for coronary disease (such as diabetes and hypertension) may also benefit from preoperative cardiac risk assessment.

Emotional support is often needed as patients may feel overwhelmed by their pre-clearance tests, imaging, and their new cancer diagnosis. Emotional support can range from answering questions, clarifying surgical terminology, helping to communicate with the surgeon, or just serving as a sounding board. Most important, though, is the navigator's critical role in assuring that preoperative tests are completed promptly so care is implemented without delay.

Preoperative Workup

Preoperative Biopsy: How and Why?

Not all lung nodules will require a biopsy. Notable guidelines have been established by the American College of Chest Physicians (ACCP) and the Fleischner Society [11]. Recommendations are based on the size and characteristics of the lung nodule. ACCP recommends nonsurgical biopsy and/or surgical resection (unless contraindicated) for a solid, indeterminate nodule that shows evidence of malignant growth on serial imaging. For a solid, indeterminate nodule >8 mm in diameter, nonsurgical biopsy is recommended when:

- The pretest probability of malignancy and findings on imaging conflict
- The probability of malignancy is low to moderate (10–60%)
- A benign diagnosis requiring specific medical treatment is likely
- A fully informed patient seeks proof of a malignant diagnosis before surgery

Sometimes, patients at high risk of a malignant lung nodule will proceed to surgery without a preoperative biopsy. This occurs when:

- The clinical probability of malignancy is high (>65%)
- The nodule has significant metabolic activity on PET (or other functional imaging test)
- Nonsurgical biopsy is suspicious for cancer
- A fully informed patient prefers having a definitive diagnostic procedure

When preoperative biopsy is required, it can be performed either percutaneously or bronchoscopically.

Noninvasive Staging

Chest CT scan (preferably with intravenous contrast) is typically the initial cross-sectional imaging study performed when evaluating a patient for lung cancer. CT scan is valuable in determining not only the size and location of the lung nodule but also its morphology (solid, subsolid, ground glass opacity) and the presence of lymphadenopathy. PET scan is indicated for noninvasive staging of nodules where malignancy is strongly suspected or known. Today's PET scan utilizes radiolabeled sugar (F18 fluorodeoxyglucose) to detect sites (from "eyes to thighs") that are metabolically active. Brain imaging (CT or MRI) is required for noninvasive staging in patients who present with neurologic signs or symptoms (see Chap. 8).

Invasive Staging

Invasive staging of the mediastinum or other areas is dictated by the results of the noninvasive staging evaluation. If the preoperative diagnostic chest CT scan and PET/CT scan suggest a clinical T1N0 tumor, then invasive staging can be omitted as the likelihood of occult metastatic disease is very low. However, if noninvasive staging suggests a tumor more advanced than T1N0, then invasive staging is required to ensure the patient receives guideline-concordant care.

When CT and/or PET/CT reveal enlarged or metabolically active mediastinal lymph nodes, then tissue sampling is required. This is most commonly performed by endobronchial ultrasound (EBUS) but can also be achieved by video-assisted mediastinoscopic lymphadenectomy (VAMLA). The decision to use EBUS versus VAMLA goes beyond the scope of this chapter, but factors such as sensitivity, negative predictive value, accuracy, and operator skill are considered when deciding between the two modalities.

When noninvasive staging detects extrathoracic disease (i.e., liver lesion, enlarged adrenal gland, or sclerotic bone mass), then that particular site should be biopsied to rule out metastatic (M1) disease.

Types of Surgical Resection

Wedge Resection/Segmentectomy

In 1995, the Lung Cancer Study Group (LCSG) published their results of a prospective, randomized study of 276 patients comparing the outcomes of limited resection (segmentectomy or wedge resection) and lobectomy. They concluded that limited resection had higher rates of death and locoregional recurrence compared to lobectomy without improvement in morbidity, mortality, or late postoperative pulmonary function [12]. There have been many criticisms of the LCSG study since its publication. These include using an earlier staging version, a limited number of patients enrolled, and the fact surgery was performed before the widespread use of thoracoscopy.

Over the past 10 years, there has been increasing data that sublobar resection is non-inferior to lobectomy in patients with early-stage lung cancer. In 2023, the results of Cancer and Leukemia Group B (CALGB) 140503 were published [13]. It was a multicenter, phase 3 trial that randomized clinically staged T1N0 NSCLC patients (nodule ≤ 2 cm) to sublobar or lobar resection (after intraoperative confirmation of node-negative disease). Altorki et al. concluded that disease-free survival was not inferior in the sublobar resection group and that overall survival was similar to the two procedures. Sublobar wedge resection or anatomic segmentectomy is also the preferred operation for patients who have moderately to severely diminished PFTs or performance status.

Lobectomy

For patients with larger (> 2 cm) or more centrally located tumors, formal lobectomy is recommended. This operation entails the anatomic dissection and division of the pulmonary artery, pulmonary vein, and lobar bronchus. Assessment of a patient's operability with PFTs (and room air arterial blood gas for COPD patients) is mandatory.

Pneumonectomy

On rare occasions, a tumor is located close to the hilum, or a large tumor may cross the fissure from one lobe to another. In these situations, a total pneumonectomy may be required. Patient selection for a pneumonectomy is more rigorous than lesser resections due to the greater physiologic impact on the body. Fewer pneumonectomies are performed than in years past due to more widespread adoption of parenchymal-sparing surgery.

Postoperative Care

Pain

Adequate postoperative analgesia is paramount for patient comfort and to avoid postoperative complications such as atelectasis, pneumonia, and venous thromboembolism. Many thoracic surgical programs utilize enhanced recovery after surgery (ERAS) protocols to ensure patients receive adequate analgesia, early mobilization, and nutrition. ERAS protocols include the use of one or more non-narcotics to minimize (but not necessarily eliminate) the need for narcotics. One such example may be to administer acetaminophen, celecoxib, and gabapentin immediately prior to as well as after surgery. Surgical teams also administer long-acting local anesthetics into the wounds and may supplement that with regional nerve blocks. Patients may have difficulty mobilizing airway secretions or using an incentive spirometer when their pain is not adequately controlled.

Pulmonary

With adequate pain control, patients can successfully adhere to instructions for lung expansion tools such as an incentive spirometer or positive expiratory pressure device. Routine usage of these devices promotes airway clearance of secretions and may avoid clinically significant atelectasis or pneumonia. Postoperative radiographs are only obtained as clinically indicated. However, when there is a concern for a postoperative infiltrate, this should be treated quickly and aggressively.

However, the most common complication following pulmonary surgery is a prolonged air leak (PAL). Air will escape from a surgical staple line or elsewhere in the parenchyma and be visible in the chest tube collection system. A postoperative air leak that persists for more than 5 days is considered to be prolonged, and this may occur in 5–25% of cases [14]. Postoperative treatment options for a PAL include watchful waiting, autologous blood patch (inserting an aliquot of the patient's own blood through the chest tube), chemical pleurodesis, endobronchial valves, and rarely reoperation.

Cardiac

In the modern era of minimally invasive thoracic surgery, postoperative cardiac complications such as arrhythmia requiring treatment or myocardial infarction are uncommon. Patients with a history of coronary artery disease, multiple risk factors for coronary disease, or those who have had prior cardiac surgery may benefit from preoperative optimization and risk stratification. When symptomatic postoperative arrhythmias are detected, medical management is initiated by the thoracic surgical team with cardiology consultation as needed.

Conclusion

Preoperative evaluation of the lung cancer patient involves numerous yet important tests. These tasks may be daunting for the lung cancer patient who may already be consumed by a new lung cancer diagnosis. The presence and support of a nurse navigator benefits the surgical patient in numerous ways. Furthermore, the principles of surgical management of lung cancer are steadfast regardless of the approach used (robotic, thoracoscopic, or open): assessment of the patient's functional status and ability to tolerate the operation; adequate preoperative staging; determination of tumor resectability; complete (R0) resection and lymph node sampling.

Key Takeaways

- Thorough preoperative assessment of the lung cancer patient includes noninvasive staging (PET/CT), invasive staging in select cases (EBUS or mediastinoscopy), measurement of pulmonary reserve (PFTs), and the selective need for formal cardiac evaluation.
- Although lobectomy had been considered the standard lung cancer operation for patients with adequate pulmonary reserve, now there is increasing evidence that sublobar resections for peripherally located <2 cm, node-negative cancers offer equivalent oncologic outcomes.
- The most common postoperative complication after pulmonary surgery is a PAL. Although various methods exist to treat PALs, the best "treatment" is avoiding injury to the lung parenchyma during surgery.
- In a multidisciplinary team approach, each discipline may have its own course of action to achieve its respective end goal. The navigator serves as a beacon to ensure that all specialty-specific plans adhere to the same overarching care plan.

Key Readings and Resources

- American Cancer Society. Cancer Facts and Figs. 2025 [1]
- NIH National Library of Medicine. National Center for Biotechnology Information [9]
- NIH National Library of Medicine. National Center for Biotechnology Information [13]

Conflict of Interest No conflicts of interest.

References

1. American Cancer Society. Cancer Facts and Figures 2024. https://www.cancer.org/content/dam/cancer-org/research/cancer-facts-and-statistics/annual-cancer-facts-and-figures/2024/2024-cancer-facts-and-figures-acs.pdf. Accessed online 22 Aug 2024.
2. Freeman HP, Rodriguez RL. History and principles of patient navigation. Cancer. 2011;117(15 Suppl):3539–42. https://doi.org/10.1002/cncr.26262.
3. Walcott-Sapp S. The history of pulmonary lobectomy: two phases of innovation. https://www.ctsnet.org/article/history-pulmonary-lobectomy-two-phases-innovation. Accessed online 22 Aug 2024.
4. Coleman F. Primary carcinoma of the lung, with invasion of the ribs: pneumonectomy and simultaneous block resection of the chest wall. Ann Surg. 1947;126(2):156–68.
5. Thomas CP. Conservative resection of the bronchial tree. J R Coll Surg Edinb. 1956;1:169–86.
6. Allison PR. Course of thoracic surgery in Groningen. Ann R Coll Surg. 1954;25:20–2.
7. Chardack WM, MacCallum JD. Pancoast syndrome due to bronchogenic carcinoma: successful surgical removal and postoperative irradiation: a case report. J Thorac Surg. 1953;25:402–12.
8. Shaw RR, Paulson DL, Kee JL. Treatment of the superior sulcus tumor by irradiation followed by resection. Ann Surg. 1961;154:29–40.
9. Rodriguez AL, Cappelletti L, Kurian SM, Passio C, Rux S. Transitional care navigation. Semin Oncol Nurs. 2024;40(2):151580. https://doi.org/10.1016/j.soncn.2024.151580.
10. Etienne H, Battilana B, Spicer J, Werner RS, Opitz I. Defining resectability: when do you try to take it out? JTCVS Open. 2024;19:338–46. https://doi.org/10.1016/j.xjon.2024.03.012. PMID: 39015436; PMCID: PMC11247203.
11. Gould M, Donington J, Lynch W, et al. Evaluation of individuals with pulmonary nodules: when is it lung cancer? Chest. 2013;143(5):e93S–e120S.
12. Ginsberg RJ, Rubinstein LV. Randomized trial of lobectomy versus limited resection for T1 N0 non-small cell lung cancer. Lung cancer study group. Ann Thorac Surg. 1995;60(3):615–22; discussion 622–3. https://doi.org/10.1016/0003-4975(95)00537-u. PMID: 7677489.
13. Altorki N, Wang X, Kozono D, et al. Lobar or sublobar resection for peripheral stage IA non-small-cell lung cancer. NEJM. 2023;388:489–98. https://doi.org/10.1056/NEJMoa2212083.
14. Aprile V, Bacchin D, Calabro F, et al. Intraoperative prevention and conservative management of postoperative prolonged air leak after lung resection: a systematic review. J Thorac Dis. 2023;15(2):878–92. https://doi.org/10.21037/jtd-22-736.

Open Access This chapter is licensed under the terms of the Creative Commons Attribution-NonCommercial 4.0 International License (http://creativecommons.org/licenses/by-nc/4.0/), which permits any noncommercial use, sharing, adaptation, distribution and reproduction in any medium or format, as long as you give appropriate credit to the original author(s) and the source, provide a link to the Creative Commons license and indicate if changes were made.

The images or other third party material in this chapter are included in the chapter's Creative Commons license, unless indicated otherwise in a credit line to the material. If material is not included in the chapter's Creative Commons license and your intended use is not permitted by statutory regulation or exceeds the permitted use, you will need to obtain permission directly from the copyright holder.

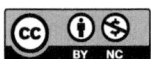

Biomarker-Directed Precision Medicine for Lung Cancer Control

14

Parth Desai and Hossein Borghaei

Contents

Navigation Vignette.	176
Introduction.	178
Strategic Considerations for Biomarker Testing in Non-small Cell Lung Cancer.	179
Types of Biospecimens: Tumor Tissue Versus Liquid Biopsy.	179
Common Types of Biomarker Tests.	181
Conclusion.	183
Key Takeaways.	183
Key Readings and Resources.	184
References.	184

Abbreviations

ALK	Anaplastic lymphoma kinase
ASCO	American Society of Clinical Oncology
CAP	College of American Pathologists
CLIA	Clinical Laboratory Improvement Amendments
CNB	Core needle biopsy
COPD	Chronic obstructive pulmonary disease
ctDNA	Circulating tumor DNA
DNA	Deoxyribonucleic acid
EBUS	Endobronchial ultrasound
EGFR	Epidermal growth factor receptor 2

P. Desai · H. Borghaei (✉)
Department of Hematology & Medical Oncology, Fox Chase Cancer Center, Philadelphia, PA, USA
e-mail: Parth.Desai@fccc.edu; Hossein.Borghaei@fccc.edu

© The Author(s) 2026
J. T. Fathi, M. F. Mortman (eds.), *Lung Cancer Navigation and Care*,
https://doi.org/10.1007/978-3-032-02200-4_14

FISH	Fluorescence in situ hybridization
FNAC	Fine needle aspiration cytology
IASLC	International Association for the Study of Lung Cancer
ICI	Immune checkpoint inhibitor
IHC	Immunohistochemistry
MDT	Multidisciplinary team
MET	Mesenchymal epithelial transition factor
NGS	Next-generation sequencing
NSCLC	Non-small cell lung cancer
NTRK	Neurotrophic tyrosine receptor kinase
ORR	Objective response rate
PCR	Polymerase chain reaction
PD-L1	Programmed cell death ligand 1
RNA	Ribonucleic acid
SCLC	Small cell lung cancer
TAT	Turnaround time
TBNA	Transbronchial needle aspiration
TKIs	Tyrosine kinase inhibitors
TTNB	Transthoracic needle biopsy
VATS	Video-assisted thoracoscopy surgery
WES	Whole-exome sequencing
WGS	Whole-genome sequencing

Navigation Vignette

Ms. A., a 62-year-old woman with no history of smoking, presented with persistent cough and fatigue. A CT scan revealed a 5 cm mass in the left upper lobe of the lung and three hepatic lesions concerning metastases. Liver biopsy confirmed non-small cell lung cancer (NSCLC), adenocarcinoma subtype. Immunohistochemistry revealed a PD-L1 tumor proportion score of 70%. Anxious to begin treatment, Ms. A. contacted the lung cancer nurse navigator, Mr. B., seeking expedited discussion with an oncologist to initiate therapy based on the available PD-L1 result since she had read on the Internet that immunotherapy is an effective treatment for lung cancer. Mr. B. empathetically reassured her, emphasizing the importance of waiting for the full biomarker profile to guide optimal treatment decisions. He followed up with the pathology laboratory to confirm that reflex next-generation sequencing (NGS) (see Table 14.1 for simplified glossary of complex medical terms) was underway and explained to Ms. A. that initiating the wrong therapy prematurely could lead to suboptimal outcomes and unnecessary toxicities. The molecular testing returned within a week and identified an EGFR exon 19 deletion mutation. After a multidisciplinary discussion, Ms. A. was started on an EGFR-targeted tyrosine kinase inhibitor (TKI). She has now been on treatment for 2 years, with minimal evidence of disease on recent imaging and excellent clinical response.

Table 14.1 Simplified glossary of terms

Technique	Description
FISH (fluorescence in situ hybridization)	A laboratory technique using fluorescent probes to detect specific DNA changes, such as gene fusions or amplifications (e.g., ALK or ROS1 rearrangements) in tumor cells.
IHC (immunohistochemistry)	Uses antibodies to detect specific proteins (e.g., PD-L1, HER2) in tissue samples, guiding treatment decisions like immunotherapy eligibility.
PCR (polymerase chain reaction)	Amplifies small DNA or RNA segments to detect mutations or fusions in tumors. Fast but less comprehensive than NGS.
FNAC (fine needle aspiration cytology)	Minimally invasive method using a thin needle to extract tumor cells for diagnosis; provides limited material for biomarker testing.
CNB (core needle biopsy)	Uses a large bore needle to collect small tissue cores, offering sufficient material for biomarker and histological analysis.
TTNB (transthoracic needle biopsy)	Needle guided through chest wall (often with CT) to sample peripheral lung tumors.
TBNA (transbronchial needle aspiration)	Performed during bronchoscopy to sample tissue from lymph nodes or central lung tumors.
EBUS (endobronchial ultrasound)	Bronchoscopy with ultrasound guidance to sample lymph nodes or central lung tumors; minimally invasive and effective for diagnosis/staging.
WES (whole-exome sequencing)	Sequences all protein-coding regions of genes, offering insights into mutations across the exome.
WGS (whole-genome sequencing)	Sequences the entire genome (coding and noncoding regions); primarily used in research settings.

This case exemplifies the critical role of patient navigators in ensuring timely, biomarker-guided treatment. Navigators can serve as strategic liaisons between patients, oncologists, and pathology or reference laboratories to reduce delays in care. Depending on institutional infrastructure, navigators may help coordinate tissue and blood sample collection, processing, and submission. They can track the progress of biomarker testing, follow up with laboratories to expedite results, and ensure proper handling of biospecimens—reinforcing adherence to testing guidelines and optimizing specimen adequacy for molecular analysis. Moreover, navigators can support patients by interpreting biomarker results in accessible language, reducing anxiety, building trust, and enhancing patient empowerment. Their communication bridges and facilitates care delivery and promotes equity by addressing gaps that may disproportionately affect underserved populations. Finally, navigators are well-positioned to provide feedback that improves biopsy techniques, supports best practices in tissue handling, and contributes to quality improvement efforts in precision oncology.

Introduction

A biomarker is a measurable biological indicator, like a gene mutation or a protein, found in blood, body fluids, or tissue that signals specific biological processes or diseases. In oncology, biomarker testing helps personalize treatment by identifying patients who are most likely to benefit from targeted therapies, minimizing unnecessary toxicity, and guiding experimental options when standard treatments fail [1]. Biomarker-guided lung cancer treatment, particularly NSCLC, has significantly improved patients' quality and quantity of lives (Fig. 14.1) [2–6]. Patients who receive target-guided therapies have significant survival advantages compared to those who do not receive such precision-guided treatments [7, 8]. It is estimated that almost 52% of patients with advanced nonsquamous histological type of NSCLC have a targetable alteration for which there is an FDA-approved therapy [9]. Biomarker identification ensures (i) selection of appropriate therapies and (ii) prevents selection of contraindicated or nonefficacious treatments [10], e.g., upfront use of immunotherapy in patients who have EGFR or ALK alterations [3]. Additionally, (iii) in patients with oncogenic drivers, concomitant or close sequential use of immunotherapy (within 3 months) followed by use of medications for molecular alterations such as EGFR/ ALK (commonly known as tyrosine kinase inhibitors-TKIs) can lead to increased risk of immunotherapy-related toxicities [11, 12] specifically, pneumonitis, hepatitis, colitis, etc. Hence, the timely completion of comprehensive biomarker testing in lung cancer treatment has become critical.

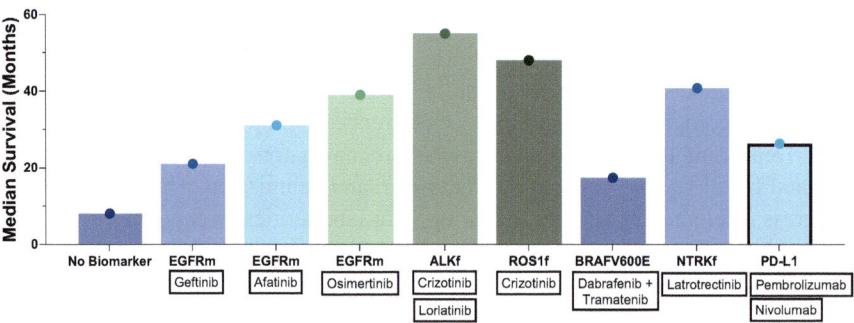

Fig. 14.1 Biomarker stratification and improvement in median survival rates (in months) for advanced/metastatic NSCLC driven by genomic and targeted therapy revolution [2–6]

Strategic Considerations for Biomarker Testing in Non-small Cell Lung Cancer

Given the continuous expansion of new targeted drugs, comprehensive biomarker testing should be strongly considered for all patients with NSCLC. However, certain patient characteristics generate a higher pretest probability of finding actionable molecular alterations. Common scenarios include a high incidence of EGFR alterations in women with East Asian ancestry, never or light smokers, and presentation at a young age. Older men with a strong history of heavy smoking have the lowest probability of finding actionable alterations; however, testing should still be performed. In terms of tumor histology, multiple guidelines recommend testing all patients with "nonsquamous" (e.g., adenocarcinomas, large cell carcinomas) and "not otherwise specified" histologies [13–15]. Testing should be considered for tumors with "squamous" histology, especially if they are young, with a light/ remote or minimal smoking history [15]. At some centers, testing is offered to all patients with any histology. In terms of stage at which biomarker testing should be initiated, with increasing integration of biomarker-adapted treatments upfront in a curative setting, testing should be considered for all stages (early and locally advanced/metastatic). Testing is commonly performed at the time of the first diagnosis [16]. Retesting during a patient's treatment journey should be considered on a case-by-case basis [17] and strongly considered at the time of disease progression, especially when patients have received EGFR-targeting treatment since retesting can help detect mechanisms of resistance and open new avenues of treatment.

Types of Biospecimens: Tumor Tissue Versus Liquid Biopsy

Tissue Biopsy

Two types of biospecimens are available for biomarker testing: (i) *Tumor tissue:* Testing has greater sensitivity (low risk of false negatives) and is considered the gold standard by many. However, it requires an invasive procedure, has longer turn-around time (TAT) (2–4 weeks), and has occasionally insufficient quantity to perform minimal essential testing. It is usually performed on residual tissue remaining after confirming the diagnosis of lung cancer and identifying NSCLC from SCLC [18]. Tumor tissue is primarily derived from two sources—diagnostic biopsy and/or surgical resection. Diagnostic biopsies are usually performed by pulmonologists who perform bronchoscopy using an ultrasound (EBUS) called TBNA and require sedation and brief intubation. Additionally, if the tumor can be accessed easily from outside (through the thorax (chest wall)), then it is performed by interventional radiologists using guidance from CT scan or ultrasound- transthoracic needle biopsy (TTNB), which can be either fine needle aspiration cytology (FNAC) or core needle biopsy (CNB) [19]. FNAC uses smaller needle diameter (22–24 gauge, 9–15 cm long), and CNB can be obtained using larger (18–20 G, 6–20 cm long) [20]. CNB provides a larger amount of tissue but can have more complications, such as pneumothorax and/or hemorrhage (5–50%) due to larger needle size; hence, the proceduralist determines the best approach [21, 22]. Degree of baseline chronic obstructive pulmonary disease (COPD), longer needle path, needle diameter, dwell time, and crossing a fissure increase odds of pneumothorax and hemorrhage. Whenever obtained, pleural fluid aspirate should also be sent for biomarker analyses if enough tumor cells are detected in the fluid. Special attention to the patient's baseline condition and medication should be addressed beforehand, specifically anticoagulation. Rarely, if biopsy is difficult to get from the above two approaches, then thoracic surgeons may be involved for a more invasive surgical approach such as VATS or mediastinoscopy.

Once tissue is obtained via FNA/CNB, it should be promptly placed in a 10% neutral buffered formalin container for fixation. Delays of no more than 1 hour are acceptable as they significantly alter RNA and DNA composition [23, 24]. Further, once in formalin, fixation time is between 6 and 48 hours and should ideally be further processed before 72 hours [23]. Usually, pathologists consider 20% of tumor cellularity and a minimum of 200 (tumor) cells as approximate minimum criteria to increase the chances of successful molecular biomarker testing [25, 26].

Pathologist-initiated reflex biomarker testing is commonly employed at most high-volume cancer centers to reduce TAT [27]. It is usually governed by a protocol defined by a multidisciplinary team (MDT). Most of these centers also have a dedicated molecular pathology division where in-house testing is commonly performed and validated. At a minimum, any laboratory performing multiple biomarker tests should be clinical laboratory improvement amendments (CLIA) certified [3].

Liquid Biopsy

(ii) *Liquid biopsy* (using circulating tumor DNA from blood) involves blood-based testing that focuses on isolating and detecting alterations in circulating tumor or cell-free deoxyribonucleic acid (DNA) circulating tumor deoxyribonucleic acid or cell-free deoxyribonucleic acid (ctDNA or cfDNA) that is shed by tumors. Liquid biopsy takes less time, is less invasive, and conserves tissue for testing biomarkers that can only be done on tissues such as immunohistochemistry (IHC) (PD-L1) [28]. It is more likely to reflect intratumoral heterogeneity (differences between tumors at various organ sites). However, it has lower sensitivity and may not be very useful in very early stages of cancer as not a lot of ctDNA is shed [28]. Half-life of ctDNA is very short in blood (2 hours) [29]. Hence, once blood is extracted, it should be immediately transferred to specialized tubes (e.g., streck tubes) [30]. It can be stored for months at −20 to −80 °C [28, 29].

In modern oncology practice, tissue and blood testing are considered complementary, with oncologists often ordering both concurrently to ensure comprehensive biomarker analysis and mitigate the limitations of each approach when used alone. Conducting both tests provides a complete picture of the tumor's molecular profile, enhancing diagnostic accuracy and therapeutic decision-making. Comprehensive testing using both approaches has been shown to improve survival outcomes [31] and, over time, may also lead to cost savings by reducing unnecessary or ineffective treatments [32]. However, ctDNA/liquid biopsy assessment should never be used in lieu of tissue testing/diagnosis [3].

Common Types of Biomarker Tests

Numerous different biomarker testing technologies/strategies are available, and usually, local/institutional resources should be considered before any particular practice pattern is adopted [33] (Table 14.2). Wherever feasible, on tumor tissues, DNA- and ribonucleic acid (RNA)-based approach that looks at a broader set of genes (NGS) should be considered as it eventually utilizes less tissue than single testing modalities.

IHC (immunohistochemistry) detects proteins relevant to pathological classification and assesses protein presence and quantification in tumor tissues. Commonly sought biomarker using this approach is PD-L1. The information is captured as a percentage of positive tumor and nontumor cells or only positive tumor cells out of the total cells. PD-L1 score can help stratify patients to determine the degree of benefit that can be obtained using immune checkpoint inhibitors (ICIs). For example, in patients with metastatic lung cancer and PD-L1 score > 50%, a common strategy is to spare the use of chemotherapy and instead use ICI alone as a treatment strategy [3]. This testing can only be performed on tumor tissues and is best interpretable on biopsy or surgical tissues as opposed to cytology (FNAC). It should be noted that for different types of approved immunotherapies, specific PD-L1 assays and antibody clones are affiliated [34]. Although PD-L1 expression can be elevated in patients with an oncogenic driver, targeted therapy for certain oncogenic drivers should take precedence over treatment with an immune checkpoint inhibitor [3]. In case of an urgent need to start systemic treatments, an initial chemotherapy-only trial is usually adopted while waiting for complete biomarker information.

Table 14.2 Common biomarker testing approaches and their characteristics [33]

Test	Biomolecule	Alteration	Biospecimen	Common biomarkers	Turnaround time
IHC	Protein	Quantification/mutation	Tissue only	PD-L1, HER2	2–3 days
PCR	DNA/RNA	Specific mutation/fusion	Tissue, blood	EGFR, ALK	3–4 days
FISH	DNA	Fusion	Tissue	ALK, ROS1	2–3 days
NGS-panel based	DNA/RNA	DNA: Mutations, deletions, insertions RNA: Fusion	Tissue, blood	Multiple	1–2 weeks
NGS-WES/WGS	DNA/RNA	Coding plus noncoding genes DNA: Mutations, deletions, insertions RNA: Fusion	Tissue, blood	Multiple	2–3 weeks

Molecular testing These advanced approaches can be performed on both tumor tissue and/or blood. They essentially utilize tumor or tumor-derived DNA or RNA to determine certain key alterations/changes in the genetic makeup of the tumors. As outlined above, various methods exist to detect these alterations, such as IHC, PCR, and FISH. However, these can usually only detect a single alteration type on a single gene at a time and hence utilize a lot of tissues despite having a faster TAT. Their use is mostly restricted to scenarios where a quick assessment of specific alterations such as EGFR or ALK is needed. Most experts currently recommend a broad panel-based NGS approach that evaluates different types of alterations across a panel of 100–500 key oncogenes, specifically focusing on alterations associated with FDA-approved treatments (Table 14.3) [3, 20]. These could be either in-house approaches developed by local molecular pathology laboratories or one of the various commercial platforms. Wherever feasible, both DNA and RNA-based NGS testing should done since actionable gene fusions (such as ROS1, RET, NTRK1/2/3 gene fusions) and structural variants (MET exon 14 skipping variants) are best detected on RNA-based NGS analyses [35, 36]. Regardless of the testing approach, these broad-based NGS panels generate complex data and need dedicated molecular

Table 14.3 Key biomarkers, testing methods, and approved drugs based on the alteration [3, 20]

Biomarker	Testing method	Commonly used drugs in first or second line
EGFR exon 19 deletion/ exon 21 p.L858R	PCR, NGS	Osimertinib, afatinib, gefitinib, dacomitinib, erlotinib, amivantamab-lazertinib
EGFR exon 20 insertion mutation	PCR, NGS	Amivantamab + chemotherapy doublet
ALK rearrangement	FISH, IHC, NGS	Alectinib, brigatinib, crizotinib, lorlatinib
ROS 1 rearrangement	FISH, IHC, NGS	Crizotinib, entrectinib, repotrectinib, lorlatinib
BRAF V600E mutation	PCR, NGS, IHC	Dabrafenib/trametinib, encorafenib/binimetinib
KRAS G12C	PCR, NGS	Sotorasib, adagrasib
MET exon 14 skipping mutations	NGS	Capmatinib, tepotinib, crizotinib
RET rearrangement	FISH, PCR, NGS	Selpercatinib, pralsetinib, cabozantinib
ERBB2/HER2 mutations	PCR, NGS	Fam-trastuzumab deruxtecan, ado-trastuzumab emtansine
NTRK1/2/3 gene fusions	FISH, IHC, NGS	Larotrectinib, entrectinib, repotrectinib
NRG1 gene fusion	NGS	Zenocutuzumab-zbco
PD-L1 IHC	IHC	Pembrolizumab, nivolumab, atezolizumab, cemiplimab-rwlc
HER2 IHC (overexpression) 3+ score	IHC	Fam-trastuzumab deruxtecan
c-MET IHC (overexpression) 3+ score	IHC	Telisotuzumab vedotin

pathology services to filter and distill the data. Many high-volume cancer centers now have molecular oncology tumor boards to discuss the nuances of these NGS results and tailor patient treatments. The majority of the genomic alterations with approved targeted drugs can be taken as oral medications, obviating the need for long-term intravenous access needed for most chemotherapies.

Conclusion

Biomarker-driven precision medicine has transformed the therapeutic landscape of lung cancer, particularly NSCLC, by enabling targeted and individualized treatment approaches that improve both survival and quality of life. Successful implementation of biomarker-guided care requires timely, comprehensive testing using tissue and liquid biopsies supported by a multidisciplinary team that includes pathologists, oncologists, and navigators. As the field continues to evolve with emerging targets and technologies, ensuring standardized workflows, minimizing delays, and integrating the expertise of allied healthcare professionals will be essential to delivering equitable and effective care to all lung cancer patients.

Key Takeaways

- Biomarker-directed treatment has significantly improved the quality and quantity of life for patients with lung cancer as it allows for personalization of care by permitting selection of therapies that are more effective and less toxic, tailored to the individual patient's tumor profile.
- Timely, comprehensive biomarker testing enables the use of optimal treatments while avoiding unnecessary or ineffective therapies, reducing associated toxicities.
- Biomarker testing is essential at diagnosis for both early-stage and advanced/metastatic lung cancer and should also be considered at the time of disease relapse.
- Comprehensive molecular-based biomarker testing is mandatory for all patients with *nonsquamous histologies* and strongly considered for squamous cell histologies with light or remote smoking history.
- Whenever possible, tissue and blood-based testing should be conducted together for optimal and timely results.
- Broad RNA and DNA-panel-based *next-generation sequencing (NGS)* is recommended to maximize the use of limited tissue samples and to test for common actionable alterations.

Key Readings and Resources

- National Comprehensive Cancer Network: The NCCN Biomarkers Compendium [37]
- Molecular Testing Guideline for the Selection of Lung Cancer Patients for Treatment with Targeted Tyrosine Kinase Inhibitors: American Society of Clinical Oncology endorsement summary of the College of American Pathologists/International Association for the Study of Lung Cancer/Association for Molecular Pathology Clinical Practice Guideline update [38]
- Updated Molecular Testing Guideline for the Selection of Lung Cancer Patients for Treatment With Targeted Tyrosine Kinase Inhibitors: Guideline From the College of American Pathologists, the International Association for the Study of Lung Cancer, and the Association for Molecular Pathology [15]

Conflicts of Interest
Parth Desai: Reports no conflicts of interest
Hossein Borghaei: Reports no conflicts of interest related to this chapter.

Disclosures:
- *Research Support* (Clinical Trials) from BMS, Lilly, Amgen
- *Advisory Board/Consultant:* BMS, Lilly, Genentech, Pfizer, Merck, EMD-Serono, Boehringer Ingelheim, Astra Zeneca, Novartis, Genmab, Regeneron, BioNTech, Amgen, Axiom, PharmaMar, Takeda, Mirati, Daiichi, Guardant, Natera, Oncocyte, Beigene, iTEO, Jazz, Janssen, Puma, BerGenBio, Bayer, Iobiotech, Grid Therapeutics, RAPT, Gilead, Abbvie, Novocure, Summit, Astellas, Systimmune
- *Data and Safety Monitoring Board:* University of Pennsylvania: CAR T Program, Takeda, Incyte, Novartis, Springworks, Servier
- *Employment:* Fox Chase Cancer Center
- *Scientific Advisory Board:* Inspirna (formerly Rgenix, Stock Options); Nucleai (stock options)
- *Honoraria:* Amgen, Pfizer, Daiichi, Regeneron, Janssen, Jazz
- *Travel:* Amgen, BMS, Merck, Lilly, EMD-Serono, Genentech, Regeneron, Mirati, Jazz, Regeneron

References

1. Passaro A, Al Bakir M, Hamilton EG, Diehn M, Andre F, Roy-Chowdhuri S, et al. Cancer biomarkers: emerging trends and clinical implications for personalized treatment. Cell. 2024;187(7):1617–35.
2. Reck M, Rodriguez-Abreu D, Robinson AG, Hui R, Csoszi T, Fulop A, et al. Updated analysis of KEYNOTE-024: Pembrolizumab versus platinum-based chemotherapy for advanced non-small-cell lung cancer with PD-L1 tumor proportion score of 50% or greater. J Clin Oncol. 2019;37(7):537–46.
3. Riely GJ, Wood DE, Ettinger DS, Aisner DL, Akerley W, Bauman JR, et al. Non-small cell lung cancer, version 4.2024, NCCN clinical practice guidelines in oncology. J Natl Compr Cancer Netw. 2024;22(4):249–74.
4. Ramalingam SS, Vansteenkiste J, Planchard D, Cho BC, Gray JE, Ohe Y, et al. Overall survival with osimertinib in untreated, EGFR-mutated advanced NSCLC. N Engl J Med. 2020;382(1):41–50.

5. Mok TS, Wu YL, Thongprasert S, Yang CH, Chu DT, Saijo N, et al. Gefitinib or carboplatin-paclitaxel in pulmonary adenocarcinoma. N Engl J Med. 2009;361(10):947–57.
6. Mok T, Camidge DR, Gadgeel SM, Rosell R, Dziadziuszko R, Kim DW, et al. Updated overall survival and final progression-free survival data for patients with treatment-naive advanced ALK-positive non-small-cell lung cancer in the ALEX study. Ann Oncol. 2020;31(8):1056–64.
7. Singal G, Miller PG, Agarwala V, Li G, Kaushik G, Backenroth D, et al. Association of patient characteristics and tumor genomics with clinical outcomes among patients with non–small cell lung cancer using a clinicogenomic database. JAMA. 2019;321(14):1391–9.
8. Bhandari NR, Hess LM, He D, Peterson P. Biomarker testing, treatment, and outcomes in patients with advanced/metastatic non-small cell lung cancer using a real-world database. J Natl Compr Cancer Netw. 2023;21(9):934–44 e1.
9. Florez Duma N, McDonald S. Updating the targeted therapy paradigm for patients with metastatic NSCLC. J Adv Pract Oncol. 2023;14(3):241–7.
10. Villaruz LC, Socinski MA, Weiss J. Guidance for clinicians and patients with non-small cell lung cancer in the time of precision medicine. Front Oncol. 2023;13:1124167.
11. Schoenfeld AJ, Arbour KC, Rizvi H, Iqbal AN, Gadgeel SM, Girshman J, et al. Severe immune-related adverse events are common with sequential PD-(L)1 blockade and osimertinib. Ann Oncol. 2019;30(5):839–44.
12. Lin JJ, Chin E, Yeap BY, Ferris LA, Kamesan V, Lennes IT, et al. Increased hepatotoxicity associated with sequential immune checkpoint inhibitor and Crizotinib therapy in patients with non-small cell lung cancer. J Thorac Oncol. 2019;14(1):135–40.
13. Cheema PK, Gomes M, Banerji S, Joubert P, Leighl NB, Melosky B, et al. Consensus recommendations for optimizing biomarker testing to identify and treat advanced EGFR-mutated non-small-cell lung cancer. Curr Oncol. 2020;27(6):321–9.
14. Lindeman NI, Cagle PT, Aisner DL, Arcila ME, Beasley MB, Bernicker EH, et al. Updated molecular testing guideline for the selection of lung cancer patients for treatment with targeted tyrosine kinase inhibitors: guideline from the College of American Pathologists, the International Association for the Study of Lung Cancer, and the Association for Molecular Pathology. Arch Pathol Lab Med. 2018;142(3):321–46.
15. Lindeman NI, Cagle PT, Aisner DL, Arcila ME, Beasley MB, Bernicker EH, et al. Updated molecular testing guideline for the selection of lung cancer patients for treatment with targeted tyrosine kinase inhibitors: guideline from the College of American Pathologists, the International Association for the Study of Lung Cancer, and the Association for Molecular Pathology. J Thor Oncol. 2018;13(3):323–58.
16. Mason C, Ellis PG, Lokay K, Barry A, Dickson N, Page R, et al. Patterns of biomarker testing rates and appropriate use of targeted therapy in the first-line, metastatic non-small cell lung cancer treatment setting. J Clin Pathw. 2018;4(1):49–54.
17. Riely GL. What, when, and how of biomarker testing in non-small cell lung cancer. J Natl Compr Cancer Netw. 2017;15(5S):686–8.
18. Kerr KM. Personalized medicine for lung cancer: new challenges for pathology. Histopathology. 2012;60(4):531–46.
19. Lee C, Guichet PL, Abtin F. Percutaneous lung biopsy in the molecular profiling era: a survey of current practices. J Thorac Imaging. 2017;32(1):63–7.
20. Leighl NB, Rekhtman N, Biermann WA, Huang J, Mino-Kenudson M, Ramalingam SS, et al. Molecular testing for selection of patients with lung cancer for epidermal growth factor receptor and anaplastic lymphoma kinase tyrosine kinase inhibitors: American Society of Clinical Oncology endorsement of the College of American Pathologists/International Association for the study of lung cancer/association for molecular pathology guideline. J Clin Oncol. 2014;32(32):3673–9.
21. Tai R, Dunne RM, Trotman-Dickenson B, Jacobson FL, Madan R, Kumamaru KK, et al. Frequency and severity of pulmonary hemorrhage in patients undergoing percutaneous CT-guided transthoracic lung biopsy: single-institution experience of 1175 cases. Radiology. 2016;279(1):287–96.

22. Nour-Eldin NE, Alsubhi M, Emam A, Lehnert T, Beeres M, Jacobi V, et al. Pneumothorax complicating coaxial and non-coaxial CT-guided lung biopsy: comparative analysis of determining risk factors and management of pneumothorax in a retrospective review of 650 patients. Cardiovasc Intervent Radiol. 2016;39(2):261–70.
23. Roy-Chowdhuri S, Dacic S, Ghofrani M, Illei PB, Layfield LJ, Lee C, et al. Collection and handling of thoracic small biopsy and cytology specimens for ancillary studies: guideline from the college of American pathologists in collaboration with the American college of chest physicians, association for molecular pathology, American society of cytopathology, American thoracic society, pulmonary pathology society, papanicolaou society of cytopathology, society of interventional radiology, and society of thoracic radiology. Arch Pathol Lab Med. 2020.
24. Compton CC, Robb JA, Anderson MW, Berry AB, Birdsong GG, Bloom KJ, et al. Preanalytics and precision pathology: pathology practices to ensure molecular integrity of cancer patient biospecimens for precision medicine. Arch Pathol Lab Med. 2019;143(11):1346–63.
25. Isla D, Lozano MD, Paz-Ares L, Salas C, de Castro J, Conde E, et al. New update to the guidelines on testing predictive biomarkers in non-small-cell lung cancer: a National Consensus of the Spanish Society of Pathology and the Spanish Society of Medical Oncology. Clin Transl Oncol. 2023;25(5):1252–67.
26. Tajarernmuang P, Ofiara L, Beaudoin S, Gonzalez AV. Bronchoscopic tissue yield for advanced molecular testing: are we getting enough? J Thorac Dis. 2020;12(6):3287–95.
27. Gosney JR, Paz-Ares L, Janne P, Kerr KM, Leighl NB, Lozano MD, et al. Pathologist-initiated reflex testing for biomarkers in non-small-cell lung cancer: expert consensus on the rationale and considerations for implementation. ESMO Open. 2023;8(4):101587.
28. Rolfo C, Mack PC, Scagliotti GV, Baas P, Barlesi F, Bivona TG, et al. Liquid biopsy for advanced non-small cell lung cancer (NSCLC): a statement paper from the IASLC. J Thorac Oncol. 2018;13(9):1248–68.
29. Chan KC, Yeung SW, Lui WB, Rainer TH, Lo YM. Effects of preanalytical factors on the molecular size of cell-free DNA in blood. Clin Chem. 2005;51(4):781–4.
30. Medina Diaz I, Nocon A, Mehnert DH, Fredebohm J, Diehl F, Holtrup F. Performance of streck cfDNA blood collection tubes for liquid biopsy testing. PLoS One. 2016;11(11):e0166354.
31. Aggarwal C, Marmarelis ME, Hwang WT, Scholes DG, McWilliams TL, Singh AP, et al. Association between availability of molecular genotyping results and overall survival in patients with advanced nonsquamous non-small-cell lung cancer. JCO Precis Oncol. 2023;7:e2300191.
32. Ezeife DA, Spackman E, Juergens RA, Laskin JJ, Agulnik JS, Hao D, et al. The economic value of liquid biopsy for genomic profiling in advanced non-small cell lung cancer. Ther Adv Med Oncol. 2022;14:17588359221112696.
33. Pennell NA, Arcila ME, Gandara DR, West H. Biomarker testing for patients with advanced non-small cell lung cancer: real-world issues and tough choices. Am Soc Clin Oncol Educ Book. 2019;39:531–42.
34. Parra ER, Villalobos P, Mino B, Rodriguez-Canales J. Comparison of different antibody clones for immunohistochemistry detection of programmed cell death ligand 1 (PD-L1) on non-small cell lung carcinoma. Appl Immunohistochem Mol Morphol. 2018;26(2):83–93.
35. Stockley TL, Lo B, Box A, Gomez Corredor A, DeCoteau J, Desmeules P, et al. Consensus recommendations to optimize the detection and reporting of NTRK gene fusions by RNA-based next-generation sequencing. Curr Oncol. 2023;30(4):3989–97.
36. Owen D, Ben-Shachar R, Feliciano J, Gai L, Beauchamp KA, Rivers Z, et al. Actionable structural variant detection via RNA-NGS and DNA-NGS in patients with advanced non-small cell lung cancer. JAMA Netw Open. 2024;7(11):e2442970.
37. National Comprehensive Cancer Network. The NCCN Biomarkers Compendium 2025. Available from: https://www.nccn.org/.
38. Kalemkerian GP, Narula N, Kennedy EB. Molecular testing guideline for the selection of lung cancer patients for treatment with targeted tyrosine kinase inhibitors: American Society of Clinical Oncology Endorsement Summary of the College of American Pathologists/International Association for the Study of Lung Cancer/Association for Molecular Pathology Clinical Practice Guideline Update. J Oncol Pract. 2018;14(5):323–7.

Open Access This chapter is licensed under the terms of the Creative Commons Attribution-NonCommercial 4.0 International License (http://creativecommons.org/licenses/by-nc/4.0/), which permits any noncommercial use, sharing, adaptation, distribution and reproduction in any medium or format, as long as you give appropriate credit to the original author(s) and the source, provide a link to the Creative Commons license and indicate if changes were made.

The images or other third party material in this chapter are included in the chapter's Creative Commons license, unless indicated otherwise in a credit line to the material. If material is not included in the chapter's Creative Commons license and your intended use is not permitted by statutory regulation or exceeds the permitted use, you will need to obtain permission directly from the copyright holder.

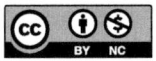

Biology and Treatment Options for Non-small Cell Lung Cancer

15

Kimberly Kish

Contents

Navigation Vignette	190
Introduction	191
Burden of Non-small Cell Lung Cancer	192
Recognizing Signs and Symptoms of Non-small Cell Lung Cancer	192
Diagnostic Workup for Lung Cancer Directs Treatment	193
Lung Cancer TNM Staging	194
Targeted Therapy for Non-small Cell Lung Cancer	195
Guideline-Directed Lung Cancer Management by Stage	195
Multimodal Treatment of NSCLC by Stage	195
Considerations and Approaches to Surgical Management of Early-Stage Lung Cancer	196
Radiotherapy in the Management of Early-Stage Lung Cancer	196
Systemic Therapy for Advanced-Stage NSCLC	197
Smoking Cessation as a Therapeutic Intervention to Improve Lung Cancer Outcomes	199
Early Lung Cancer Detection as a Means for Improving Lung Cancer Outcomes	200
Conclusion	200
Key Takeaways	201
Key Readings and Resources	201
References	201

Abbreviations

ACCP   American College of Chest Physicians
ACS   American Cancer Society
AJCC   American Joint Committee on Cancer
ALK   Anaplastic lymphoma kinase

K. Kish (✉)
M. D. Anderson Cancer Center, Houston, TX, USA
e-mail: kkish@mdanderson.org

© The Author(s) 2026
J. T. Fathi, M. F. Mortman (eds.), *Lung Cancer Navigation and Care*,
https://doi.org/10.1007/978-3-032-02200-4_15

BRAF	B-Raf proto-oncogene
CT	Computed tomography
DNA	Deoxyribonucleic acid
EBUS	Endobronchial ultrasound
EGFR	Epidermal growth factor receptor
ERBB2	erb-B2 receptor tyrosine kinase 2
FISH	Fluorescence in situ testing
HER2	Human epidermal growth factor receptor 2
IASLC	International Association for the Study of Lung Cancer
IR	Interventional radiology
KRAS	Kirsten rat sarcoma
LDCT	Low-dose computed tomography
MET	Mesenchymal–epithelial transition
MOA	Mechanism of action
MRI	Magnetic resonance imaging
NCCN	National Comprehensive Cancer Network
NLST	National Lung Cancer Screening Trial
NSCLC	Non-small cell lung cancer
NTRK	Neurotrophic tyrosine receptor kinase
PD-L1	Program death-ligand 1
PET	Positron emission tomography
PFT	Pulmonary function testing
QOL	Quality of life
RNA	Ribonucleic acid
ROS1	ROS proto-oncogene 1
RT	Radiation therapy
SBRT	Stereotactic body radiation therapy
SCLC	Small cell lung cancer
TKI	Tyrosine kinase inhibitor
USPSTF	United States Preventive Services Task Force

Navigation Vignette

A 57-year-old female with no tobacco use history presented to her local doctor with a persistent nonproductive cough and was treated for allergy-induced asthma. Chest X-ray revealed a left lower lung opacity, followed by a chest computed tomography (CT) scan, which showed a 5.0 cm left lower lobe mass with a satellite nodule. The patient was introduced to a navigator, who assisted her with new patient appointments and secured multidisciplinary visits with medical, radiation, and thoracic surgery oncologists.

Her biopsy and staging studies ultimately revealed stage IIIA NSCLC. In addition, the molecular profiling of her tumor revealed an epidermal growth factor receptor (EGFR) mutation, and program death-ligand 1 (PD-L1) was 50%, indicating potential response to immunotherapy. The navigator was instrumental in explaining indications for certain tests and consultations and providing emotional support, access to social workers, and other resources.

The patient was noted to have excellent performance status with normal pulmonary function testing. Thus, she was deemed to be a candidate for surgical resection. In the setting of stage IIIA disease, the multidisciplinary tumor board recommended neoadjuvant (before surgery) chemo-immunotherapy, followed by surgery, then 3 years of EGFR targeted therapy. The navigator stayed in touch with the patient throughout the entire treatment process to ensure she understood each step, and the navigator also assisted the clinical teams with the coordination of care.

The patient tolerated three cycles of chemo-immunotherapy very well with no interruptions to treatment. Following a restaging evaluation, she underwent a left lower lobectomy. Final surgical pathology revealed 10% residual tumor in the lower lobe. She continues to receive EGFR targeted therapy in her second postoperative year with no evidence of disease recurrence.

Introduction

This chapter will discuss the biology and treatment options for NSCLC. The major types of NSCLC are adenocarcinoma, squamous cell carcinoma, and large cell carcinoma. The risk factors for NSCLC include smoking, environmental exposures such as radon and air pollution, and genetic predispositions. Accurate diagnosis and staging are crucial initial steps toward developing a treatment plan. The histological type of NSCLC, as well as the biological aspects of the tumor (i.e., degree of differentiation, presence of lymphovascular invasion), drives the personalized treatment plan, unique to each patient and their cancer.

Best practice for NSCLC may involve a single line of therapy or a combination of chemotherapy, immunotherapy, targeted therapy, surgery, and radiotherapy, depending on stage and performance status. Recent advances have been made in identifying targeted genetic mutations, such as EGFR mutations, anaplastic lymphoma kinase (ALK) rearrangements, and Kirsten rat sarcoma (KRAS) mutations. It is well established that these genetic identifiers can drive tumor growth and influence treatment efficacy as well as survival outcomes [1]. Understanding the PD-L1 expression of a patient's tumor is also crucial in predicting the immune evasion mechanisms of the tumor and how the patient's tumor will respond to immunotherapy [1].

Early detection through lung cancer screening or incidental discovery has improved survival outcomes and highlights the importance of low-dose CT (LDCT) screening programs [1]. Smoking cessation not only decreases the risk of developing lung cancer but may also decrease disease progression even after diagnosis [2].

Burden of Non-small Cell Lung Cancer

Lung cancer is the leading cause of cancer-related deaths in the United States. In 2024, there were an estimated 234,580 new cases of lung cancer and 125,070 lung cancer deaths [3]. Lung cancer is irrefutably connected to smoking patterns. However, people who have never smoked may also develop lung cancer attributed to exposure to radon gas, secondhand smoke, asbestos, or other chemical, environmental, and occupational exposures [3]. NSCLC comprises approximately 87% of diagnosed lung cancer cases. The median age of diagnosis is 70 for both men and women, which indicates that lung cancer is primarily a disease of older people [4]. Mortality rates have declined by 59% since 1990 for men and by 36% since 2002 for women [3]. Recent advances and earlier detection have contributed to a 4% decrease in mortality in men and women from 2017 to 2021 [3]. The overall 5-year survival (all patients alive 5 years after diagnosis, regardless of stage) is 25%. When lung cancer is detected, diagnosed, and treated early, the 5-year survival rate greatly improves to 63% [3].

Recognizing Signs and Symptoms of Non-small Cell Lung Cancer

Lung cancer is not typically high on the diagnostic considerations when a patient presents with a new onset or persistent cough. However, a persistent cough nonresponsive to evidence-based therapeutic interventions, including clinically indicated pharmacotherapy, may be due to a more serious diagnosis such as pneumonia or lung cancer. Early and accurate diagnosis requires an astute clinician to recognize when the often-subtle clinical presentation points to lung cancer as the primary diagnosis. For a summary of early and more advanced signs and symptoms of lung cancer, please refer to Table 15.1 and Chap. 11 of this text.

The earlier a lung cancer diagnosis is, the better the expected clinical outcomes are. Signs and symptoms can be subtle but are clinical indications of the presence of

Table 15.1 Common signs and symptoms of early and advanced disease [5]

Early disease	Advanced disease
Persistent cough, bronchitis, or pneumonia illness	Back or hip pain
Bloody or rust-colored sputum	Headache
Persistent non-heart/cardiac-related chest pain	Extremity weakness or numbness
Unexplained hoarseness	Dizziness, imbalance, or seizures
Appetite or weight loss	Lymph node swelling
Shortness of breath	Jaundice, representing spread to the liver
New onset weakness or fatigue	

lung cancer and important to identify to make the right diagnosis. Coupling these clinical findings with the patient's past medical, family, and social history, including their age, cigarette smoking history, and occupational and environmental exposures, is a key consideration when lung cancer is suspected.

Diagnostic Workup for Lung Cancer Directs Treatment

Once a lung nodule or mass is detected and deemed concerning based on size, quality, characteristics, and growth pattern over time, a definitive diagnosis must be made by obtaining a tissue sample.

When a lung cancer diagnosis is determined, further testing is required to determine the stage of the disease. Timeliness and accuracy of lung cancer staging and biomarker testing are crucial to ensuring patients receive current guideline-directed and personalized treatment plans. Furthermore, staging aids in discussing prognosis, surveillance, survival care plans, and, in some situations, palliative care.

Diagnostic Imaging and Procedures

Diagnostic and staging studies may include any combination of the following imaging and procedures:

- CT chest (preferably with intravenous contrast)
- PET/CT imaging
- MRI brain
- Interventional radiology (IR) CT-guided percutaneous lung biopsy
- Navigational bronchoscopic lung biopsy
- Endobronchial ultrasound (EBUS) nodal sampling
- Mediastinoscopy

Biomarker Testing for Personalized Treatment

Equally important in the initial lung cancer workup is tumor biomarker profiling and PD-L1 status (see Chap. 14). Tumor biomarkers refer to genes expressed by the tumor cells, such as EGFR and KRAS [6]. There are FDA-approved medications that target these genes to kill the cancer cells. PD-L1 receptors on the surface of tumor cells can bind with immune cells and turn off the immune cell response to the tumor. It is important, therefore, to know what percentage of tumor cells have this PD-L1 receptor. The higher the percentage, the higher the probability that immunotherapy will be effective [7]. These results can also drive decisions about which systemic therapies will be most effective and contribute to offering more personalized cancer care [6]. This is an evolving area of lung cancer treatment, and new updates to standard of care are introduced frequently. The National Comprehensive

Cancer Network (NCCN) routinely updates its guidelines with the latest targeted therapy recommendations, reflecting the most recent published evidence. To learn more, please refer to these guidelines periodically [8]. A link below has been provided in Key Readings and Resources.

Current guidelines recommend routinely testing the following molecular targets at the time of tissue acquisition in diagnostic workup [9].

- EGFR
- ALK
- ROS proto-oncogene 1 (ROS1)
- B-Raf proto-oncogene (BRAF)
- KRAS
- Mesenchymal–epithelial transition (MET)
- Rearranged during transection (RET)
- erb-B2 receptor tyrosine kinase 2 (ERBB2)
- Human epidermal growth factor receptor 2 (HER2) protein overexpression
- Neurotrophic tyrosine receptor kinase (NTRK1/2/3) [9]

Lung Cancer TNM Staging

The accuracy and completeness of staging NSCLC are crucial to guideline-directed treatment and high-quality cancer outcomes. Staging of NSCLC is based on the TNM staging system, where "T" refers to the tumor size, "N" refers to nodal involvement, and "M" refers to any evidence of metastatic lesions. The International Association for the Study of Lung Cancer (IASLC) and the American Joint Committee on Cancer (AJCC) are two organizations that utilize the same widely adopted staging system for NSCLC. The staging system is derived from a database of cases submitted from 25 countries worldwide [8]. With the introduction of immunotherapy and targeted therapies in the last few years, new versions of the staging system have been released, so it is pertinent to utilize the most recent one [10] (Chaps. 12 and 14, offers more detail on this topic)

Invasive staging of mediastinal lymph nodes, especially when there's evidence or a high index of suspicion that lung cancer has spread to the lymph nodes, is performed in select situations via mediastinoscopy or endobronchial ultrasound (EBUS). Combined with a PET/CT scan and a brain MRI, these tests complete the staging workup for the newly diagnosed NSCLC patient [10].

The navigator can be a helpful resource through each step of the staging process to help ensure understanding of the indications for each test or procedure and assist with obtaining timely results from the medical team.

Targeted Therapy for Non-small Cell Lung Cancer

Targeted therapy is essential for treating NSCLC, particularly for patients whose tumors harbor genetic mutations [11]. Unlike traditional chemotherapy, which affects both cancerous and healthy cells, targeted therapies work by inhibiting molecular pathways critical to cancer cell survival and proliferation. Such treatments are predominantly clinically indicated in advanced-stage NSCLC and earlier stages where neoadjuvant or adjuvant treatment may be beneficial [11]. The testing and treatment landscape is ever evolving. Thus, referring to professional organization guidelines routinely for the most up-to-date management recommendations, including lung cancer treatment, is prudent.

Guideline-Directed Lung Cancer Management by Stage

Once diagnostic workup, lung cancer staging, and biomarker testing have been achieved, the therapeutic management plan for NSCLC can be determined. Therapeutic management is based not only on the type and stage of NSCLC but also on appropriateness for surgery, determined by underlying and concomitant comorbidities and preoperative performance status. This upfront determination of surgical candidacy and proper patient selection must occur to ensure safe, high-quality health outcomes [12].

Current evidence serves as the foundation for the diagnostic workup and management of lung cancer, with numerous professional societies regularly updating guidelines to reflect evolving research. These include, but are not limited to, the American Thoracic Society, American College of Chest Physicians (ACCP), American Society of Clinical Oncology, American Society for Radiation Oncology, and the NCCN [8]. The guidelines are quite complex, and algorithms are laid out to address each stage from diagnosis to surveillance. This section provides a basic overview of the multimodal treatment for effectively managing NSCLC by stage, understanding that recommendations continually change.

Multimodal Treatment of NSCLC by Stage

Determination of the definitive cancer diagnosis and stage is crucial when deciding on a treatment plan. For stage IA NSCLC, treatment options are surgery or radiation in the form of stereotactic body radiation therapy (SBRT). For all other stages, there are many options, and the treatment plan depends on several factors unique to each patient. Directed therapies lead to a personalized treatment plan to improve survival while maintaining quality of life [13]. Biomarker testing and PD-L1 status contribute to optimizing the treatment plan, including when clinical trials are considered a treatment option.

Considerations and Approaches to Surgical Management of Early-Stage Lung Cancer

Surgical resection is the standard of care for early-stage (stage I) lung cancer. When surgery is not an option (i.e., the patient prefers an alternative to surgery, or has been deemed medically inoperable), SBRT is a treatment alternative. SBRT directs radiation therapy targeting the lesion (lung cancer) and a small margin of healthy tissue around the lesion, delivering a maximum dose for consecutive days over 1–2 weeks [13].

Once a patient is deemed appropriate for surgery, the surgeon will decide the most appropriate surgical approach (or technique) for lung cancer resection. Minimally invasive surgery includes both video-assisted and robotic-assisted techniques. Both methods offer smaller incisions, lower complication rates, and can potentially decrease total admission time [14]. A well-trained thoracic surgeon should provide these minimally invasive techniques to ensure that the tumor is completely resected and that hilar and mediastinal lymph nodes are removed. Open thoracotomy is typically used in the setting of very large tumors or when deemed necessary by the surgeon [15].

Preoperative evaluation includes testing of pulmonary functional status and review of past medical history with special attention to heart disease, autoimmune conditions, renal disease, and uncontrolled type 2 diabetes mellitus. Pulmonary function testing (PFT) is one of the most important factors in determining surgical candidacy. The ACCP, the European Respiratory Society/European Society of Thoracic Surgeons, and the British Thoracic Society all have guidelines to help determine pulmonary preoperative risk assessment for patients needing a lung cancer resection [16, 17].

For an in-depth review of surgical therapy for NSCLC, please refer to Chap. 13.

Radiotherapy in the Management of Early-Stage Lung Cancer

Radiation therapy (RT) plays a pivotal role in both curative and palliative treatment for NSCLC. SBRT is preferred for medically inoperable early-stage NSCLC and is increasingly recognized as a viable alternative to surgery [18]. As described earlier, SBRT delivers a full dose of targeted radiation therapy to the tumor and a surrounding margin of healthy tissue. The CT simulation before the treatment specifies the contours of treatment. Treatment is delivered in consecutive daily treatments ranging from 3–14 days, depending on the location and size of the tumor [19].

Conventionally fractionated radiation therapy is typically used for advanced-stage, inoperable patients using doses of 45–66 Gy in daily fractions over 6 weeks [15].

Proton therapy is an emerging modality for NSCLC utilizing protons instead of photons to deliver radiation. The unique physical properties of protons allow for precise energy deposition within the tumor, minimizing exposure to surrounding healthy tissues. This is particularly beneficial for patients with tumors near critical structures such as the heart and spinal cord. Proton therapy may be advantageous in reducing long-term toxicities, especially in patients with poor pulmonary function [20].

In summary, for operable early-stage NSCLC, surgery is the standard of care, but SBRT provides an alternative if surgery is not an option. In the advanced stage of NSCLC, combination therapy is utilized with conventional RT or proton RT.

Systemic Therapy for Advanced-Stage NSCLC

Now that we have discussed treatment recommendations for early-stage NSCLC, this next section will cover the management of advanced-stage NSCLC with systemic therapy. Overall, treatment of advanced NSCLC is palliative (or noncurative), and the goal is to prolong survival and maintain quality of life (QOL). Given the tremendous advances in immunotherapy and targeted therapy, patients are maintaining a better QOL and surviving longer.

Chemotherapy

The main drug classes for treating advanced NSCLC are platinum-based doublet regimen chemotherapy, immune checkpoint inhibitors or immunotherapy, and targeted therapy (Table 15.2). Doublet regimen chemotherapy refers to two chemotherapy drugs intended to be administered at the same time or concurrently. Chemotherapy is typically given every 2–3 weeks for four to six cycles and can be

Table 15.2 Mechanism of action (MOA) and key tests for systemic therapies

NSCLC systemic treatment options	Chemotherapy	Immunotherapy	Targeted therapy
MOA	Platinum binds to the tumor cell DNA, causing damage, preventing the cell cycle, and inducing apoptosis or cell death in rapidly dividing tumor cells [29]	Immune checkpoint inhibitors block the checkpoint protein from binding to its partner on the T cell, allowing the T cell to kill the tumor cell [30]	Agent targets specific genetic or molecular pathways in cancer cells that disrupt pathways for tumor growth [28]
Key tests	Biopsy and histology to determine the type of NSCLC	Specialized pathology test using a PD-L1 clone assay using monoclonal anti-PD-L1, clone 22C3	DNA sequencing DNA allele-specific testing DNA, RNA, and next-generation sequencing Fluorescence in situ testing (FISH) Liquid biopsy

administered at the same time as immunotherapy. Platinum-based doublet regimen chemotherapy use is supported by evidence that shows this regimen is associated with increased tumor response and a higher survival rate [21, 22].

Reviewing the two main types, or histologies, of NSCLC, adenocarcinoma and squamous cell carcinoma, is important. The tumor histology assists in determining the optimal choice for the combination of chemotherapy regimen selected by the oncologist. For example, phase III trials have previously reported that prognosis and survival in patients with adenocarcinoma were statistically superior when given a cisplatin/pemetrexed combination. Whereas if a patient had squamous histology, there was a significant improvement in survival with a cisplatin/gemcitabine regimen [23, 24].

Immunotherapy

As discussed earlier in this chapter under biomarker testing, the PD-L1 status is important before treatment planning. The PD-L1 expression is documented as a percentage, and research has shown that if PD-L1 is 50% or more, immunotherapy is associated with longer progression-free interval, increased overall survival, and fewer adverse events [25]. If PD-L1 expression is less than 50%, a combination of two chemotherapy agents with immunotherapy is the preferred initial therapy [25].

Targeted Therapy

The presence of tumor biomarkers indicating mutations of the cancer cells is equally important as histology, stage, surgical candidacy, and PD-L1 expression. Patients with advanced NSCLC should routinely have their tumor assessed for these mutations, also called driver mutations. Therapies that target specific molecular pathways in cancer cells are engineered to avoid the destruction of healthy normal cells [26]. Driver mutations typically initiate the transformation of noncancerous cells to malignant ones and alter cancer cell biology to the extent that the tumor becomes dependent on these signals for survival [27].

Discussion of targeted therapy must also include that of tyrosine kinase and tyrosine kinase inhibitors (TKIs). Tyrosine kinases are enzymes that can lead cancer cells to uncontrolled growth. TKIs specifically target these enzymes, disrupting cancer cells' transformation, growth, proliferation, and survival [28]. The different mutations can be DNA rearrangements, translocations, fusions, or amplifications [27].

This area of NSCLC therapy is rapidly evolving; the professional guidelines are an excellent resource for the most up-to-date target agents for each mutation.

Table 15.2 summarizes each systemic therapy treatment for NSCLC, its MOA, and key tests required (see section on Biomarkers and Chap. 14).

Neoadjuvant Versus Adjuvant Systemic Therapy

In the case of advanced-stage NSCLC in a patient deemed to be a surgical candidate, there is often a discussion of neoadjuvant versus adjuvant systemic therapy. Neoadjuvant therapy takes place before surgery, and adjuvant treatment occurs after surgery. The recommendations for each may vary based on tumor size, proximity of tumor to vital structures, and presence of nodal involvement [31].

The Society of Thoracic Surgeons recently published a consensus document on managing locally advanced (stage II–III) NSCLC [32]. The 19 recommendations in the consensus statement addressed resectability, multidisciplinary management, neoadjuvant therapy, and adjuvant therapy. Imperative to the treatment decision is deciding if the patient is operable and the tumor resectable, determining the extent of nodal involvement, and testing PD-L1 and biomarker status [32].

Stage IV Non-small Cell Lung Cancer

We now turn to stage IV NSCLC, characterized by metastatic disease where lung cancer has spread to distant organs such as the other lung, brain, bones, or liver. When there are multiple metastatic lesions or organs involved, surgery is not typically offered. Stage IV disease commonly requires molecular profiling followed by systemic treatment with or without radiation therapy. Treatment algorithms also consider performance status and whether the metastasis is in a single or multiple locations. NCCN guidelines outline chemotherapy, immunotherapy, and targeted therapy options [8].

Additionally, palliative and supportive care should be incorporated, and clinical trials should be discussed. There should also be discussions around prognosis, QOL, and patient goals of care early in treatment decisions. Early integration of palliative care has been shown to enhance overall QOL, improve mood, and support longer survival with less aggressive care at the end of life [33].

Smoking Cessation as a Therapeutic Intervention to Improve Lung Cancer Outcomes

Cigarette smoking represents the primary risk factor for developing lung cancer [34]. Quitting smoking has been shown to reduce the risk of developing lung cancer, after 10 years, by 30–50% compared to people who continue to smoke [35]. In the setting of a lung cancer diagnosis, smoking cessation with sustained abstinence is increasingly recognized as a primary, secondary, and tertiary prevention method. Recent studies have demonstrated this, showing that abstinence from smoking, especially in the first 3–6 months following a lung cancer diagnosis, is associated with improved cancer control, increased survival, and reduced overall mortality [36, 37]. Cinciripini et al. found that individuals who were currently smoking and diagnosed with lung cancer experienced a 22–26% reduction in cancer-related mortality with sustained abstinence within 3–6 months of diagnosis [36]. The study further found that abstinence from smoking within 3 months of diagnosis increased survival from 2.1 to 3.9 years [36]. All patients should be screened for tobacco use at the time of diagnosis, advised to quit, and aided to quit as early as possible, regardless of stage or planned treatment [34].

Early Lung Cancer Detection as a Means for Improving Lung Cancer Outcomes

Many seminal studies have shown great benefit from low-dose CT imaging in the early detection of lung cancer. To name a few, the International Early Lung Cancer Action Program (I-ELCAP) study found that early detection through annual low-dose CT screening can lead to a high cure rate. This study reported a 20-year lung cancer-specific survival rate of 81%, with cure rates as high as 92% for patients with stage I lung cancer who undergo surgical treatment [38]. The National Lung Cancer Screening Trial (NLST) showed that screening by LDCT can achieve as much as a 20% mortality reduction compared to screening with chest radiography [39]. The NELSON trial revealed that in men and women between the ages of 50 and 74, LDCT screening also significantly reduces lung cancer mortality [40]. Over the past three decades, these studies have demonstrated the benefit of lung cancer screening by LDCT scan in detecting lung cancer earlier. Many professional organizations, including the United States Preventive Services Task Group, the NCCN, and the American Cancer Society (ACS), have published guidelines and recommended screening criteria.

Conclusion

Multiple factors, including disease stage, patient eligibility for specific treatments, and individual care goals, influence the therapeutic management of NSCLC. Early-stage NSCLC is associated with favorable outcomes, particularly with surgical resection or stereotactic body radiotherapy (SBRT). In advanced stages, treatment strategies increasingly rely on comprehensive biomarker testing, critical in guiding therapy and predicting prognosis. Identifying actionable driver mutations and the advent of immunotherapy have significantly improved survival outcomes, even in advanced disease. Furthermore, lung cancer screening facilitates detection of early-stage disease, contributing to better treatment responses and enhanced survival rates. Finally, successful abstinence from cigarette smoking plays a key role in the primary, secondary, and tertiary prevention of lung cancer and related morbidity and mortality. Every step of the way, navigators support and encourage our NSCLC patients as they shift their mindset from the dread of the diagnosis to a hopeful future due to the numerous treatment options we have today.

Key Takeaways

- Patients should be advised to stop smoking, and if qualified, lung cancer screening with a low-dose CT chest should be obtained and followed annually.
- Early detection of lung cancer has been proven to increase the prognosis and survival of lung cancer.
- Biomarkers should be evaluated in all NSCLC patients eligible for systemic therapy, as these can increase disease-free intervals.
- Frequent consultation of professional clinical guidelines for the most up-to-date recommendations for management of NSCLC is highly recommended.
- Management of NSCLC should be data-driven and guided by histology, stage, and biomarker studies.
- The involvement of a navigator can significantly improve the patients' experience both at the time of diagnosis and throughout treatment.

Key Readings and Resources

- National Comprehensive Cancer Network (NCCN) Guidelines: Lung Cancer Screening [41]
- National Comprehensive Cancer Network (NCCN) Guidelines: Non-Small Cell Lung Cancer [8]
- Lung Cancer Surveillance After Definitive Curative-Intent Therapy: American Society of Clinical Oncology (ASCO) Guideline [42]
- International Association for the Study of Lung Cancer (IASLC) Staging Manual, third edition [10]
- International Association for the Study of Lung Cancer (IASLC) ATLAS for Molecular Testing for Targeted Therapy in Lung Cancer [43]
- Pearson's General Thoracic Surgery – STS Cardiothoracic Surgery E-Book Accessed [44]

Conflict of Interest Author reports no conflicts of interest.

References

1. Herbst RS, Morgensztern D, Boshoff C. The biology and management of non-small cell lung cancer. Nature. 2018;553(7689):446–54.
2. Sheikh M, Mukeriya A, Shangina O, Brennan P, Zaridze D. Postdiagnosis smoking cessation and reduced risk for lung cancer progression and mortality: a prospective cohort study. Ann Intern Med. 2021;174(9):1232–9.
3. American Cancer Society Cancer Facts & Figures 2024. American Cancer Society; 2024. Available from https://www.cancer.org/research/cancer-facts-statistics/all-cancer-facts-figures/2024-cancer-facts-figures.html. Accessed 17 Jan 2025.
4. American Cancer Society Lung Cancer Statistics | How Common is Lung Cancer? 2024. Available from: https://www.cancer.org/cancer/types/lung-cancer/about/key-statistics.html. Accessed 17 Jan 2025.

5. American Cancer Society Lung Cancer Signs & Symptoms. 2025. Available from: https://www.cancer.org/cancer/types/lung-cancer/detection-diagnosis-staging/signs-symptoms.html. Accessed 27 Feb 2025.
6. Godoy LA, Chen J, Ma W, Lally J, Toomey KA, Rajappa P, Sheridan R, Mahajan S, Stollenwerk N, Phan CT, Cheng D, Knebel RJ, Li T. Emerging precision neoadjuvant systemic therapy for patients with resectable non-small cell lung cancer: current status and perspectives. Biomark Res. 2023;11(1):7.
7. Chen JA, Ma W, Yuan J, Li T. Translational biomarkers and rationale strategies to overcome resistance to immune checkpoint inhibitors in solid tumors. Cham: Springer; 2020.
8. National Comprehensive Cancer Network. NCCN clinical practice guidelines in oncology non-small cell lung cancer, National Comprehensive Cancer Network; 2025. Available from: https://www.nccn.org/guidelines/guidelines-detail?category=1&id=1450 Accessed January 14.
9. Sholl L, Cooper W, Kerr K, Tan DS, Tsao M, Yang JC. IASLC Atlas of molecular testing for targeted therapy in lung cancer.pdf. Denver: IASLC; 2023. Available from: https://www.iaslc.org/iaslc-atlas-molecular-testing-targeted-therapy-lung-cancer Accessed 4 Feb 2025.
10. Asamura H. IASLC staging manual in thoracic oncology, 3rd ed. 2024. Denver: International Association for the Study of Lung Cancer.
11. Neal J. Personalized, genotype-directed therapy for advanced non-small cell lung cancer - UpToDate. 2025, March 31. Available from: https://www.uptodate.com/contents/personalized-genotype-directed-therapy-for-advanced-non-small-cell-lung-cancer?search=non%20small%20cell%20lung%20cancer&topicRef=4607&source=see_link. Accessed 27 Feb 2025.
12. DeVita VT, Jr., Lawrence TS, Rosenberg SA. Devita, Hellman, and Rosenberg's cancer: principles and practice of oncology, 11e. Lippincott Williams & Wilkins, a Wolters Kluwer Business; 2019.
13. Lilenbaum R. Overview of the initial treatment of advanced non-small cell lung cancer - UpToDate. 2024, December 3. Available from: https://www.uptodate.com/contents/overview-of-the-initial-treatment-of-advanced-non-small-cell-lung-cancer?search=non%20small%20cell%20lung%20cancer&topicRef=4630&source=see_link. Accessed 27 Feb 2025.
14. Cai Y, Fu X, Xu Q, Sun W, Zhang N. Thoracoscopic lobectomy versus open lobectomy in stage I non-small cell lung cancer: a meta-analysis. PLoS One. 2013;8(12):e82366.
15. Vallieres E, Schild S. Management of stage I and stage II non-small cell lung cancer - UpToDate. 2025, January 17. Available from: https://www.uptodate.com/contents/management-of-stage-i-and-stage-ii-non-small-cell-lung-cancer?search=lung%20cancer%20surgery&topicRef=4639&source=see_link#H3. Accessed 27 Feb 2025.
16. Brunelli A, Charloux A, Bolliger CT, Rocco G, Sculier J, Varela G, Licker M, Ferguson MK, Faivre-Finn C, Huber RM, Clini EM, Win T, De Ruysscher D, Goldman L. ERS/ESTS clinical guidelines on fitness for radical therapy in lung cancer patients (surgery and chemo-radiotherapy). Eur Respir J. 2009;34(1):17–41.
17. Brunelli A, Kim AW, Berger KI, Addrizzo-Harris DJ. Physiologic evaluation of the patient with lung cancer being considered for resectional surgery: Diagnosis and management of lung cancer, 3rd ed: American College of Chest Physicians evidence-based clinical practice guidelines. Chest 2013;143(5 Suppl):e166S–e90S.
18. Chang JY, Mehran RJ, Feng L, Verma V, Liao Z, Welsh JW, Lin SH, O'Reilly MS, Jeter MD, Balter PA, McRae SE, Berry D, Heymach JV, Roth JA. Stereotactic ablative radiotherapy for operable stage I non-small-cell lung cancer (revised STARS): long-term results of a single-arm, prospective trial with prespecified comparison to surgery. Lancet Oncol. 2021;22(10):1448–57.
19. Heinzerling J, Timmerman R. Stereotactic body radiation therapy for lung tumors - UpToDate. 2024, June 4. Available from: https://www.uptodate.com/contents/stereotactic-body-radiation-therapy-for-lung-tumors?search=sbrt&source=search_result&selectedTitle=1%7E68&usage_type=default&display_rank=1#H12. Accessed 27 Feb 2025.

20. Dupuy D. Image-guided ablation of lung tumors - UpToDate. 2023, November 6. Available from: https://www.uptodate.com/contents/image-guided-ablation-of-lung-tumors?search=radiotherapy%20for%20non%20small%20cell%20lung%20cancer&topicRef=4642&source=see_link. Accessed 27 Feb 2025.
21. Azzoli CG, Baker S, Temin S, Pao W, Aliff T, Brahmer J, et al. American Society of Clinical Oncology Clinical Practice Guideline update on chemotherapy for stage IV non-small-cell lung cancer. J Clin Oncol. 2009;27(36):6251–66.
22. Delbaldo C, Michiels S, Syz N, Soria J, Le Chevalier T, Pignon J. Benefits of adding a drug to a single-agent or a 2-agent chemotherapy regimen in advanced non-small-cell lung cancer: a meta-analysis. JAMA. 2004;292(4):470–84.
23. Scagliotti GV, Parikh P, von Pawel J, Biesma B, Vansteenkiste J, Manegold C, Serwatowski P, Gatzemeier U, Digumarti R, Zukin M, Lee JS, Mellemgaard A, Park K, Patil S, Rolski J, Goksel T, de Marinis F, Simms L, Sugarman KP, Gandara D. Phase III study comparing cisplatin plus gemcitabine with cisplatin plus pemetrexed in chemotherapy-naive patients with advanced-stage non-small-cell lung cancer. J Clin Oncol. 2008;26(21):3543–51.
24. Syrigos KN, Vansteenkiste J, Parikh P, von Pawel J, Manegold C, Martins RG, Simms L, Sugarman KP, Visseren-Grul C, Scagliotti GV. Prognostic and predictive factors in a randomized phase III trial comparing cisplatin-pemetrexed versus cisplatin-gemcitabine in advanced non-small-cell lung cancer. Ann Oncol. 2010;21(3):556–61.
25. Reck M, Rodríguez-Abreu D, Robinson AG, Hui R, Csőszi T, Fülöp A, Gottfried M, Peled N, Tafreshi A, Cuffe S, O'Brien M, Rao S, Hotta K, Leiby MA, Lubiniecki GM, Shentu Y, Rangwala R, Brahmer JR. Pembrolizumab versus Cchemotherapy for PD-L1-positive non-small-cell lung cancer. N Engl J Med. 2016;375(19):1823–33.
26. Barlesi F, Mazieres J, Merlio J, Debieuvre D, Mosser J, Lena H, Ouafik L, Besse B, Rouquette I, Westeel V, Escande F, Monnet I, Lemoine A, Veillon R, Blons H, Audigier-Valette C, Bringuier PP, Lamy R, Beau-Faller M, Pujol JL, Sabourin JC, Penault-Llorca F, Denis MG, Lantuejoul S, Morin F, Tran Q, Missy P, Langlais A, Milleron B, Cadranel J, Soria JC, Zalcman G. Routine molecular profiling of patients with advanced non-small-cell lung cancer: results of a 1-year nationwide programme of the French Cooperative Thoracic Intergroup (IFCT). Lancet. 2016;387(10026):1415–26.
27. Neal JW. Initial systemic therapy for advanced non-small cell lung cancer lacking a driver mutation - UpToDate. 2024, September 30. Available from: https://www.uptodate.com/contents/initial-systemic-therapy-for-advanced-non-small-cell-lung-cancer-lacking-a-driver-mutation?sectionName=FACTORS+IN+CHOOSING+INITIAL+THERAPY&search=non+small+cell+lung+cancer&topicRef=4607&anchor=H3447715580&source=see_link#H3447715580. Accessed 27 Feb 2025.
28. Min H, Lee H. Molecular targeted therapy for anticancer treatment. Exp Mol Med. 2022;54(10):1670–94.
29. Shiny PJ, Mukherjee A, Chandrasekaran N. DNA damage and mitochondria-mediated apoptosis of A549 lung carcinoma cells induced by biosynthesised silver and platinum nanoparticles. RSC Adv. 2016;6(33):27775–87.
30. National Institutes of Health (NIH) National Cancer Institute Immune Checkpoint Inhibitors. 2019. Available from: https://www.cancer.gov/about-cancer/treatment/types/immunotherapy/checkpoint-inhibitors. Accessed 2 May 2025.
31. Lim E, Harris G, Patel A, Adachi I, Edmonds L, Song F. Preoperative versus postoperative chemotherapy in patients with resectable non-small cell lung cancer: systematic review and indirect comparison meta-analysis of randomized trials. J Thorac Oncol. 2009;4(11):1380–8.
32. Kim SS, Cooke DT, Kidane B, Tapias LF, Lazar JF, Awori Hayanga JW, et al. The society of thoracic surgeons expert consensus on the multidisciplinary management and resectability of locally advanced non-small cell lung cancer. Ann Thorac Surg. 2025;119(1):16–33.
33. Temel JS, Greer JA, Muzikansky A, Gallagher ER, Admane S, Jackson VA, et al. Early palliative care for patients with metastatic non-small-cell lung cancer. N Engl J Med 2010–08-19;363(8):733–742.

34. Caliri AW, Tommasi S, Besaratinia A. Relationships among smoking, oxidative stress, inflammation, macromolecular damage, and cancer. Mutat Res Rev Mutat Res. 2021;787:108365.
35. Park E, Kang H, Lim MK, Kim B, Oh J. Cancer risk following smoking cessation in Korea. JAMA Netw Open. 2024;7(2):e2354958.
36. Cinciripini PM, Kypriotakis G, Blalock JA, Karam-Hage M, Beneventi DM, Robinson JD, et al. Survival outcomes of an early intervention smoking cessation treatment after a cancer diagnosis. JAMA Oncol. 2024;10(12):1689–96.
37. Fathi J, Sheikh M. New, Indisputable Data Demonstrate Smoking Cessation Should be Considered a First-Line Therapeutic Intervention for Thoracic Malignancies. 2025, January 21. Available from: https://www.ilcn.org/new-indisputable-data-demonstrate-smoking-cessation-should-be-considered-a-first-line-therapeutic-intervention-for-thoracic-malignancies/ Accessed 4 Feb 2024.
38. Henschke CI, Yip R, Shaham D, Markowitz S, Cervera Deval J, Zulueta JJ, et al. A 20-year follow-up of the International Early Lung Cancer Action Program (I-ELCAP). Radiology. 2023;309(2):e231988.
39. Aberle DR, Adams AM, Berg CD, Black WC, Clapp JD, Fagerstrom RM, et al. Reduced lung-cancer mortality with low-dose computed tomographic screening. N Engl J Med. 2011;365(5):395–409.
40. de Koning HJ, van der Aalst CM, de Jong PA, Scholten ET, Nackaerts K, Heuvelmans MA, et al. Reduced lung-cancer mortality with volume CT screening in a randomized trial. N Engl J Med. 2020;382(6):503–13.
41. National Comprehensive Cancer Network. NCCN Clinical Practice Guidelines in Oncology Lung Cancer Screening. 2024, October 14. Available from: https://wwwnccnorg/guidelines/guidelines-detail?category=1&id=1450. Accessed 2 Feb 2025.
42. Schneider BJ, Ismaila N, Aerts J, Chiles C, Daly ME, Detterbeck FC, et al. Lung cancer surveillance after definitive curative-intent therapy: ASCO guideline. J Clin Oncol. 2020;38(7):753–66.
43. International Association for the Study of Lung Cancer. IASLC Atlas of Molecular Testing for Targeted Therapy in Lung Cancer 2023. Available from: https://www.iaslc.org/iaslc-atlas-molecular-testing-targeted-therapy-lung-cancer. Accessed 17 Feb 2025.
44. Meyerson SL, Baumgartner WA, Jacobs JP. Pearson's General Thoracic Surgery - STS Cardiothoracic Surgery E-Book. 2024. Available from: https://www.sts.org/education/education/sts-cardiothoracic-surgery-e-book Accessed 20 Jan 2025

Open Access This chapter is licensed under the terms of the Creative Commons Attribution-NonCommercial 4.0 International License (http://creativecommons.org/licenses/by-nc/4.0/), which permits any noncommercial use, sharing, adaptation, distribution and reproduction in any medium or format, as long as you give appropriate credit to the original author(s) and the source, provide a link to the Creative Commons license and indicate if changes were made.

The images or other third party material in this chapter are included in the chapter's Creative Commons license, unless indicated otherwise in a credit line to the material. If material is not included in the chapter's Creative Commons license and your intended use is not permitted by statutory regulation or exceeds the permitted use, you will need to obtain permission directly from the copyright holder.

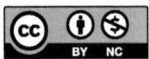

Biology and Treatment Options for Small Cell Lung Cancer and Other Lung Neuroendocrine Neoplasm

16

Lei Deng

Contents

Navigation Vignette.	206
Introduction.	206
Pathology and Incidence.	207
Clinical Presentation and Staging of Small Cell Lung Cancer.	207
Therapeutic Options for Small Cell Lung Cancer.	208
Other Thoracic Neuroendocrine Malignancy.	210
Conclusion.	211
Key Takeaways.	211
Key Readings and Resources.	211
References.	212

Abbreviations

AJCC	American Joint Committee on Cancer
CRS	Cytokine release syndrome
LCNEC	Large cell neuroendocrine carcinoma
NSCLC	Non-small cell lung cancer
SCLC	Small cell lung cancer
SIADH	Syndrome of inappropriate antidiuretic hormone
SVC	Superior vena cava
TNM	Tumor size, lymph node involvement, and metastasis
WHO	World Health Organization

L. Deng (✉)
Division of Hematology and Oncology, Department of Medicine, University of Washington, Seattle, WA, USA

Clinical Research Division, Fred Hutchinson Cancer Center, Seattle, WA, USA
e-mail: LDeng1@FredHutch.org

© The Author(s) 2026
J. T. Fathi, M. F. Mortman (eds.), *Lung Cancer Navigation and Care*,
https://doi.org/10.1007/978-3-032-02200-4_16

Navigation Vignette

A 70-year-old man who formerly smoked with a heavy smoking history (50 pack-year) presented to the emergency room with chest heaviness. Workup showed a 4 cm left hilar mass and mediastinal lymphadenopathy. Bronchoscopy of mediastinal lymph nodes showed small cell carcinoma.

Upon his diagnosis, an oncology nurse navigator introduced herself to the patient and his family, offering emotional support and education about this condition and treatment options. She explained the next steps in his care plan, provided printed resources, and ensured he understood his diagnosis and the potential treatment side effects.

He presented to a medical oncologist's office 2 weeks later and was found to be dyspneic and hypoxemic with SpO2 of 90% on room air and down to 85% on ambulation. He was also found to have swelling of his bilateral neck veins and swelling of his arms. The navigator facilitated his immediate admission to the hospital, coordinating with the medical team to expedite care.

The medical oncologist started carboplatin + etoposide on day 1. In the following several days, he had symptomatic relief with reduced edema of his arms and veins. He was able to wean off supplemental oxygen. Inpatient imaging showed no distant metastases. Radiation oncology was consulted and felt that one radiation field can cover his disease.

The patient was eventually discharged home and started radiation therapy in the clinic. The navigator maintained regular contact and phone check-ins to ensure he attended scheduled appointments, assisted in managing side effects, and helped him stay informed of current goals of care and treatment plan.

Three weeks later, he called the office, reporting a new cough, dyspnea, and fever. The navigator triaged his symptoms and directed him to the emergency room where he was found to have neutropenic fever and pneumonia. He started on antibiotics. Of note, daily radiation therapy continued inpatient. Eventually, the patient was discharged home and completed the rest of the prescribed chemoradiation as planned.

Prophylactic brain irradiation was discussed, but he declined due to concerns of cognitive decline. Finally, he was started on durvalumab infusion. The navigator continued to follow up with him, monitoring for side effects and serving as his point of contact for ongoing concerns. The navigator's involvement ensured the patient felt supported and empowered throughout his cancer diagnosis and treatment.

Introduction

Neuroendocrine cells are a type of cell that receive nervous signals and respond by secreting hormones. This is how our body's hormone secretions are regulated by nervous systems. This type of cell is therefore widely distributed through the human body, including lung, gastrointestinal tract, and pancreas. When these cells become cancerous in the lung, they are called lung neuroendocrine neoplasm [1]. However, this term consists of a wide variety of malignant entities, with strikingly different clinical courses, treatment modality and response, and prognosis. The understanding of these differences is critical in determining the urgency of diagnostic workup and treatment initiation to save patients' lives.

According to 2021 World Health Organization (WHO) classification of lung tumors, neuroendocrine lung neoplasms are broadly classified into two subtypes, neuroendocrine carcinomas and neuroendocrine tumors [1]. The former includes small cell lung cancer (SCLC) and large cell neuroendocrine carcinoma (LCNEC), which are of high-grade and more aggressive, often warranting urgent treatment initiation, particularly the former. In contrast, neuroendocrine tumors include carcinoids, which are low- and intermediate-grade with relatively less aggressive clinical behavior.

Pathology and Incidence

SCLC is the most common type of lung neuroendocrine malignancy, accounting for about 15% of all lung cancers [2]. It is strongly associated with cigarette smoking, but in extremely rare situations, it can be found in patients without any smoking history [3]. Occasionally, SCLCs can also be transformed from other lung histologies—for example, adenocarcinoma after targeted therapies treatment [4].

LCNEC of the lung used to be classified under non-small cell lung cancer (NSCLC). It was unclear at that time whether it was a subtype of NSCLC or a variant of SCLC. In the 2015 WHO classification, LCNEC of the lung became a separate entity independent of NSCLC and was grouped into high-grade neuroendocrine carcinoma with SCLC [5]. It is reported to account for less than 4% of resected lung cancers. It generally confers a poor prognosis similar to SCLC.

Lung neuroendocrine tumors are classified into typical and atypical carcinoids. The latter is histologically and clinically more aggressive than the former, but both are generally associated with a relatively indolent course compared SCLC and LCNEC [6]. They account for approximately 1–2% of lung tumors with typical carcinoid being more common. Its etiology is unclear, and the vast majority appears to be sporadic. In rare cases, it can occur in MEN1 syndrome.

Sometimes, the pathological classification of a particular case can be challenging, as one tumor may harbor features of at least two of the above. A consultation with a lung pathologist would be important to ensure the diagnostic accuracy.

Clinical Presentation and Staging of Small Cell Lung Cancer

SCLC typically presents as a large hilar mass and bulky mediastinal lymphadenopathy with possible airway compromise [2]. Therefore, clinical symptoms and signs are generally due to the mass effect of the growing cancer, including cough, dyspnea, hemoptysis, and postobstructive pneumonia. When the tumor mass obstructs the superior vena cava (SVC), patients may experience a sensation of general fullness in the head, dilated neck veins, and edema of the upper extremities, face, and neck. SVC syndrome is a clinical diagnosis and an oncologic emergency, requiring prompt recognition and treatment initiation.

One of the inherent functions of neuroendocrine cells is to secrete various hormones under physiological conditions. Therefore, malignancies arising from these cells may maintain some of these endocrine features. With the uncontrolled growth of SCLCs, excess hormones and autoantibodies can lead to several distinct paraneoplastic syndromes [7]. Some of the well-known ones are syndrome of inappropriate antidiuretic hormone (SIADH), Cushing syndrome, and Lambert-Eaton myasthenic syndrome. Some rare neurological syndromes may also be seen due to antibodies. Consultation with neurology specialists is recommended due to the subtleties of these symptoms. Typically, paraneoplastic syndrome improves with treatment, but not always.

Although the staging of SCLC can follow the same American Joint Committee on Cancer (AJCC) tumor size, lymph node involvement, and metastasis, (TNM) staging as non-small cell lung cancer, clinically SCLCs are just staged as in two categories: limited and extensive stage [2]. Limited stage is defined as disease limited to one hemithorax and regional nodes that can be included in a single radiation field. Treatment intent for limited stage SCLC is generally curative. In contrast, other SCLCs are considered as extensive stage, and treatment is usually with palliative intent.

Therapeutic Options for Small Cell Lung Cancer

Treatment for Limited-Stage SCLC

Patients with limited stage SCLC are generally treated with concurrent chemoradiation first. This has been the standard of care for more than four decades. The total duration of treatment in this period typically spans 1–2 months [8]. Because radiation is typically administered every day and radiation interruption may lead to inferior outcome, it is critical to have sufficient transportation and lodging support for patients to be close to the treatment center. Nausea/vomiting, mucositis, and infection are some of the known adverse events during treatment. Early recognition and intervention are important measures to support patients. However, growth factor support is generally not given due to lack of survival benefit, and potentially reduced efficacy and increased toxicities [9].

After the completion of concurrent chemoradiation, recently consolidative immunotherapy, durvalumab for 2 years has been approved by the US FDA and is a new standard of care [10]. The ADRIATIC trial demonstrates that durvalumab improves both progression-free survival and overall survival [10]. This is the first drug approval for limited stage SCLC in the past four decades.

Surgery generally has a limited role in the management of SCLC. However, in highly selected early-stage SCLC without mediastinal lymphadenopathy with a small primary tumor, surgery could be an option after multidisciplinary discussions. It is important to offer adjuvant chemotherapy if the plan is to offer surgical resection, even for stage I disease [11].

Treatment for Extensive-Stage SCLC

The treatment of extensive-stage SCLC is generally not curable, and the goal of treatment is to palliate symptoms. SCLC is unique in that it often responds to initial treatment quickly. Patient's symptoms from SCLC can rapidly improve. Therefore, prompt initiation of treatment is of critical importance and can be given in the inpatient setting if one is sick. Early consultation with an oncologist is needed.

The current standard of care of extensive-stage SCLC is a combination of platinum + etoposide + immune checkpoint inhibitor [12, 13]. Even with the addition of immune checkpoint inhibitor, the prognosis remains poor with an overall survival around a year in large phase 3 clinical trials.

After progression from first-line treatment, if there was a long gap between the last platinum + etoposide chemotherapy dose from disease progression, rechallenge with the same chemotherapy can be considered. Otherwise, the options used to be limited to single agent chemotherapy with limited efficacy.

However, it is very exciting that recently, tarlatamab, a DLL-3 bispecific T cell engager was recently approved by US FDA for its durable response [12]. However, due to the high incidence of cytokine release syndrome (CRS) and inpatient dosing requirements in the first 2 doses, this has posed significant challenges for the healthcare system [13]. Luckily, unlike CAR-T therapy, most CRS is low or moderate grade, which can be monitored or managed with supportive care. Grade 3 and above immune effector cell-associated neurotoxicity syndromes (ICANS) were not reported in the FDA-approved dosage in this trial. It is anticipated that with the healthcare team's familiarity of tarlatamab and its associated adverse events, outpatient administration would be possible under appropriate monitoring protocols.

Currently, tarlatamab is approved after progression of first-line therapy. Ongoing studies are investigating its role to be given early in the course, and results are eagerly awaited.

Role of Prophylactic Brain Radiation

Because of the high tendency of brain metastases, prophylactic brain radiation has been investigated to prevent SCLC metastatic to the brain. Older studies without advanced brain imaging like MRI generally showed delayed brain disease and overall survival improvement [14, 15]. However, brain radiation is associated with severe long-term cognitive impairment. With the more readily access to brain MRI and more advanced stereotactic radiosurgery, the use of prophylactic brain radiation is less favored in modern era [16].

Other Thoracic Neuroendocrine Malignancy

Large Cell Neuroendocrine Carcinoma

The treatment of nonmetastatic large cell neuroendocrine carcinoma largely follows NSCLC with surgery and radiation in combination with systemic chemotherapy. The optimal systemic regimen for large cell neuroendocrine carcinoma (LCNEC) is not well defined, due to its heterogeneity and rarity. Typically, there are two approaches: (1) to treat like small cell lung cancer or (2) to treat like non-small cell lung cancer [17]. Molecular studies have shown that LCNEC can be classified to SCLC-like or NSCLC-like, but it is unknown whether molecular-guided treatment approach is superior to one-size-fits-all in terms of patient's survival [18]. Further studies are needed. When an actionable biomarker is detected, it is reasonable to consider targeted therapy.

Carcinoids

Carcinoids are considered as well- and moderately differentiated neuroendocrine tumors [19]. Compared to LCNEC and SCLC, they are on the other spectrum of this neuroendocrine lung tumor. They are generally less aggressive with a favorable prognosis. Carcinoids consist of two subtypes—typical and atypical carcinoid, based on their mitotic index and presence of necrosis. Typical carcinoid has favorable prognosis while atypical carcinoid is slightly more aggressive. Although most carcinoids are not as aggressive as the NSCLC, LCNEC, and SCLC, in some cases, an accurate pathological diagnosis cannot be entirely clear, particularly in small biopsy samples.

Compared to neuroendocrine tumors arising from the gastrointestinal tract, lung carcinoids are much less likely to have secretary endocrine hormones from tumors and are less likely to have carcinoid symptoms.

Surgical resection is the main treatment for nonmetastatic disease. The systemic treatment of carcinoids is, however, largely different from other lung neuroendocrine cancers and non-small cell lung cancer. In general, the first-line systemic treatment is extrapolated from well-differentiated gastrointestinal neuroendocrine tumors. Somatostatin analogs, e.g., injectable octreotide and lanreotide are commonly used for patients with indolent disease course. Somatostatin analogs are not tumoricidal but are associated with durable disease control. After somatostatin analogs, peptide receptor radionuclide therapy or chemotherapy could be considered depending on the clinical situations.

Conclusion

Lung neuroendocrine neoplasm is a diverse group of lung cancer entities that have distinct outcomes. An accurate pathological diagnosis and vigilance on clinical presentation are vital for decisions on treatment urgency. SCLC is aggressive but typically responds to the initial rounds of chemotherapy. Unfortunately, SCLC tends to recur despite the initial response, and the long-term prognosis is unfavorable. Lung carcinoids are more indolent, and chemotherapy is used much less often. However, occasionally, the pathological distinction among these entities may not be clear, and clinical presentation should also be taken into account for treatment planning.

Key Takeaways

- Lung neuroendocrine neoplasm consists of a highly heterogenous group of malignancies, ranging from aggressive SCLC and LCNEC to relatively indolent typical and atypical carcinoid.
- The clinical presentation, urgency of diagnostic workup, treatment, and prognosis vary significantly.
- Although SCLC is aggressive, it tends to respond very well to chemotherapy in treatment-naïve patients. Therefore, prompt diagnosis of SCLC and initiation of treatment can be lifesaving.
- Occasionally, pathological classification can be challenging, and more than one entity can be seen in the same diagnostic specimen. Consultation with oncology experts is important for optimal management.

Key Readings and Resources

- The 2021 WHO Classification of Lung Tumors: Impact of Advances Since 2015 [1]
- Small cell lung cancer [2]
- NCCN Guidelines for patients: Small cell lung cancer 2024 [20]
- NCCN Guidelines for patients: Neuroendocrine tumors 2022 [21]

Conflicts of Interest Lei Deng has received research funds from BridgeBio Oncology Therapeutics, received consulting feeds from Bristol Myers Squibb, and Regeneron, and received travels from Merck.

References

1. Nicholson AG, Tsao MS, Beasley MB, Borczuk AC, Brambilla E, Cooper WA, et al. The 2021 WHO classification of lung tumors: impact of advances since 2015. J Thorac Oncol. 2022;17(3):362–87.
2. Rudin CM, Brambilla E, Faivre-Finn C, Sage J. Small-cell lung cancer. Nat Rev Dis Primer. 2021;7(1):3.
3. Früh M, De Ruysscher D, Popat S, Crinò L, Peters S, Felip E. Small-cell lung cancer (SCLC): ESMO clinical practice guidelines for diagnosis, treatment and follow-up. Ann Oncol. 2013;24:vi99–105.
4. Ferrer L, Giaj Levra M, Brevet M, Antoine M, Mazieres J, Rossi G, et al. A brief report of transformation from NSCLC to SCLC: molecular and therapeutic characteristics. J Thorac Oncol. 2019;14(1):130–4.
5. Travis WD, Brambilla E, Nicholson AG, Yatabe Y, Austin JHM, Beasley MB, et al. The 2015 World Health Organization classification of lung tumors. J Thorac Oncol. 2015;10(9):1243–60.
6. Robelin P, Hadoux J, Forestier J, Planchard D, Hervieu V, Berdelou A, et al. Characterization, prognosis, and treatment of patients with metastatic lung carcinoid tumors. J Thorac Oncol. 2019;14(6):993–1002.
7. Soomro Z, Youssef M, Yust-Katz S, Jalali A, Patel AJ, Mandel J. Paraneoplastic syndromes in small cell lung cancer. J Thorac Dis. 2020;12(10):6253–63.
8. Faivre-Finn C, Snee M, Ashcroft L, Appel W, Barlesi F, Bhatnagar A, et al. Concurrent once-daily versus twice-daily chemoradiotherapy in patients with limited-stage small-cell lung cancer (CONVERT): an open-label, phase 3, randomised, superiority trial. Lancet Oncol. 2017;18(8):1116–25.
9. Bunn PA, Crowley J, Kelly K, Hazuka MB, Beasley K, Upchurch C, et al. Chemoradiotherapy with or without granulocyte-macrophage colony-stimulating factor in the treatment of limited-stage small-cell lung cancer: a prospective phase III randomized study of the southwest oncology group. J Clin Oncol. 1995;13(7):1632–41.
10. Cheng Y, Spigel DR, Cho BC, Laktionov KK, Fang J, Chen Y, et al. Durvalumab after Chemoradiotherapy in limited-stage small-cell lung cancer. N Engl J Med. 2024;391(14):1313–27.
11. Yang CFJ, Chan DY, Speicher PJ, Gulack BC, Wang X, Hartwig MG, et al. Role of adjuvant therapy in a population-based cohort of patients with early-stage small-cell lung cancer. J Clin Oncol. 2016;34(10):1057–64.
12. Ahn MJ, Cho BC, Felip E, Korantzis I, Ohashi K, Majem M, et al. Tarlatamab for patients with previously treated small-cell lung cancer. N Engl J Med. 2023;389(22):2063–75.
13. Sands JM, Champiat S, Hummel HD, Paulson KG, Borghaei H, Alvarez JB, et al. Practical management of adverse events in patients receiving tarlatamab, a delta-like ligand 3-targeted bispecific T-cell engager immunotherapy, for previously treated small cell lung cancer. Cancer. 2025;131(3):e35738.
14. Aupérin A, Arriagada R, Pignon JP, Le Péchoux C, Gregor A, Stephens RJ, et al. Prophylactic cranial irradiation for patients with small-cell lung cancer in complete remission. Prophylactic cranial irradiation overview collaborative group. N Engl J Med. 1999;341(7):476–84.
15. Le Péchoux C, Dunant A, Senan S, Wolfson A, Quoix E, Faivre-Finn C, et al. Standard-dose versus higher-dose prophylactic cranial irradiation (PCI) in patients with limited-stage small-cell lung cancer in complete remission after chemotherapy and thoracic radiotherapy (PCI 99-01, EORTC 22003-08004, RTOG 0212, and IFCT 99-01): a randomised clinical trial. Lancet Oncol. 2009;10(5):467–74.
16. Rusthoven CG, Kavanagh BD. Prophylactic cranial irradiation (PCI) versus active MRI surveillance for small cell lung cancer: the case for equipoise. J Thorac Oncol. 2017;12(12):1746–54.
17. Lindsay CR, Shaw EC, Moore DA, Rassl D, Jamal-Hanjani M, Steele N, et al. Large cell neuroendocrine lung carcinoma: consensus statement from the British thoracic oncology group and the Association of Pulmonary Pathologists. Br J Cancer. 2021;125(9):1210–6.

18. George J, Walter V, Peifer M, Alexandrov LB, Seidel D, Leenders F, et al. Integrative genomic profiling of large-cell neuroendocrine carcinomas reveals distinct subtypes of high-grade neuroendocrine lung tumors. Nat Commun. 2018;9(1):1048.
19. Rekhtman N. Lung neuroendocrine neoplasms: recent progress and persistent challenges. Mod Pathol. 2022;35(Suppl 1):36–50.
20. National Comprehensive Cancer Network. NCCN Guidelines for patients: Small cell lung cancer 2024 [Internet]. Available from: https://www.nccn.org/patients/guidelines/content/PDF/SCLC-patient-guideline.pdf
21. National Comprehensive Cancer Network. NCCN Guidelines for patients: Neuroendocrine tumors 2022. [Internet]. Available from: https://www.nccn.org/patients/guidelines/content/PDF/neuroendocrine-patient.pdf

Open Access This chapter is licensed under the terms of the Creative Commons Attribution-NonCommercial 4.0 International License (http://creativecommons.org/licenses/by-nc/4.0/), which permits any noncommercial use, sharing, adaptation, distribution and reproduction in any medium or format, as long as you give appropriate credit to the original author(s) and the source, provide a link to the Creative Commons license and indicate if changes were made.

The images or other third party material in this chapter are included in the chapter's Creative Commons license, unless indicated otherwise in a credit line to the material. If material is not included in the chapter's Creative Commons license and your intended use is not permitted by statutory regulation or exceeds the permitted use, you will need to obtain permission directly from the copyright holder.

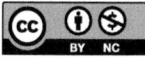

Clinical Trials in Lung Cancer

17

Andrew Ciupek and Brittney Nichols

Contents

Navigation Vignette	216
Introduction	216
Phases and Stages of Clinical Trials	217
Patient Journey Through Clinical Trial Enrollment	218
Recommendations for Communication	220
Suggested Topics for Clinical Trial Discussions with Prospective Trial Participants	220
Intersectionality and Disparities	221
Psychosocial and Historical Barriers	221
Data-Based Barriers	222
Financial Barriers	222
Geographic Barriers	223
Conclusion	223
Key Takeaways	223
Key Readings and Resources	224
References	224

Abbreviations

ADLs	Activities of daily living
EGFR	Epidermal growth factor receptor
FDA	U.S. Food and Drug Administration
LGBTQ	Lesbian, Gay, Bisexual, Transgender, Queer
NCCN	National Comprehensive Cancer Network
PHI	Protected health information
SDoH	Social determinants of health
SGM	Sexual gender minority

A. Ciupek (✉) · B. Nichols
GO2 for Lung Cancer, Washington, DC, USA
e-mail: aciupek@go2.org; bnichols@go2.org

© The Author(s) 2026
J. T. Fathi, M. F. Mortman (eds.), *Lung Cancer Navigation and Care*,
https://doi.org/10.1007/978-3-032-02200-4_17

Navigation Vignette

Mrs. E. is a 54-year-old woman who was diagnosed with stage IV epidermal growth factor receptor (EGFR)-positive non-small cell lung cancer 18 months ago. Her disease had remained stable during this time with daily oral targeted therapy. However, following her most recent surveillance CT scan, she was informed of new progression (growth) within her primary tumor, as well as new brain lesions. When Mrs. E. asked her oncologist what her options were, her oncologist recommended a triplet therapy regimen including an EGFR targeted therapy and platinum-based chemotherapy agent. Mrs. E. is concerned about this regimen, as she has two grown children, one about to graduate college and another who is soon to be married; she is worried about feeling too sick to attend these milestones. Mrs. E. asked if she would be eligible for clinical trials that may be less intensive, but her oncologist shared that since they are a stand-alone rural hospital, they do not have an active research program, and therefore, there are no available trials.

Following the conversation with the oncologist, Mrs. E. was introduced to KD, a nurse navigator at the cancer center. KD met with Mrs. E the same afternoon at the oncology clinic to review her treatment plan and provide education about side effect management. KD also referred Mrs. E. to the nearest major medical center with a clinical trials unit. Once there, Mrs. E. connected with a research navigator who carefully reviewed her records and matched her with a clinical trial tailored for patients with her specific mutation and progression pattern. The research navigator then guided her through the eligibility screening, coordinated necessary testing, and ensured that all enrollment paperwork was completed efficiently. Thanks to this coordinated effort, Mrs. E. was successfully enrolled in the clinical trial, enabling her to achieve her goal of receiving less intensive treatment.

Introduction

Clinical trials are a valid alternative for patients at every step of their cancer journey, and the National Comprehensive Cancer Network (NCCN) recommends that all patients consider participation [1]. Like other therapeutic options, clinical trials have risks and benefits that patients should discuss with their providers [2]. Patients must know their options to make the best choice for themselves, including understanding if they are eligible for clinical trials. However, only 7% of cancer patients in the United States (U.S.) are enrolled to participate in a clinical trial; lack of awareness of trials as a care option contributes to this low enrollment [3]. A 2001 survey of nearly 6000 cancer patients in the U.S. indicated that 85% were unaware of or unsure that a trial was an option [4]. Numerous studies indicate that healthcare providers play an important role in spreading trial awareness—they are the most cited source for learning about a trial, and their involvement in discussing and providing support is a key factor for successfully joining trials [5]. Thus, providers consistently presenting trials alongside other care options and supporting patients by considering their needs and preferences may increase trial participation.

Lung cancer navigators can support patients who are considering trials in many ways. They can gauge patient awareness and interest in trials, provide education on trials and how they work, assist with locating trials for the patient to review with their treatment team, and help the patient to think about what questions to ask regarding trial options [6]. This chapter will provide an overview of clinical trials, focusing on oncology, and considerations for providers helping to navigate patients making decisions about or going through the clinical trial process.

Phases and Stages of Clinical Trials

Clinical trials are research studies where people are assigned to receive specific interventions to understand how they affect health-related outcomes [7]. These interventions are not limited to medicines and can include medical procedures, medical devices, or different care protocols or models. Before trials are allowed to begin, the "preclinical phase" is required. This is where new interventions must be evaluated in a laboratory setting with experiments to understand if and how an intervention works and the potential unwanted effects it may cause. For many interventions, this also involves first seeing how it works in animal models of the condition being treated.

Treatment-based trials then move through ordered phases, the characteristics of which can be informative when comparing options (see Tables 17.1 and 17.2). Late-stage clinical trials (phase III) often involve randomization of participants to a new intervention or the current standard of care (SOC). Patients are sometimes concerned that when they are in a trial comparing one drug to another, they may receive a "placebo drug" in place of treatment [8]. However, the only time a placebo (or "sugar pill") is used alone (no treatment used) in an oncology trial with randomization is if the current standard of care outside of the trial would be observation only/no treatment.

Table 17.1 Clinical trial phases

Phase	Purpose	Sample size
Phase I	Determining the safety and dosage of the new intervention	Few participants, often less than 30
Phase II	Determining the overall efficacy of the new intervention	Still relatively small, generally less than 100 participants
Phase III	Comparison of the new intervention's efficacy and side effect profile to the current standard of care (SOC). Will often see groups "randomized" to receive the new intervention or SOC	Larger, usually seeking several hundred participants

Table 17.2 Clinical trial status guide

Trial status	Definition
Active/not recruiting	The study is ongoing, but patient accrual has ended.
Active/recruiting	The study is actively accepting new patients.
Not yet recruiting	The study is in the start-up process and has not yet opened to subject accrual.
Withdrawn	Study halted prior to enrolling the first subject.
Suspended	Study has stopped, but activities/recruitment may resume in the future.

Patient Journey Through Clinical Trial Enrollment

Before a person enrolls in a clinical trial, they must go through several steps:

Prescreening

An initial meeting where a study team member completes a preliminary check to determine if they meet the study eligibility requirements, providing study details and an opportunity for questions [9].

Informed Consent

Interested people who meet study requirements are provided with an in-depth study overview, including an informed consent form with detailed trial information that must be signed to join the trial. People may ask the study team questions, take the form home, and spend as much time considering participation as needed [9, 10].

Screening

The final step before joining is an in-depth evaluation that could involve medical record review, physical examinations, and laboratory tests to determine if a person meets all participation requirements. All clinical trials include some inclusion and exclusion criteria, ensuring that volunteer trial participants are good candidates regarding their health and related factors. The eligibility criteria can consist of having a certain medical history, treatment history, lab values, histology, or stage of disease, location, and more [9].

For most trials, the presteps must be completed at the trial center. Once a person completes all presteps, they will officially join the trial, a process called "*enrollment.*"

The experience a trial participant has after enrollment will vary from study to study but may involve several of the following:

- *Treatment*: The participant will receive any trial treatments; usually, they must be administered at the trial center.
- *Medical or laboratory assessments*: During trial appointments, physical examinations, lab tests, or imaging may be required. Some trials may ask for or require additional tissue biopsies.
- *Nonmedical assessments*: Trials may ask participants to complete surveys, interviews, or experience journals.
- *Remote follow-up or monitoring*: Trials may phone or email participants to follow up and remotely monitor or assess them. Some trials may ask participants to use a wearable or other device for remote information collection.

A person may choose to end their active trial participation for several reasons. While the list below is not all-encompassing, it illuminates several of the more common reasons that a participant may elect to withdraw from the trial:

- *Voluntary*: All trial participants are volunteers and may choose to leave the trial at any time and for any reason. The informed consent form will describe the process for leaving a trial.
- *Side effects*: If side effects (called *"adverse events"* by trials) are too severe, intolerable, or deemed unsafe for a participant's health, a treating clinician may recommend leaving the trial. Some participants worry that experiencing side effects may force them to withdraw, but side effects in trials can often be managed while maintaining active participation:
  - *Palliative care*: Participants can be referred for supportive care while enrolled in the trial to help manage side effects. Some trials, anticipating potential side effects, may provide educational resources or "take-home kits" to prepare participants and support them with at-home care.
  - *Dose adjustments*: Some trials allow treating clinicians to lower treatment dose or temporarily delay dosing cycles to resolve side effects.
- *Progression or worsening health*: If disease progression (lung cancer growth) occurs or a participant's health declines severely, trial researchers or clinicians may recommend withdrawing from the trial. Trials define disease progression (e.g., percentage change in tumor size) and monitoring procedures to be followed within study protocols. These decisions may also be left to the treating and/or study clinicians' discretion to promote the welfare of the individual.
- *Completion of trial activities*: If participants complete all required activities (i.e., all treatment cycles and follow-up assessments), they are transitioned out of the trial.

When patients end active trial participation, they usually return to regular care with their original treatment team. There may be basic follow-up assessments or activities for months or years after this in the "Long-Term Follow-Up" stage. This may include direct follow-up, where trial team members may phone or otherwise contact past participants for updates on their current condition (these may also be requested electronically). Follow-up assessments may be conducted through surveys or other means to ask about the impact of the trial on participants' long-term quality of life or health. In addition, trial team members may request medical records from a participant's treating clinician to document disease progression, treatment changes, or other events occurring after trial participation ends.

Recommendations for Communication

Navigators can play a key role in helping patients (and caregivers or family members) understand trial options and address concerns. However, it is also important to emphasize to the patient that the decision to participate is theirs alone and they may withdraw at any time.

When engaging in discussions about clinical trials, it is important to cultivate a setting in which open and honest communication is encouraged and where there is freedom to ask questions. It is important to ensure that the environment is free from distractions and allows enough time to address concerns. While meeting with individuals, learning what they already know about clinical trials and their attitudes towards participation is helpful. This allows for the conversation to be adapted to their level of knowledge and focused on their specific interests or concerns [10]. It can also be helpful to use a *shared decision-making* model. This is a collaborative model of care where clinicians and patients work together to identify a solution that will be medically and ethically sound while also meeting the needs of the patient and their loved ones [11].

Due to the complexity of clinical trials, it is essential that navigators consider the *health literacy* level of their patients when discussing such things as trial goals and eligibility criteria for trial participation, related procedures and trial schedule, the informed consent, compensation and costs of study participation, privacy and confidentiality, and follow-up care. Even those with a high degree of literacy may still have low health literacy. Best practice is to use clear, simple terms and to ensure that materials provided are written at a 4th to 6th grade reading level [12]. When selecting materials for the patient, try to determine how they prefer to receive information (visually, auditory, by reading, etc.) and provide a preferred format when possible [13]. If the patient's primary language is one other than English, provide translated materials when available. During face-to-face encounters, ensure a certified medical interpreter is available for patients with limited English proficiency.

Suggested Topics for Clinical Trial Discussions with Prospective Trial Participants

- *Health*: Is the patient healthy enough to participate? What could the potential impacts of this trial be on their health and their ability to carry out activities of daily living (ADLs)? [14]
- *Financial*: What costs associated with this trial will be covered by the trial sponsors or insurance? What costs will the patient be responsible for, and do they

have the resources for this? Are there support programs that the patient may qualify for? How could this impact the patient's finances and/or work life? [14]
- *Logistical*: How far and how often will the patient need to travel for this trial? Do they have transportation available? What tasks will the patient be required to complete? What new care team members will be included? [14]
- *Values/goals of care*: How will this impact the patient's quality of life? What are their goals of care, and how would this trial fit into these? Is there any curative intent associated with the trial? [14]

Intersectionality and Disparities

Clinical trials exhibit disparities, just as in other areas of healthcare, with several populations being underrepresented [15]. This may be exacerbated by the already-existing inequalities within the lung cancer community. Lung cancer is a disease fraught with stigma due to the association with tobacco usage [16] (for more information on stigma, please see Chap. 1). In addition to this base stigma, lung cancer is more prevalent among certain marginalized and minoritized populations that have already experienced historical mistreatment or biases [17]. For example, the tobacco industry has a history of directing marketing to historically marginalized groups, such as racial/ethnic minorities and the LGBTQIA+ community, exposing these communities to lung cancer risk [18]. Therefore, navigators, especially in the area of lung cancer, should be aware of these clinical trial disparities, as well as the history of medical mistrust and structural racism that contributed to them. This can help inform conversations about clinical trial participation with patients who have concerns or are having impacts from these disparities.

Psychosocial and Historical Barriers

Although the way clinical trials are conducted has changed over the past several decades, many people still have negative connotations regarding medical research. For many, the thought of clinical trials calls to mind experiments such as the human subjects research conducted during World War II or the infamous Tuskegee Syphilis Study (in which hundreds of African American men were deprived of treatment). From the 1940s to the 1970s, regulations were introduced to ensure that people would not be harmed during medical research and that they would volunteer freely without coercion or force (such as the Nuremberg Code, the Declaration of Helsinki, and the Belmont Report) [19, 20].

Despite these strides, navigators may still find themselves in a position where the patient does not trust them, the researchers, or the healthcare system. For instance, some people may want to know why they are being asked to share personal information in a trial. They may be worried that this data will be used to marginalize them further or shared with others without their consent [21]. A navigator could help by reassuring them that the information they share is considered protected health information (PHI) and will be de-identified so it cannot be traced back to them [6, 22]. Recognizing and directly addressing concerns may lead to more effective trial conversations.

Generational trauma, unconscious bias, stigma, and a lack of transparency are all contributing factors to mistrust [20]. Medical mistrust has been shown to have a negative impact on care, leading to delayed screenings, which can in turn lead to late-stage diagnosis and limited treatment options [21]. Acknowledging the events that have led to these feelings and actively listening to a patient's concerns can be helpful. Navigators can build rapport and learn what specific worries a person may have.

Data-Based Barriers

Data drives evidence-based decisions in science and medicine, but certain patient populations are not adequately represented in clinical trial data, making it difficult at times to draw conclusions about broad applicability [22]. For example, despite many minorities facing a higher burden of disease and/or death, most clinical trial participants are non-Hispanic whites [23]. Another example is evidenced by the dearth of clinical research data from individuals who identify as being part of a sexual gender minority (SGM). Many studies do not ask questions that allow participants to identify their sexual orientation or gender identity and ask only about a person's physical sex [24].

In response to these issues, the U.S. Food and Drug Administration (FDA) issued guidance in 2024 regarding diversity action plans detailing how they may facilitate more equal representation in their pivotal clinical trials [25]. While there are no current regulations around this subject, the diversity of a patient's experiences and backgrounds impacts how they may come to the clinical trial discussion and should be considered during the navigation process. People who support and navigate patients considering clinical trials will play a key role in forming community connections and can help educate patients on the importance of trial participation to ensure we can learn more about how interventions affect people like them [6].

Financial Barriers

Social determinants of health (SDoH), such as where a person lives, their education, their insurance status, and their finances, all play an important role in a person's decision-making and can affect the type of care they receive, including what clinical trials they can access. While clinical trials often provide treatments free of charge, there are many overlooked costs to consider. Clinical trials can require additional diagnostic tests such as scans, biopsies, and/or laboratory work that may or may not be covered. If a study requires additional visits for routine lab draws or infusions, this can also equate to time off and lost wages. Extra travel costs and time due to living far from a trial location may create financial barriers for patients and can cause added stress and costs. Some trials may reimburse these additional expenses [26]. The availability of such resources can be determined by contacting the clinical trial personnel directly. Identifying and conversing with patients about their potential participation barriers can help ensure realistic expectations for the clinical trial experience. For example, utilizing a screening tool for financial toxicity can identify individuals who may be at risk for financial hardship over the course of their trial treatment [27].

Geographic Barriers

Due to isolation and resource scarcity, people in rural areas face unique challenges regarding healthcare and research participation. Fifteen percent of people in the U.S. live in rural zones, and these individuals tend to be older, with higher rates of tobacco and alcohol consumption, and lower rates of preventive healthcare utilization [28]. Thus, this group faces a higher disease burden and limited accessibility. This is a particular problem for clinical trials, as the majority are hosted through larger, urban academic medical centers. When providing navigation to rural residents, the travel distance, their frequency, and whether patients have a reliable means of transportation should be considered. Rural residents are also more likely to be uninsured than their urban counterparts [28], so a discussion about coverage of trial participation costs is important.

Conclusion

Clinical trials represent a recommended therapeutic option of high-quality care for all people who are at risk or living with lung cancer. Despite this, a person may face many barriers to learning about and enrolling in a clinical trial. From personal misunderstandings and misgivings, social determinants of health, and structural biases, to the many nuances of enrollment and consent, numerous hurdles exist to overcome. Fortunately, a lung cancer navigator can guide the patient through difficulties on this path. By using clear, evidence-based information and effective communication, navigators can empower patients to make the best choice for themselves.

Key Takeaways

- There are many types of clinical trials and a wide variety of factors to consider, which underscores the important role of the lung cancer navigator in the clinical trial process.
- The choice to participate and to remain in a trial is solely that of the patient; they may withdraw at any time for any reason.

- Clinical trials are a valid option for patients at any step of their journey, and many patients report that they would be interested in participating if asked by their healthcare provider.
- There are many reasons that a person may be wary of joining a trial. Navigators should explore these further through empathy and active listening.

Key Readings and Resources

- National Institutes of Health: Participate in Cancer Research [29]
- Strategies to Maximize Patient Participation in Clinical Trials [30]
- National Institutes of Health: Clinical Research Trials and You [31]
- GO2 for Lung Cancer Research [32]

Conflicts of Interest Andrew Ciupek reports the following disclosures: Novartis—Consulting Fees (paid to organization), Genentech, Inc.—Consulting Fees (paid to organization), Seagen, Inc.—Consulting Fees (paid to organization), Gilead Sciences, Inc.—Consulting Fees (paid to organization), Daiichi Sankyo, Inc.—Consulting Fees (paid to organization), GlaxoSmithKline, Inc.—Advisory Board participation

Brittney Nichols reports the following disclosures: Novartis—Consulting Fees (paid to organization), AstraZeneca—Advisory Board participation, Daiichi Sankyo—Advisory Board participation, Boehringer Ingelheim—Consulting Fees (paid to organization), AbbVie—Consulting Fees (paid to organization)

References

1. National Institutes of Health (NIH). National Institutes of Health (NIH) Clinical research trials and you: the basics. Available at: https://www.nih.gov/health-information/nih-clinical-research-trials-you/basics. Accessed 17 Mar 2025.
2. National Institutes of Health (NIH). National Cancer Institute Center for Cancer Research: Clinical trials frequently asked questions. 2025. Available at: https://ccr.cancer.gov/clinical-trials/patients/faq. Accessed 19 Mar 2025.
3. Unger JM, Shulman LN, Facktor MA, Nelson H, Fleury ME. National estimates of the participation of patients with cancer in clinical research studies based on commission on cancer accreditation data. J Clin Oncol. 2024;42(18):2139–48.
4. Taylor H. Misconceptions and lack of awareness greatly reduce recruitment for cancer, Clinical trials. Harris Interactive Healthcare News. 2001:1–3.
5. Comis RL, Miller JD, Colaizzi DD, Kimmel LG. Physician-related factors involved in patient decisions to enroll onto cancer clinical trials. J Oncol Pract. 2009;5(2):50–6.
6. Grady C, Edgerly M. Science, technology, and innovation: nursing responsibilities in clinical research. Nurs Clin North Am. 2009;44(4):471–81.
7. National Institutes of Health. National library of medicine: learn about studies. National Centers for Biotechnology Information. Available at: https://clinicaltrials.gov/study-basics/learn-about-studies. Accessed 17 Mar 2025.
8. National Institutes of Health (NIH). National Institute on Aging: Clinical research: benefits, risks, and safety. 2023, May 18. Available at: https://www.cancer.gov/research/participate/clinical-trials/what-to-expect. Accessed 17 Mar 2025.

9. National Institutes of Health. National Cancer Institute Clinical Trials: What to expect. 2024. Available at: https://www.cancer.gov/research/participate/clinical-trials/what-to-expect. Accessed 17 Mar 2025.
10. National Institutes of Health (NIH). Talking to your patient about a clinical trial. 2015. Available at: https://www.nih.gov/health-information/nih-clinical-research-trials-you/talking-your-patient-about-clinical-trial. Accessed 17 Feb 2025.
11. Shickh S, Leventakos K, Lewis MA, Bombard Y, Montori VM. Shared decision making in the care of patients with cancer. Am Soc Clin Oncol Educ Book. 2023;43:e389516.
12. Paasche-Orlow MK, Taylor HA, Brancati FL. Readability standards for informed-consent forms as compared with actual readability. N Engl J Med. 2003;348(8):721–6.
13. Bakerjian D. Personal health literacy. Patient Safety Network; 2023, August 30.
14. American Cancer Society (ACS). Deciding whether to be part of a clinical trial. 2022. Available at: https://www.cancer.org/cancer/managing-cancer/making-treatment-decisions/clinical-trials/what-you-need-to-know/who-does-clinical-trials.html. Accessed 17 Mar 2025.
15. Food and Drug Administration. FDA Clinical Investigator Training Course (CITC). 2024. 2025 Fri, 01/17/ - 09:36. Available at: https://www.fda.gov/drugs/news-events-human-drugs/fda-clinical-investigator-training-course-citc-2024-12102024. Accessed 17 Jan 2025.
16. Hamann HA, Williamson TJ, Studts JL, Ostroff JS. Lung cancer stigma then and now: continued challenges amid a landscape of Progress. J Thorac Oncol. 2021;16(1):17–20.
17. Zavala VA, Bracci PM, Carethers JM, Carvajal-Carmona L, Coggins NB, Cruz-Correa MR, et al. Cancer health disparities in racial/ethnic minorities in the United States. Br J Cancer. 2021;124(2):315–32.
18. Jackler R, Ramamurthi D, Willett J, Chau C, Muoneke MN, Zeng A, et al. Advertising created & continues to drive the menthol tobacco market: methods used by the industry to target youth. Women, & Black Americans. SRITA Paper; 2022.
19. Barksdale A. Overcoming barriers of distrust. Fam Pract Manag. 2022;29(2):40.
20. Jaiswal J, Halkitis PN. Towards a more inclusive and dynamic understanding of medical mistrust informed by science. Behav Med. 2019;45(2):79–85.
21. Fiala MA. Discrimination, medical mistrust, and delaying cancer screenings and other medical care. JCO Oncol Pract. 2023;19(11).
22. Institute of Medicine of The National Academies. Chapter 2: Sharing clinical trial data: maximizing benefits, minimizing risk. In: Guiding principles for sharing clinical trial data.
23. Alarcón Garavito GA, Gilchrist K, Ciurtin C, Khanna S, Chambers P, McNally N, et al. Enablers and barriers of clinical trial participation in adult patients from minority ethnic groups: a systematic review. Trials. 2025;26(1):65.
24. Ndugga N, Pillai D, Published SA. Racial and ethnic disparities in access to medical advancements and technologies. KFF. 2024, February 22. Available at: https://www.kff.org/racial-equity-and-health-policy/issue-brief/racial-and-ethnic-disparities-in-access-to-medical-advancements-and-technologies/. Accessed 17 Feb 2025.
25. Office of the Commissioner. U.S. Food & Drug Administration (USFDA). Diversity action plans to improve enrollment of participants from underrepresented populations in clinical studies. 2024 June. Available at: https://www.fda.gov/regulatory-information/search-fda-guidance-documents/diversity-action-plans-improve-enrollment-participants-underrepresented-populations-clinical-studies. Accessed 2 Apr 2025.
26. Unger JM, Cook E, Tai E, Bleyer A. The role of clinical trial participation in cancer research: barriers, evidence, and strategies. Am Soc Clin Oncol Educ Book. 2016;35:185–98.
27. Samaha NL, Mady LJ, Armache M, Hearn M, Stemme R, Jagsi R, et al. Screening for financial toxicity among patients with cancer: a systematic review. J Am Coll Radiol. 2024;21(9):1380–97.
28. Bhatia S, Landier W, Paskett ED, Peters KB, Merrill JK, Phillips J, et al. Rural-urban disparities in cancer outcomes: opportunities for future research. J Natl Cancer Inst. 2022;114(7):940–52.

29. National Institutes of Health. National Cancer Institute Participate in Cancer Research. 2023. Available at: https://www.cancer.gov/research/participate. Accessed 15 Jan 2025.
30. Rubin EH, Scroggins MJ, Goldberg KB, Beaver JA. Strategies to maximize patient participation in clinical trials. American Society of Clinical Oncology Educational Book; 2017, p. 37.
31. National Institutes of Health. National Institutes of Health (NIH) Clinical Trials and you: for healthcare providers. 2015. Available at: https://www.nih.gov/health-information/nih-clinical-research-trials-you/health-care-providers. Accessed 15 Jan 2025.
32. GO2 for Lung Cancer. GO2 for Lung Cancer: Research. 2025; Available at: https://go2.org/research/. Accessed 17 Jan 2025.

Open Access This chapter is licensed under the terms of the Creative Commons Attribution-NonCommercial 4.0 International License (http://creativecommons.org/licenses/by-nc/4.0/), which permits any noncommercial use, sharing, adaptation, distribution and reproduction in any medium or format, as long as you give appropriate credit to the original author(s) and the source, provide a link to the Creative Commons license and indicate if changes were made.

The images or other third party material in this chapter are included in the chapter's Creative Commons license, unless indicated otherwise in a credit line to the material. If material is not included in the chapter's Creative Commons license and your intended use is not permitted by statutory regulation or exceeds the permitted use, you will need to obtain permission directly from the copyright holder.

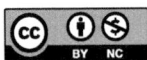

Evaluation and Management of Lung Cancer and Treatment-Related Side Effects and Symptoms

18

Christopher R. Pallas and Kathryn F. Mileham

Contents

Navigation Vignette	229
Introduction	229
Approach to History-Taking	229
Components of the Clinical History	230
Clinical Presentation	232
Diagnostic Considerations	233
Tissue Evaluation and Genomic Profiling	234
Initial Staging Evaluation	234
Key Components of Staging	235
Approaches to the Management of Lung Cancer	236
Treatment of Resectable Disease in Non-small Cell Lung Cancer	236
Treatment of Unresectable Locally Advanced NSCLC	238
Treatment for Advanced or Metastatic Non-small Cell Lung Cancer	239
Small Cell Lung Cancer Treatment Considerations	239
Limited-Stage Small Cell Lung Cancer	239
Extensive-Stage Small Cell Lung Cancer	240
Prevention and Screening	241
Identification of Common Treatment-Related Side Effects by Therapeutic Class	241
Cytotoxic Chemotherapy	242
Immunotherapy	245
Targeted Therapies	246
Radiation Therapy	247
When to Escalate Management Interventions	247

C. R. Pallas (✉) · K. F. Mileham
Department of Solid Tumor Oncology and Investigational Therapeutics,
Levine Cancer Institute, Atrium Health, Charlotte, NC, USA
e-mail: christopher.pallas@atriumhealth.org; kathryn.mileham@atriumhealth.org

© The Author(s) 2026
J. T. Fathi, M. F. Mortman (eds.), *Lung Cancer Navigation and Care*,
https://doi.org/10.1007/978-3-032-02200-4_18

Patient-Centered Approach to Management and Education.................................... 248
Patient Support and Quality of Life.. 249
Long-Term Surveillance for Recurrence... 250
Conclusion.. 250
Key Takeaways... 251
Key Readings and Resources.. 251
References... 251

Abbreviations

AJCC	American Joint Committee on Cancer
ALK	Anaplastic lymphoma kinase
ANC	Absolute neutrophil count
BiTE	Bispecific T cell engager
BMP	Basic metabolic panel
C. Diff	Clostridioides difficile
CBC	Complete blood count
CBT	Cognitive behavioral therapy
CT	Computed tomography
EBUS	Endobronchial ultrasound
ECOG	Eastern Cooperative Oncology Group
EGFR	Epidermal growth factor receptor
EKG	Electrocardiogram
ESAs	Erythropoiesis-stimulating agents
EUS	Endoscopic ultrasound
FDG	Fluorodeoxyglucose
G-CSF	Granulocyte colony-stimulating factor
ILD	Interstitial lung disease
irAEs	Immune-related adverse events
KPS	Karnofsky Performance Status
LDCT	Low-dose computed tomography
LFTs	Liver function tests
MRI	Magnetic resonance imaging
NSCLC	Non-small cell lung cancer
PCI	Prophylactic cranial irradiation
PD-L1	Programmed death-ligand 1 (a protein expressed on the surface of the tumor cells and immune cells)
PET	Positron emission tomography
SCLC	Small cell lung cancer
SVC	Superior vena cava
VALG	Veterans Administration Lung Cancer Study Group
VEGF	Vascular endothelial growth factor

Navigation Vignette

Ms. J., a 62-year-old female who formerly smoked cigarettes, presented with a persistent cough and unintentional weight loss over 2 months. Imaging revealed a right upper lobe lung mass and liver lesions. A biopsy confirmed metastatic non-small cell lung cancer (adenocarcinoma). Staging brain MRI was negative for metastasis. A patient navigator was introduced to Ms. J. as she began her diagnostic workup, assisting her by setting up appointments, advocating for testing, and helping to educate her throughout the process.

Her initial oncology consultation emphasized biomarker testing, including broad molecular profiling and PD-L1 testing. The tumor PD-L1 expression was low at 1%, and no driver mutation was identified. She began combination chemotherapy and immunotherapy with carboplatin, pemetrexed, and pembrolizumab, accompanied by an early referral to palliative care.

Ms. J. encountered challenges, including arranging transportation for appointments. Her navigator coordinated transportation services and connected her with financial assistance resources. During a routine phone check-in, Ms. J. reported worsening shortness of breath and a nonproductive cough. The navigator alerted her oncologist, which led to imaging that revealed pneumonitis. Prompt initiation of prednisone therapy resolved her symptoms, and follow-up scans demonstrated the resolution of the inflammatory changes.

Introduction

Lung cancer is the leading cause of cancer-related death worldwide, with significant associated morbidity [1]. The management of lung cancer requires a comprehensive and multidisciplinary approach across the disease spectrum, from early diagnosis and survivorship care to advanced disease and therapeutic interventions [2, 3]. Patient navigation has emerged as an essential strategy for ensuring timely patient access to the full continuum of cancer care from screening to detection, diagnosis, treatment, and beyond. This chapter aims to provide patient navigators and allied healthcare professionals with a broad overview of the essential steps in lung cancer evaluation, therapeutic approaches, management of treatment-related side effects, and strategies to improve patient quality of life.

Approach to History-Taking

History-taking should be patient-centered and empathetic, as patients may experience significant anxiety related to potential diagnoses. Open-ended questions allow patients to elaborate on their symptoms and concerns. Providers should follow up with targeted questions to refine the clinical picture. Incorporating active listening, empathy, and clear communication helps foster trust with the patient, which is important as patients and their care providers navigate the diagnostic and treatment journey [4].

When lung cancer is suspected, a thorough clinical history is essential. While there are no specific symptoms that are pathognomonic for lung cancer, most patients will present at an advanced stage and with symptomatic disease, highlighting the need to identify risk factors for disease progression [5]. A cancer-specific social history should investigate deeper into aspects of the patient's lifestyle that could influence the body's performance while undergoing treatment. For instance, understanding the patient's daily routine provides valuable insight into the potential impact of cancer-directed therapies.

Traditional questions about tobacco, alcohol, and recreational drug use remain important. Notably, patients may experience feelings of self-blame related to lifestyle choices. Approaching these conversations with empathy rather than judgment helps create a supportive environment and acknowledges the emotional challenges the patient may be facing [4]. This information may provide an opportunity for cessation assistance.

Components of the Clinical History

The components of the clinical history should include the following:

Patient Demographics

Age and sex at birth can be helpful. The incidence of lung cancer rises significantly with age. While men have historically had a higher incidence of lung cancer, the rate in women is decreasing at a slower rate compared to males [6]. Ethnicity and socioeconomic status may also help assess for disparities, impact access to care, and play a role in outcomes [7]. Understanding these demographic variables helps providers identify high-risk patients and address potential health inequities.

Symptomatology

Care should be taken to document the onset, duration, and severity of symptoms, which may provide diagnostic clues and aid in differentiating types of lung cancer or other pulmonary conditions. Respiratory symptoms such as persistent cough, hemoptysis (coughing up blood), dyspnea (shortness of breath), and chest pain may be encountered in both non-small cell lung cancer (NSCLC) and small cell lung cancer (SCLC). However, the rapid onset of symptoms over weeks would favor possible small cell lung cancer and the need for an expedited evaluation. Constitutional symptoms, including unexplained weight loss, anorexia, muscle weakness, and fatigue, may suggest more advanced disease or an underlying paraneoplastic syndrome. Organ-specific symptoms of bone pain or headaches may also be suggestive of underlying metastatic disease.

Providers must remain vigilant for potential oncologic emergencies [2]. For example, superior vena cava syndrome may present with facial and neck swelling related to tumor compression of the superior vena cava (SVC), or the development of fever with change in sputum production is indicative of associated infection related to obstruction from a tumor. Identifying such emergencies early is crucial to prevent life-threatening complications and improve patient outcomes.

Medical History

Obtaining a comprehensive medical history can reveal conditions that predispose patients to lung cancer or complicate its management. Preexisting medical conditions such as chronic obstructive pulmonary disease and interstitial lung disease (ILD) are independent risk factors for lung cancer [3]. A history of a growing lung nodule should increase suspicion for the development of malignancy. A prior history of malignancy raises the question of secondary lung cancer or metastatic disease. Cardiovascular disease and the need for anticoagulation may be a complicating factor when considering surgical evaluation and should be documented.

Tobacco History

Current or prior smoking remains the single most important risk factor for all types of lung cancer [8]. Counseling and assistance with tobacco cessation should be addressed at each visit, as active tobacco leads to reduced treatment efficacy, increased recurrence rates, and worse prognosis [9, 10]. Secondhand smoke should also be assessed with an increased risk of developing lung cancer by 20–30% [11]. Similar to active smoking, the risk of developing lung cancer rises with both the duration and intensity of exposure to secondhand smoke. Notably, the absence of a smoking history does not exclude the possibility of lung cancer, particularly as the incidence of lung cancer in nonsmokers is rising. This trend is often seen in younger patients, more often female than male, and more likely to be associated with driver mutations, such as EGFR or ALK alterations, which may guide the use of targeted therapies [12]. Recognizing this subgroup is critical for ensuring accurate diagnosis and appropriate evaluation and management.

Occupational and Environmental Exposures

While tobacco use remains the most common risk factor for lung cancer, other risk factors can cause changes in the lung cells, leading to abnormal cell growth and cancer. Environmental factors may increase the risk of lung cancer, with radon gas exposure as the leading cause among people who do not smoke. Occupational exposure to carcinogens should also be addressed. There is usually a lag period of 10–30 years from initial exposure to development of lung cancer [13].

Performance Status

The assessment of functional ability using the validated scales of the Eastern Cooperative Oncology Group (ECOG) or Karnofsky Performance Status (KPS) is essential to document each visit. Measuring patients' capacity to perform daily activities and care for themselves offers insight into their overall fitness for treatment and the ability to track response or toxicity to therapy [14]. Recognizing patients with compromised performance status underscores the importance of a multidisciplinary approach that includes evaluating the need for physical or occupational rehabilitation, nutritional support, or psychosocial care.

Psychosocial and Other Lifestyle Factors

A comprehensive history should include psychosocial and lifestyle factors. Understanding a patient's background, mental health, work commitments, literacy and language, caregiver responsibilities, and support systems helps healthcare providers tailor treatment plans and supportive measures to better meet the patient's unique needs. Moreover, this helps to identify potential barriers to care, such as transportation challenges, mistrust in healthcare, or financial difficulties. If recognized, patients should be referred for counseling or social services [7]. Lifestyle details, including exercise habits and dietary patterns, provide additional context regarding a patient's fitness and disease burden.

Clinical Presentation

Unfortunately, many cases of lung cancer are diagnosed at advanced stages, with metastatic disease being common at presentation, highlighting the significance of screening to identify the disease earlier when it may be more amenable to curative treatment. Patients with lung cancer typically present with symptomatic disease, which may provide important diagnostic clues.

Signs and symptoms of lung cancer arise from various mechanisms, including local tumor growth, invasion into surrounding structures, regional lymphatic spread, distant metastases, or the effects of paraneoplastic syndromes. Medical emergencies such as hypercalcemia, syndrome of inappropriate antidiuretic hormone secretion, tumor lysis syndrome, spinal cord compression, brain metastases with increased intracranial pressure, SVC syndrome, and malignant pericardial effusion can occur and require immediate intervention [5].

Local primary tumor growth may cause respiratory symptoms such as cough from endobronchial irritation or compression, hemoptysis from central or cavitary lesions, wheezing due to partially obstructed airways, fever, and dyspnea resulting from bronchial obstruction, pneumonia, or pleural effusion.

When the primary tumor invades adjacent structures or spreads regionally, symptoms may include hoarseness from left vocal cord paralysis caused by recurrent laryngeal nerve involvement, hemidiaphragm elevation due to phrenic nerve compression, dysphagia from esophageal compression, chest pain related to pleural or chest wall involvement, and life-threatening conditions like SVC syndrome or pericardial effusion with tamponade. Cervical or supraclavicular lymph node enlargement may also be present, providing a visible clue to the underlying disease.

Extrathoracic metastases produce varied symptoms depending on the site of involvement. Brain metastases may manifest as headaches, focal neurological deficits, confusion, slurred speech, or gait instability, and leptomeningeal carcinomatosis (cancer cells spread to the thin layers covering the brain and spinal cord) can cause cranial nerve palsies, diplopia, or radicular back pain. Adrenal metastases may present with mid-back or flank pain and tenderness, and liver metastases can lead to right upper quadrant pain, jaundice, fatigue, or hepatomegaly. Bone metastases frequently cause localized pain and may result in spinal cord compression, presenting as back pain, muscle weakness, numbness, or loss of bowel and bladder control. Systemic symptoms such as anorexia, cachexia, and fatigue reflect the widespread effects of advanced disease.

Diagnostic Considerations

The diagnostic and staging evaluation of lung cancer aims to gather sufficient clinical, radiographic, and tissue information to guide timely treatment decisions. The process should involve a multidisciplinary team with the preferred approach considering individual patient characteristics, the size and location of the tumor, the presence of mediastinal or distant metastases, and the available local expertise and resources [2, 3].

Lung cancer may initially be suspected and detected on chest imaging by either chest X-ray or CT scan. All current chest imaging should be compared to prior scans, as measurable growth in any nodule or mass raises suspicion for underlying malignancy. However, tissue biopsy remains the gold standard for diagnosis, with histologic and molecular analyses guiding diagnosis and treatment decisions. Depending on the size, location, and stage for disease isolated to the chest, biopsy through one of the following procedures is typically pursued: bronchoscopy with or without endobronchial ultrasound and biopsy, image-guided biopsy, or surgical biopsy [15].

Concomitant staging during diagnostic workup (see Chaps. 8 and 12) is often beneficial, particularly when malignancy is strongly suspected, as it avoids unnecessary delays in treatment planning. For patients with early-stage disease, surgical options may proceed without preoperative biopsy in cases of high clinical suspicion. Intraoperative biopsy or VATS wedge resection can confirm malignancy, leading to subsequent definitive resection. Central masses are typically biopsied via bronchoscopy, while peripheral lesions may be more amenable to CT-guided biopsy. For suspected nodal involvement, methods like endobronchial ultrasound (EBUS) or mediastinoscopy (lymph node sampling) are employed. The finding of a pleural effusion warrants thoracentesis with cytologic evaluation and should be prioritized, as a positive result (cancer cells present in the pleural fluid) indicates stage IV disease. Similarly, biopsy of distant metastases (growths outside the lung that could represent cancer spread) is preferred, when possible, since it provides the most advanced stage information [15]. Patients with advanced disease benefit from tailored systemic therapies informed by molecular profiling (biomarker testing) and staging results.

Tissue Evaluation and Genomic Profiling

Tissue sampling is essential for lung cancer diagnosis. The evaluation involves histologic, immunophenotypic, and genomic profiling (see Chap. 6). Histology distinguishes between the four most common subtypes of lung cancer (adenocarcinoma, squamous cell carcinoma, large cell carcinoma [collectively referred to as NSCLC], and SCLC) [3].

Molecular profiling has transformed lung cancer care. Testing for actionable genomic alterations, preferably with broad molecular profiling and PD-L1 status, is necessary for treatment determination in NSCLC when a systemic agent, whether immunotherapy or targeted therapy, is being considered. While blood-based genomic testing offers a less invasive alternative, its limitations (possibility for false negatives) necessitate confirmatory tissue testing when negative [15] (see Chap. 14).

Initial Staging Evaluation

Lung cancer staging plays a vital role in guiding treatment decisions and predicting patient outcomes. The American Joint Committee on Cancer (AJCC) criteria provide a standardized system for classification encompassing three key components: the size and extent of the primary tumor (T), lymph node involvement (N), and the presence of distant metastases (M) [16]. Based on these components, lung cancer can be classified into four different stages, from I (early disease) to IV (metastatic). While AJCC criteria stage SCLC, terminology from the Veterans Administration Lung Cancer Study Group (VALG) staging system is often referenced, using limited-stage disease (involvement restricted to ipsilateral hemothorax with no extrathoracic metastases and can be encompassed within safe radiation treatment plan) or extensive stage disease (any disease beyond ipsilateral hemothorax, including malignant pleural or pericardial effusion or hematogenous metastases) [17]. Ultimately, staging evaluates the extent of disease to determine treatment options and prognostic factors.

Key Components of Staging

Systemic Evaluation

Comprehensive history and physical examination, including performance status and weight loss assessment, may not impact the actual TNM staging yet are prognostic indicators. Laboratory tests, including complete blood count (CBC), basic metabolic panel (BMP), and liver function tests (LFTs), provide baseline data and may reveal evidence of metastatic involvement.

Mediastinal Evaluation

Pathologic assessment of mediastinal lymph nodes is critical, particularly for enlarged nodes on imaging or those positive on positron emission tomography (PET) scans. EBUS/EUS and mediastinoscopy remain gold standards for confirming nodal metastases, as PET imaging alone can yield false-positive or false-negative results.

Pleural Evaluation

Malignant pleural effusions are considered metastatic disease and preclude curative options. Single thoracentesis has limited sensitivity and repeat procedures or thoracoscopic evaluation may be necessary.

Metastatic Disease Evaluation

Biopsy of suspected distant disease is required to confirm metastatic involvement. PET/CT is particularly useful in identifying clinically unsuspected metastases. Radiographically, contrasted CT scans of the chest and abdomen (lymph nodes, liver, adrenal glands), PET/CT, and brain MRI are key elements to staging.

Please refer to Table 18.1 for staging evaluation in lung cancer.

Table 18.1 Staging evaluation

All patients
Biopsy with tissue diagnosis
History and physical: Include performance status and weight loss
Labs: CBC, BMP, LFTs
Imaging: CT scan of the chest and upper abdomen with IV contrast (including liver and bilateral adrenal glands) and PET/CT, especially if consideration of curative intent therapy (assess mediastinum and for distant disease)
Brain imaging: Any patient with neurologic symptoms and all patients with stage II–IV NSCLC (stage IB optional), and all patients with SCLC
Supportive: Smoking cessation guidance, counseling, pharmacotherapy
Limited-stage or early-stage disease (assess for surgical candidacy)
Pulmonary function testing and pathologic mediastinal lymph node evaluation

Approaches to the Management of Lung Cancer

The treatment of lung cancer is highly nuanced, depending on the histologic subtype, stage at diagnosis, and molecular profile. Therapeutic approaches include surgery, radiation therapy, systemic therapies (such as chemotherapy, immunotherapy, and targeted therapy), and frequently, a combination of these modalities. Treatment plans should be tailored to the individual patient for optimal outcomes, incorporating evidence-based strategies and a multidisciplinary approach. Participation in clinical trials is encouraged at every stage of lung cancer management.

Treatment of Resectable Disease in Non-small Cell Lung Cancer

Surgical Treatment

Surgery remains the cornerstone for treatment of patients with resectable NSCLC, particularly stages I–IIIA. Surgical approaches include lobectomy, segmentectomy, or pneumonectomy with mediastinal lymph node dissection for accurate staging. Lobectomy is typically preferred if the patient can tolerate the procedure due to its balance of efficacy and safety (see Chap. 13). For patients with early-stage NSCLC who are not surgical candidates, definitive radiation therapy is an alternative [3].

In patients with NSCLC, approximately 25–30% of patients will present with potentially curable and resectable disease [18]. Unfortunately, many patients will have tumor recurrence within 5 years after surgery, posing a significant clinical challenge due to the propensity for distant metastasis and early relapse. For decades, treatment of early-stage NSCLC has remained largely unchanged. Adjuvant platinum-based doublet chemotherapy has been the standard of care for completely resected higher-risk early-stage NSCLC (tumor ≥4 cm or lymph node positive) with the goal to treat microscopic metastases (micrometastasis) and prevent recurrence.

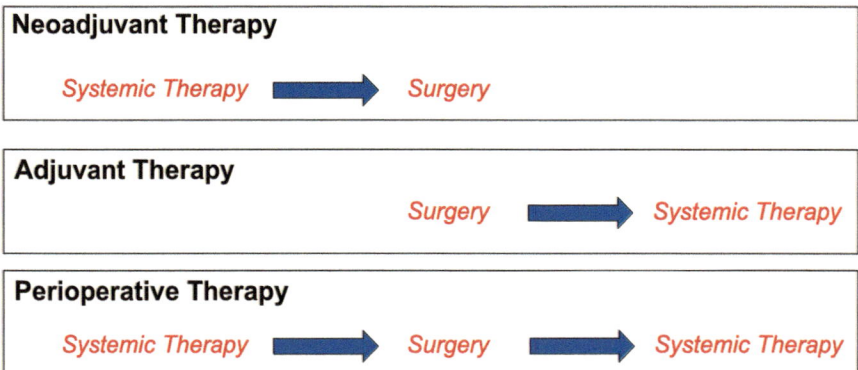

Fig. 18.1 Approaches in resectable NSCLC (tumor ≥4 cm or lymph node positive)

However, the 5-year survival rates with adjuvant chemotherapy are ~4–5% higher than with observation, indicating a large unmet need for improvement [19].

Immunotherapy and targeted therapies have revolutionized the management of advanced and metastatic NSCLC, leading to their consideration in earlier stages of the disease. The study of new adjuvant, neoadjuvant, and perioperative systemic strategies has demonstrated encouraging results and led to multiple recent FDA approvals (Fig. 18.1).

Adjuvant Therapy

Following surgery, adjuvant therapy is used to reduce recurrence risk and improve patient survival. Platinum-based chemotherapy is standard of care for stage II–III disease. More recent advances include the use of immunotherapy for 1 year after platinum-based chemotherapy (atezolizumab for PD-L1-positive tumors or pembrolizumab), osimertinib for 3 years after optional adjuvant chemotherapy in EGFR-mutant tumors, and alectinib for 2 years without adjuvant chemotherapy in ALK-positive tumors [3].

Neoadjuvant Therapy

Preoperative therapy aims to reduce tumor burden, allow a more complete surgical resection, and treat micrometastasis that may have already spread, thereby potentially improving patient survival rates. There is the additional benefit of pathologic response evaluation, which provides information on the tumor's response to treatment by examining the resected tissue after surgery. Neoadjuvant chemotherapy plus immunotherapy followed by surgery should be considered in stage II–III NSCLC (tumor ≥4 cm or lymph node positive) [3].

Perioperative Therapy

Neoadjuvant chemotherapy plus immunotherapy followed by surgery and adjuvant therapy should be considered in stage II–III NSCLC (tumor ≥4 cm or lymph node positive). This approach provides a combination of neoadjuvant and adjuvant treatments with the advantage of both approaches [3].

Importantly, before initiating a neoadjuvant or perioperative treatment approach, the patient should be evaluated by a thoracic surgeon to confirm the tumor is resectable at diagnosis. This means the tumor is considered operable without evidence of contraindications. Establishing resectability upfront ensures that the treatment plan, including preoperative systemic therapy, is being pursued with the clear goal of proceeding to curative-intent surgery, thereby avoiding unnecessary delays or exposure to ineffective interventions. Multidisciplinary discussion is essential to align treatment goals, assess surgical risk, and determine the optimal sequence of therapy to maximize long-term outcomes.

Treatment of Unresectable Locally Advanced NSCLC

For patients with unresectable stage III NSCLC, the goal of therapy remains curative intent utilizing a multimodal approach. Multidisciplinary evaluation is recommended for all patients.

Definitive Chemoradiation

The use of chemotherapy and radiation at the same time (concurrent chemoradiation) with platinum-based chemotherapy is the standard treatment for unresectable stage III disease and superior to radiation alone or chemotherapy for two to four cycles followed by radiation therapy (sequential chemoradiation) [3].

Consolidation Immunotherapy

The addition of the immunotherapy agent, durvalumab, after chemotherapy and radiation is recommended for non-EGFR-mutated tumors after being shown to help people live longer and significantly reduce the chance of lung cancer spreading [20].

Targeted Therapy

Treatment with osimertinib after chemoradiation reduced the risk of progression or death by 84% compared to placebo for EGFR-mutated, unresectable stage III NSCLC. For patients with tumors containing EGFR exon 19 deletion or exon 21

L858R mutation, osimertinib should be offered over durvalumab, as these malignancies are typically less responsive to immunotherapy [21].

Treatment for Advanced or Metastatic Non-small Cell Lung Cancer

For patients with stage IV NSCLC, systemic therapy guided by biomarker testing is the primary approach with a palliative intent focused on improving survival and quality of life (see Chap. 15). Early integration of palliative care should be offered with a focus on collaborative discussions and shared decision-making with the patient, family, and caregivers to align treatment goals, develop care plans, and prioritize quality of life [22].

The choice of systemic therapy between chemotherapy, immunotherapy, targeted therapy, or a combination of these approaches is guided by histology, programmed death ligand 1 (PD-L1) status, and comprehensive molecular testing. Broad molecular profiling with the goal of identifying driver mutations, for which effective drugs may already be available, should be performed in metastatic adenocarcinoma and considered for squamous cell carcinoma. Molecular testing includes assessment for genomic alterations in EGFR, ALK, KRAS, ROS1, BRAF, NTRK1/2/3, METex 14 skipping, RET, NRG1, ERBB2 (HER2), and HER2 (immunohistochemistry) [3, 15].

Palliative radiation may be considered for symptomatic metastasis and brain metastasis. In cases with oligometastatic disease, defined by a limited number of metastases in a limited number of organ sites, a more definitive approach with the incorporation of surgery or radiation therapy may be considered in highly selected patients after multidisciplinary care review [3].

Small Cell Lung Cancer Treatment Considerations

The management of SCLC is based on stage but more simply determined by extent and distribution of disease (see Chap. 16).

Limited-Stage Small Cell Lung Cancer

The goal is curative in intent for disease confined to one hemithorax (one side of the chest) and amenable to a single radiation field.

Surgical Resection

While uncommon, in clinical stage I-IIA disease (T1-2, N0, M0), surgical resection with lobectomy and mediastinal lymph node dissection is preferred [17].

Definitive Chemoradiation

Most patients' standard of care is combining cisplatin (or carboplatin if not a cisplatin candidate) with etoposide and thoracic radiation therapy [17].

Consolidation Immunotherapy

In patients without disease progression following definitive chemoradiation, 2 years of durvalumab treatment significantly improves both overall survival and progression-free survival compared to placebo. Durvalumab should be considered after chemoradiotherapy [23].

Prophylactic Cranial Irradiation

For patients achieving a complete or partial response following primary treatment, prophylactic cranial irradiation (PCI) is considered with the intent to eliminate potential microscopic cancer cells that may have spread to the brain and thus reduce the risk of brain metastases development. If planned, PCI should be completed prior to initiation of durvalumab. Regardless of PCI status, all patients should have brain MRI surveillance [17].

Extensive-Stage Small Cell Lung Cancer

For disease that has spread beyond one hemithorax, treatment is palliative, focusing on prolonging life and balancing quality of life. Despite advancements in systemic therapy, the prognosis remains poor and clinical trial participation is encouraged.

Systemic Chemoimmunotherapy

Platinum-based chemotherapy combined with etoposide and an immune checkpoint inhibitor (atezolizumab or durvalumab) is the standard first-line treatment [24, 25]. Treatment is given every 21 days for four cycles, although some patients may receive up to six cycles based on response and tolerability. At time of progression, rechallenge of platinum doublet therapy may be considered depending on time from the initial treatment in addition to subsequent line chemotherapy (e.g., topotecan, lurbinectedin) or immunotherapy with tarlatamab [26]. Tarlatamab is a type of immunotherapy known as a bispecific T cell engager (BiTE). Due to the risk of serious side effects such as cytokine release syndrome and nervous system problems, close monitoring in a healthcare setting is expected for about 24 h after the first two infusions and for at least several hours after later treatments.

Maintenance Immunotherapy

Immunotherapy is continued after completion of four to six cycles of chemoimmunotherapy until dose-limiting toxicity, patient preference, or disease progression.

Radiation Therapy

While systemic therapy is the primary treatment modality, radiation therapy has a potential role in the management of extensive-stage SCLC. For patients who achieve a complete or partial response following initial systemic therapy, consolidative thoracic radiation and PCI may be considered to reduce thoracic recurrences and risk of brain metastases, respectively. MRI brain surveillance is an alternative to PCI, and the decision should be individualized with radiation oncology involvement. Palliative radiation may also be employed to alleviate symptoms caused by localized disease progression, such as shortness of breath from bronchial obstruction, pain from bone metastases, or management of brain metastases or spinal cord compression. The goal in this setting is to provide rapid symptom relief and improve quality of life [17].

Prevention and Screening

The therapeutic landscape for lung cancer continues to evolve with more personalized and effective treatment strategies. While these advancements have significantly improved outcomes for many patients, early detection is essential to improved outcomes. Lung cancer screening with low-dose CT scans has been shown to reduce mortality by detecting lung cancer at an earlier and more curable stage [27]. For patients aged 50–80 years and who have a smoking history of 20 or more pack-years, screening for lung cancer with annual low-dose computed tomography (LDCT) scan of the chest is recommended [28] (see Chap. 9). Moreover, continued tobacco use has multiple adverse effects on lung cancer outcomes, and smoking cessation interventions should be incorporated into visits for those with an active history of smoking [3] (see Chap. 10 for more information on therapeutic approaches to smoking cessation). Expanding access to screening programs and increasing awareness among high-risk populations is critical to achieving better long-term outcomes and reducing the burden of this disease [7].

Identification of Common Treatment-Related Side Effects by Therapeutic Class

The side effects of systemic therapy are of particular concern due to the potential negative effects on quality of life for patients both during and after treatment. Toxicities vary depending on the therapeutic regimen.

Cytotoxic Chemotherapy

Chemotherapy remains a cornerstone of lung cancer treatment. Management strategies focus on proactive and supportive care.

Myelosuppression

Chemotherapy-induced bone marrow suppression can cause hematologic toxicity, including anemia leading to fatigue, neutropenia with an increased risk of infection, and thrombocytopenia with risk of bleeding and bruising.

Neutropenia

Fever in neutropenic patients requires urgent and immediate evaluation. Febrile neutropenia is defined as an absolute neutrophil count (ANC) of less than 500–1000/mm^3 and is considered a medical emergency with simultaneous infectious evaluation and broad-spectrum antibiotics recommended. Administration of granulocyte colony-stimulating factor (G-CSF), such as filgrastim or pegfilgrastim, may be considered as part of the treatment for (therapeutic) or prevention of (prophylactic) febrile neutropenia. G-CSF should only be used prophylactically when the risk of febrile neutropenia is at least 20%. Bone pain can be seen with the use of G-CSF. Naproxen and similar nonsteroidal anti-inflammatory drugs or loratadine can be used for 5–7 days after G-CSF administration to help alleviate this pain. For patients who are receiving palliative systemic therapy, alternative chemotherapy or dose reductions may be preferred over the addition of G-CSF [29].

Anemia and Thrombocytopenia

Further evaluation may be helpful depending on the clinical history and chemotherapy used. This can involve assessment for associated hemolysis (breakdown of red blood cells), bleeding, or nutritional deficiencies (e.g., iron, vitamin B12, and folate), which should be repleted if found. Erythropoiesis-stimulating agents (ESAs) may be considered in anemic patients who are symptomatic and on palliative therapy for an incurable malignancy. However, benefits should be weighed against the risks of venous thromboembolism, reduced survival, and burdens of therapy. In severe cases, supportive care with red blood cells or platelet transfusions may be performed [30].

Gastrointestinal Symptoms

Nausea, vomiting, and diarrhea are common side effects of many chemotherapies, and severity can vary greatly between individuals. Symptoms may begin shortly following treatment (acute) or occur starting more than 24 h after treatment (delayed). With proactive therapy and monitoring, nausea and vomiting can usually be prevented or managed effectively.

Management
- Administration of antiemetics is the primary management of nausea and vomiting. Depending on the emetogenic potential of the anticancer agent(s), the prophylactic use of antiemetics, such as ondansetron, aprepitant, and olanzapine, may be considered [31].
- Anticipatory nausea and vomiting should be considered in patients who have previously received therapy treatment and experience symptoms shortly before the next infusion or upon thinking about an upcoming treatment. Behavioral treatment techniques, such as systematic desensitization, have been shown to be effective, and medications like benzodiazepines may be used. However, the most effective way to avoid development is to ensure adequate prophylaxis from the very first exposure to therapy [32].
- Diarrhea may be managed with loperamide to avoid volume depletion [33]. When loperamide is ineffective, diphenoxylate atropine ("Lomotil") or other agents may be considered. For patients at risk for infection and recent antibiotic exposure, evaluation to rule out infections like Clostridioides difficile (C. diff) should be performed before using antidiarrheal.

Mucositis

Inflammation and ulceration of the mucous membranes in the mouth and digestive tract can cause pain and difficulty eating.

Management
- Encourage patients on oral hygiene with soft-bristle toothbrushes and nonalcoholic mouthwashes.
- Dietary modifications, with soft and non-irritating foods, can reduce discomfort.
- Symptom management with topical analgesics, including viscous lidocaine, may be considered [34].

Nephrotoxicity

Nephrotoxicity, particularly with chemotherapy regimens containing cisplatin, can lead to acute kidney injury and be severe.

Management
- Monitoring of renal function (serum creatinine and glomerular filtration).
- Dose adjustment for patients with preexisting renal impairment or consideration of alternative agents with lower nephrotoxic potential, if appropriate.
- For certain regimens, like cisplatin, intensive hydration is required, including adequate pre- and posthydration protocols [35].

Neurotoxicity

Chemotherapy-induced peripheral neuropathy is more common with agents like cisplatin and taxanes (paclitaxel, docetaxel).

Management
- Dose modification may be necessary, or therapy may be discontinued in severe cases. After therapy is discontinued, neurotoxicity is usually at least partially reversible.
- Symptom relief may be achieved with medications, such as gabapentin or duloxetine, exercise therapy, or acupuncture.
- For patients with mobility or balance issues, referral to physical and occupational therapy should be considered [36].

Fatigue

Fatigue is a common symptom in patients and may be due to chemotherapy or the cancer itself.

Management
- Underlying causes such as anemia, sleep disturbances, or depression should be considered and addressed if present.
- Exercise, cognitive behavioral therapy (CBT), mindfulness-based programs, and tai chi or qigong are recommended to reduce the severity of fatigue during cancer treatment. Psychoeducation and American ginseng may also be considered [37].

Anorexia and Weight Loss

Similar to fatigue, appetite suppression and unintentional weight loss may be due to chemotherapy or the cancer itself.

Management
- Nutrition counseling and the involvement of dieticians should be considered. A calorie-dense, high-protein supplementation can be recommended [38].
- Consider appetite stimulants such as olanzapine [39].

Alopecia

Hair loss is a common side effect of many chemotherapies. Alopecia is highly visible and may be a distressing side effect for many patients.

Management
- Inform patients about the likelihood of hair loss and provide resources for wigs.
- Scalp cooling may be considered to reduce the risk of hair loss but is limited by logistical issues, including availability of devices, inconsistent insurance coverage, and the incorporation of use into typical infusion center workflow [40].

Fertility Issues

Cytotoxic chemotherapy can impair fertility in both men and women.

Management
- Counsel patients on the risk of infertility.
- Offer referrals to reproductive specialists as part of a multidisciplinary approach with discussion of fertility preservation options before initiation of treatment, including sperm banking for men and cryopreservation (freezing embryos or eggs) for women [41].

Infusion Reactions

Some individuals may experience infusion-related reactions while receiving chemotherapy. These reactions resemble allergic responses and may include fever, chills, facial flushing, rash, itching, dizziness, wheezing, or difficulty breathing.

Management
- Closely monitoring patients during infusions, especially when using agents associated with high reaction risk, such as taxane chemotherapy (paclitaxel and docetaxel), etoposide, and platinum chemotherapy.
- If a reaction occurs, depending on the severity, the infusion may be paused with the administration of antihistamines, corticosteroids, or epinephrine as needed.
- Slowing the rate of an infusion and premedication with antihistamines or corticosteroids may help reduce the risk in subsequent infusions [42].

Immunotherapy

Immune checkpoint inhibitors, such as PD-1/PD-L1 (e.g., pembrolizumab, durvalumab, cemiplimab, atezolizumab, and nivolumab) or CTLA-4 inhibitors (e.g., ipilimumab), have transformed the treatment of NSCLC and SCLC. However, they can cause immune-related adverse events (irAEs), which may affect any organ system. These drugs function by inhibiting the immune system's natural checks and balances. In some cases, this can lead the immune system to mistakenly attack healthy tissues, potentially causing severe or life-threatening complications. Corticosteroids, such as prednisone, are commonly used for managing irAEs and act as the brakes for the immune system, helping to control overactive immune responses. Doses are tailored to the severity of the reaction with higher doses required for more severe cases. For severe or refractory cases, additional immunosuppressive therapies may be required, and management should involve a multidisciplinary team. Prompt recognition and intervention are key to minimizing complications and ensuring patient safety [43].

Common Immune-Related Adverse Events

Dermatologic
Rash and pruritus are usually first managed with topical corticosteroids or antihistamines. Warning signs of severe dermatologic toxicity include extensive blistering, painful sores, or involvement of large areas of skin, which require prompt evaluation and escalation to systemic corticosteroids and/or specialist referral.

Gastrointestinal
Diarrhea and colitis may require corticosteroids like prednisone for moderate to severe cases, while milder symptoms can be cautiously managed first with hydration, dietary modifications with a lactose-free and low-fiber diet, and close monitoring. Infectious evaluation, including C. diff, should be considered in all cases.

Endocrinopathies
Hypothyroidism and pituitary dysfunction are addressed with hormone replacement. Regular monitoring of thyroid function tests while on immunotherapy is essential for early diagnosis and management.

Pulmonary
Immune-related pneumonitis is a less common but serious adverse reaction. Corticosteroids are the mainstay of treatment, with infliximab or other immunosuppressive agents used in refractory cases.

The choice to rechallenge immunotherapy depends on multiple factors, including the nature and severity of the initial irAE and the degree of responsiveness to immunosuppression. Careful discussion of the risks and benefits of restarting immunotherapy should be performed with patients who are candidates for retreatment.

Targeted Therapies

Targeted therapies for lung cancer, including inhibition of EGFR, ALK, ROS1, BRAF, RET, MET, TRK, HER2, KRAS, and angiogenesis, work differently from standard chemotherapy and are associated with side effects related to their mechanism of action [44] (see Chap. 14). For example, rash and diarrhea are common among EGFR inhibitors. Rashes may be managed with emollients, topical steroids, and oral antibiotics (e.g., doxycycline). Diarrhea may be managed with dietary adjustments and loperamide. The VEGF inhibitors, bevacizumab and ramucirumab, can lead to hypertension, proteinuria, and delayed wound healing. Blood pressure is managed with antihypertensive medications, and patients should be counseled about risk of surgical procedures requiring holding of the drug. Each drug class has a unique side effect profile that should be known by the prescribing team and reviewed with the patient and care provider. Package inserts detail known side effects, monitoring parameters, and dose adjustments.

Rare but serious side effects among some targeted therapies may include QTc prolongation (necessitating EKG monitoring), cardiotoxicity (with baseline echocardiogram at treatment start), ILD/pneumonitis (monitoring for respiratory changes including dry cough and shortness of breath), and mental status changes, such as confusion and mood changes.

Radiation Therapy

Used in both the curative and palliative settings, radiation therapy can cause localized side effects depending on the area treated. Esophagitis is common in thoracic radiation, and management includes soft diets, topical anesthetics, and proton pump inhibitors. Inflammation in the lung from radiation pneumonitis is a serious side effect presenting with shortness of breath, cough, and/or fever and requires corticosteroid treatment [45].

When to Escalate Management Interventions

The escalation of care is necessary when side effects become severe or refractory to initial management, symptoms worsen, or disease progresses. Situations requiring intervention include patients experiencing uncontrolled pain or nausea, significant weight loss, fevers, persistent shortness of breath, psychological distress, new neurologic deficits, or abrupt changes in their condition. Regular monitoring allows healthcare providers to identify issues early and intervene before they progress. Equally important to ensure continuity of care is addressing logistical and psychosocial barriers, such as difficulty with transportation or lack of caregiver support. Clear communication among the care team, structured symptom reporting mechanisms, and regular patient follow-up are essential to guide escalation decisions. These strategies enable timely interventions and help maintain a patient-centered approach while optimizing clinical outcomes and quality of life.

Patient-Centered Approach to Management and Education

Symptom Monitoring and Reporting

Essential for early intervention and improved outcomes is educating patients to monitor and report symptoms promptly. Patients may keep a daily log of symptoms, such as fatigue, pain, nausea, or respiratory changes, noting their severity and frequency. They should be informed about specific symptoms to watch for, including fever, changes in appetite and weight, new or increased pain, or worsening shortness of breath. Clear instructions should be provided on how and when to contact their healthcare team, emphasizing the importance of timely communication to address issues before they escalate.

Self-Management Strategies

Patients should be empowered with self-management strategies to enhance their comfort and quality of life. These may include managing nausea with prescribed antiemetics, eating small but more frequent meals, and staying hydrated. Patients experiencing fatigue may benefit from scheduling activities during times of higher energy. Pain management strategies, including the use of prescribed medications, should be clearly explained. Setting goals to work on can help patients feel more in control of their care.

Lifestyle Modifications

Encouraging lifestyle modifications can improve overall health and treatment outcomes. Patients should be guided to maintain a nutritious diet rich in fruits, vegetables, lean proteins, and whole grains to support their immune system and overall well-being. Smoking cessation is critical for lung cancer patients, as it can improve treatment effectiveness and reduce complications. Moderating alcohol intake, engaging in appropriate physical activity, and maintaining adequate hydration are also beneficial. Stress management techniques such as mindfulness, yoga, or counseling can further support emotional well-being [46].

When to Seek Help

Patients must be provided with well-defined guidelines on when to seek immediate medical attention. Symptoms warranting urgent evaluation include high fever, persistent vomiting, severe or intractable pain, sudden shortness of breath, confusion, or any sudden or concerning changes in their condition. Patients should be advised to report early signs of infection, such as redness, swelling, warmth, or pus around any wound or port site. Providing a list of emergency contact numbers and a plan for accessing care during after-hours or weekends ensures patients feel supported and prepared for any situation.

Patient Support and Quality of Life

The management of lung cancer extends beyond the disease itself and involves comprehensive support to address the physical and emotional challenges patients face.

Supportive Oncology

Early integration of palliative care into the disease-specific therapies for patients with advanced NSCLC has been shown to significantly improve both quality of life and mood and prolong patient survival [22]. Palliative care teams work collaboratively with oncology providers to enhance well-being throughout the cancer journey. Effective symptom management, including pain control, fatigue reduction, and addressing treatment-related side effects, is critical. Symptom palliation may include pain management with use of opioids, nerve blocks, or short courses of palliative radiation therapy. Establishing clear goals of care through shared decision-making, including discussions about hospice services when appropriate, ensures that treatment aligns with the patient's values, preferences, and overall well-being [47].

Psychological Support

For patients and their families, a diagnosis of lung cancer can be emotionally overwhelming. Counseling services with psychology can aid in coping with anxiety, depression, and stress associated with a cancer diagnosis and treatment. Tailored interventions like CBT and mindfulness-based practices may be considered [46]. Patients often rely on family and friends at home for caregiving needs, including help with activities of daily living and instrumental activities of daily living (e.g., managing finances and medications, food preparation, and housekeeping). Caregivers for a loved one are at risk for significant emotional, physical, and financial stress. Attention should be paid to the patient and their family for psychological, spiritual, and social needs. Open communication should be encouraged regarding emotional needs with healthcare providers [48].

Social Support

Social workers can assist with practical challenges, including financial concerns, navigating insurance, and transportation to medical appointments [47]. Peer support groups from cancer survivors can provide encouragement and valuable insights. A strong network of family and friends is important to patient resilience.

Nutritional Support

Patients and caregivers should be educated on the patient's condition, potential for cancer, anorexia, and risk of treatment side effects on appetite. A consultation with a registered dietitian may be considered for nutritional counseling to optimize energy and overall health [38]. Medications, including olanzapine, may be considered for chemotherapy-associated anorexia [49].

Rehabilitation and Survivorship

Survivorship programs address long-term effects of cancer and its treatment. Patients are guided in reintegration into daily activities and work with programs that often include ongoing monitoring for late effects of treatment and support for managing chronic conditions. Rehabilitation programs aim to help patients regain physical strength, mobility, and confidence, focusing on exercise regimens tailored to individual capabilities [50] (see Chap. 20).

Long-Term Surveillance for Recurrence

Lung cancer survivors are at risk for recurrence of their primary (original) cancer and the development of second primary lung cancers, particularly those related to smoking. Surveillance is vital for survivors to detect such malignancies at an early stage. Depending on the stage and histologic subtype, a history, physical examination, and chest computed tomography (CT), including the adrenals, are guideline recommended every 3–6 months for at least the first 2 years to evaluate for recurrence and every 6–12 months for up to 5 years. Annual low-dose CT screening is reasonable after 5 years due to risk of recurrence. In patients with SCLC, a brain MRI is routinely performed every 3 months during the first year, then every 6 months for the second year for surveillance for new or recurrent brain metastases (regardless of PCI status). FDG-PET/CT is not routinely warranted in surveillance, and chest X-ray is insufficient [51].

Conclusion

The field of thoracic oncology has undergone remarkable advancements, transforming the diagnosis and treatment of lung cancer. Patient outcomes have improved significantly in the last decade, from lung cancer screening to the introduction of innovative therapeutic options, including immune checkpoint inhibition and personalized targeted therapies for oncogene-driven tumors. The management of lung cancer requires a multidisciplinary approach that integrates these recent advances. By emphasizing patient-centered care and fostering open communication, providers can ensure that patients receive comprehensive and individualized management.

Key Takeaways

- A multidisciplinary approach plays a crucial role in the management of lung cancer and is essential to optimal outcomes.
- Remember lung cancer screening, especially with the emergence of exciting new treatment approaches for our patients with early-stage lung cancer.
- Broad molecular profiling and immune testing play a pivotal role in guiding personalized treatment strategies in lung cancer.
- Educating patients about their diagnosis, treatment options, and potential side effects is fundamental to empowering the patient in their cancer journey.
- The proactive management of treatment-related side effects enhances patient quality of life, and early involvement of palliative care is critical to addressing symptom burden and supporting patients and their families through the cancer continuum.

Key Readings and Resources

- American Cancer Society lung cancer guide [52].
- National Comprehensive Cancer Network (NCCN) guidelines for lung cancer [53, 54].
- American Society of Clinical Oncology (ASCO) guidelines for thoracic oncology and supportive care and treatment-related issues [55].

Conflict of Interests Christopher Pallas reports no conflicts of interest.
Kathryn Mileham discloses receiving consultant honoraria from AstraZeneca, Bayer, Genentech, Merck, Nuvation Bio, and Takeda.

References

1. Bray F, Laversanne M, Sung H, Ferlay J, Siegel RL, Soerjomataram I, et al. Global cancer statistics 2022: GLOBOCAN estimates of incidence and mortality worldwide for 36 cancers in 185 countries. CA Cancer J Clin. 2024 May;74(3):229–63.
2. Kim J, Lee H, Huang BW. Lung cancer: diagnosis, treatment principles, and screening. Am Fam Physician. 2022;105(5):487–94.
3. Hendriks LEL, Remon J, Faivre-Finn C, Garassino MC, Heymach JV, Kerr KM, et al. Non-small-cell lung cancer. Nat Rev Dis Primers. 2024;10:71.
4. Rosenzweig MQ, Gardner D, Griffith B. The history and physical in cancer care: a primer for the oncology advanced practitioner. J Adv Pract Oncol. 2014;5(4):262–8.

5. Shim J, Brindle L, Simon M, George S. A systematic review of symptomatic diagnosis of lung cancer. Fam Pract. 2014 Apr;31(2):137–48.
6. MacRosty CR, Rivera MP. Lung cancer in women: a modern epidemic. Clin Chest Med. 2020;41(1):53–65.
7. Kearney L, Nguyen T, Steiling K. Disparities across the continuum of lung cancer care: a review of recent literature, vol. 30. Current Opinion in Pulmonary Medicine. Lippincott Williams and Wilkins; 2024. p. 359–67.
8. Barta JA, Powell CA, Wisnivesky JP. Global epidemiology of lung cancer, vol. 85. Annals of Global Health. Ubiquity Press; 2019.
9. Cinciripini PM, Kypriotakis G, Blalock JA, Karam-Hage M, Beneventi DM, Robinson JD, et al. Survival outcomes of an early intervention smoking cessation treatment after a cancer diagnosis. JAMA Oncol. 2024;10(12):1689.
10. Sheikh M, Mukeriya A, Shangina O, Brennan P, Zaridze D. Postdiagnosis smoking cessation and reduced risk for lung cancer progression and mortality. Ann Intern Med. 2021 Sep;174(9):1232–9.
11. Department of Health U, Services H. The Health Consequences of Smoking—50 Years of Progress: A Report of the Surgeon General [Internet]. Available from: www.cdc.gov/tobacco
12. LoPiccolo J, Gusev A, Christiani DC, Jänne PA. Lung cancer in patients who have never smoked—an emerging disease. In: Nature reviews clinical oncology, vol. 21. Springer; 2024. p. 121–46.
13. Spyratos D, Zarogoulidis P, Porpodis K, Tsakiridis K, Machairiotis N, Katsikogiannis N, et al. Occupational exposure and lung cancer. Journal of Thoracic Disease Pioneer Bioscience Publishing. 2013;5
14. Sehgal K, Gill RR, Widick P, Bindal P, McDonald DC, Shea M, et al. Association of performance status with survival in patients with advanced non-small cell lung cancer treated with pembrolizumab monotherapy. JAMA Netw Open. 2021;4(2)
15. Alexander M, Kim SY, Cheng H. Update 2020: management of non-small cell lung cancer. Lung. 2020 Dec;198(6):897–907.
16. Detterbeck FC, Boffa DJ, Kim AW, Tanoue LT. The eighth edition lung cancer stage classification. Chest. 2017 Jan;151(1):193–203.
17. Rudin CM, Brambilla E, Faivre-Finn C, Sage J. Small-cell lung cancer. Nat Rev Dis Primers. 2021;7(1):3.
18. Le Chevalier T. Adjuvant chemotherapy for resectable non-small-cell lung cancer: where is it going? vol. 21. In: Annals of Oncology; 2010.
19. Pignon JP, Tribodet H, Scagliotti GV, Douillard JY, Shepherd FA, Stephens RJ, et al. Lung adjuvant cisplatin evaluation: a pooled analysis by the LACE collaborative group. J Clin Oncol. 2008;26(21):3552–9.
20. Spigel DR, Faivre-Finn C, Gray JE, Vicente D, Planchard D, Paz-Ares L, et al. Five-year survival outcomes from the PACIFIC trial: Durvalumab after chemoradiotherapy in stage III non-small-cell lung cancer. J Clin Oncol [Internet]. 2022;40:1301–11.
21. Lu S, Kato T, Dong X, Ahn MJ, Quang LV, Soparattanapaisarn N, et al. Osimertinib after chemoradiotherapy in Stage III EGFR-mutated NSCLC. N Engl J Med. 2024;391(7):585–97.
22. Temel JS, Greer JA, Muzikansky A, Gallagher ER, Admane S, Jackson VA, et al. Early palliative care for patients with metastatic non-small-cell lung cancer A bs tr ac t. N Engl J Med. 2010;363:733.
23. Cheng Y, Spigel DR, Cho BC, Laktionov KK, Fang J, Chen Y, et al. Durvalumab after chemoradiotherapy in limited-stage small-cell lung cancer. New England Journal of Medicine [Internet]. 2024;391(14):1313–27. Available from: http://www.nejm.org/doi/10.1056/NEJMoa2404873
24. Paz-Ares L, Dvorkin M, Chen Y, Reinmuth N, Hotta K, Trukhin D, et al. Durvalumab plus platinum–etoposide versus platinum–etoposide in first-line treatment of extensive-stage small-cell lung cancer (CASPIAN): a randomised, controlled, open-label, phase 3 trial. Lancet. 2019;394(10212):1929–39.

25. Horn L, Mansfield AS, Szczęsna A, Havel L, Krzakowski M, Hochmair MJ, et al. First-line Atezolizumab plus chemotherapy in extensive-stage small-cell lung cancer. N Engl J Med. 2018;379(23):2220–9.
26. Ahn MJ, Cho BC, Felip E, Korantzis I, Ohashi K, Majem M, et al. Tarlatamab for patients with previously treated small-cell lung cancer. N Engl J Med. 2023;389(22):2063–75.
27. Adams SJ, Stone E, Baldwin DR, Vliegenthart R, Lee P, Fintelmann FJ. Lung cancer screening, vol. 401. The Lancet. Elsevier B.V; 2023. p. 390–408.
28. Krist AH, Davidson KW, Mangione CM, Barry MJ, Cabana M, Caughey AB, et al. Screening for lung cancer: US preventive services task force recommendation statement. JAMA. 2021;325(10):962–70.
29. Smith TJ, Bohlke K, Lyman GH, Carson KR, Crawford J, Cross SJ, et al. Recommendations for the use of WBC growth factors: American society of clinical oncology clinical practice guideline update. J Clin Oncol. 2015;33(28):3199–212.
30. Bohlius J, Bohlke K, Castelli R, Djulbegovic B, Lustberg MB, Martino M, et al. Management of Cancer-Associated Anemia with Erythropoiesis-Stimulating Agents: ASCO/ASH clinical practice guideline update. J Clin Oncol [Internet]. 2019;37:1336–51.
31. Hesketh PJ, Kris MG, Basch E, Bohlke K, Barbour SY, Rebecca, et al. Antiemetics: ASCO guideline update [Internet]. J Clin Oncol. 2020. Available from: www.asco.org/supportive-care-guidelines;38:2782.
32. Roscoe JA, Morrow GR, Aapro MS, Molassiotis A, Olver I. Anticipatory nausea and vomiting. Supportive Care in Cancer. 2011;19:1533–8.
33. Akbarali HI, Muchhala KH, Jessup DK, Cheatham S. Chemotherapy induced gastrointestinal toxicities. In: Advances in cancer research. Academic Press Inc.; 2022. p. 131–66.
34. Brown TJ, Gupta A. Management of cancer therapy-associated oral mucositis. JCO Oncol Pract [Internet]. 2020;16:103–9.
35. Chiruvella V, Annamaraju P, Guddati AK. Management of nephrotoxicity of chemotherapy and targeted agents: 2020. Am J Cancer Res. 2020;10(12):4151–64.
36. Loprinzi CL, Lacchetti C, Bleeker J, Cavaletti G, Chauhan C, Hertz DL, et al. Prevention and management of chemotherapy-induced peripheral neuropathy in survivors of adult cancers: ASCO guideline update [Internet]. J Clin Oncol. 2020. Available from: www.cancer.net;38:3325.
37. Bower JE, Lacchetti C, Alici Y, Barton DL, Bruner D, Canin BE, et al. Management of fatigue in adult survivors of cancer: ASCO-Society for integrative oncology guideline update. J Clin Oncol. 2024;42(20):2456–87.
38. Roeland EJ, Bohlke K, Baracos VE, Bruera E, del Fabbro E, Dixon S, et al. Management of cancer cachexia: ASCO Guideline [Internet]. J Clin Oncol. 2020;38. Available from: www.asco.org/guidelines-methodology
39. Roeland EJ, Bohlke K, Baracos VE, Smith TJ, Loprinzi CL, Bruera E, et al. Cancer cachexia: ASCO guideline rapid recommendation update. J Clin Oncol. 2023;41(25):4178–9.
40. Kruse M, Abraham J. Management of chemotherapy-induced Alopecia with scalp cooling. J Oncol Pract. 2018;14(3):149–54.
41. Santaballa A, Márquez-Vega C, Rodríguez-Lescure A, Rovirosa, Vázquez L, Zeberio-Etxetxipia I, et al. Multidisciplinary consensus on the criteria for fertility preservation in cancer patients. Clin Transl Oncol. 2022;24(2):227–43.
42. Barroso A, Estevinho F, Hespanhol V, Teixeira E, Ramalho-Carvalho J, Araújo A. Management of infusion-related reactions in cancer therapy: strategies and challenges, vol. 9. ESMO Open. Elsevier B.V; 2024.
43. Schneider BJ, Naidoo J, Santomasso BD, Lacchetti C, Adkins, Sherry, Anadkat M, et al. Management of immune-related adverse events in patients treated with immune checkpoint inhibitor therapy: ASCO guideline update. J Clin Oncol [Internet]. 2021;39:4073–126.
44. Shyam Sunder S, Sharma UC, Pokharel S. Adverse effects of tyrosine kinase inhibitors in cancer therapy: pathophysiology, mechanisms and clinical management, vol. 8. Signal Transduction and Targeted Therapy. Springer Nature; 2023.

45. Family A, Berkey FJ. Managing the adverse effects of radiation therapy [Internet] Vol. 82. 2010. Available from: www.aafp.org/afp
46. Antoni MH, Moreno PI, Penedo FJ. Stress management interventions to facilitate psychological and physiological adaptation and optimal health outcomes in cancer patients and survivors. Ann Rev Psychol. 2023;74:423–55.
47. Smith CB, Phillips T, Smith TJ. Using the new ASCO clinical practice guideline for palliative care concurrent with oncology care using the TEAM approach. Am Soc Clin Oncol Educ Book. 2017;37:714–23.
48. Sanders JJ, Temin S, Ghoshal A, Alesi ER, Ali ZV, Chauhan C, et al. Palliative care for patients with cancer: ASCO guideline update. J Clin Oncol. 2024;42(19):2336–57.
49. Sandhya L, Nirmala, Sreenivasan D, Goenka L, Dubashi B, Kayal S, et al. Randomized double-blind placebo-controlled study of olanzapine for chemotherapy-related anorexia in patients with locally advanced or metastatic gastric, hepatopancreaticobiliary, and lung cancer. J Clin Oncol [Internet]. 2023;41:2617–27.
50. Ligibel JA, Bohlke K, May AM, Clinton SK, Demark-Wahnefried W, Gilchrist SC, et al. Exercise, diet, and weight management during cancer treatment: ASCO Guideline [Internet]. J Clin Oncol. 2022;40. Available from: www.asco.org/guideline-methodology
51. Schneider BJ, Ismaila N, Aerts J, Chiles C, Daly ME, Frank, et al. Lung cancer surveillance after definitive curative-intent therapy: ASCO guideline. J Clin Oncol [Internet]. 2019;38:753–66.
52. American Cancer Society. Lung cancer [Internet]. Available from: https://www.cancer.org/cancer/types/lung-cancer.html
53. Buffett Cancer Center P, Loo BW, Chair V, Badiyan S, Bassetti M, Bestvina C, et al. NCCN Guidelines Version 4.2025 Small Cell Lung Cancer [Internet]. 2025. Available from: https://www.nccn.org/guidelines/category_1
54. Kristina Gregory N, Lisa Hang M, Aisner DL, Akerley W, Bauman JR, Chang JY, et al. NCCN Guidelines Version 3.2025 Non-Small Cell Lung Cancer Continue [Internet]. 2025. Available from: https://www.nccn.org/guidelines/category_1
55. American Society of Clinical Oncology. ASCO Clinical Practice Guidelines [Internet]. Available from: https://ascopubs.org/jco/special/guidelines

Open Access This chapter is licensed under the terms of the Creative Commons Attribution-NonCommercial 4.0 International License (http://creativecommons.org/licenses/by-nc/4.0/), which permits any noncommercial use, sharing, adaptation, distribution and reproduction in any medium or format, as long as you give appropriate credit to the original author(s) and the source, provide a link to the Creative Commons license and indicate if changes were made.

The images or other third party material in this chapter are included in the chapter's Creative Commons license, unless indicated otherwise in a credit line to the material. If material is not included in the chapter's Creative Commons license and your intended use is not permitted by statutory regulation or exceeds the permitted use, you will need to obtain permission directly from the copyright holder.

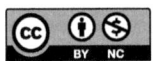

Supportive, Palliative, and Hospice Care

19

Jennifer E. Jacky and Angie Larsh

Contents

Introduction	255
Navigation Vignette	256
Planning from the Beginning: Initial Meetings and Assessment	256
Reassessment	260
Multidisciplinary Team: Supportive and Palliative Care	261
Conclusion	265
Key Takeaways	265
Key Readings and Resources	265
References	265

Introduction

Though the number of anticancer treatments has grown, and survival has improved, lung cancer remains a deadly disease with complex symptoms and significant impact on patients and their community. Every year, approximately 235,000 Americans are diagnosed, with 125,000 succumbing to lung cancer [23]. The 5-year survival rate for people with lung cancer is 25.2% [23]. Healthcare providers and caregivers are often caring for lung cancer patients at the end of their lives. A structured assessment and ongoing reassessment along the continuum of care optimally care for patients from diagnosis to end of life.

J. E. Jacky (✉) · A. Larsh
Fred Hutch Cancer Center, University of Washington School of Medicine, Seattle, WA, USA
e-mail: jjacky@fredhutch.org; alarsh@fredhutch.org

© The Author(s) 2026
J. T. Fathi, M. F. Mortman (eds.), *Lung Cancer Navigation and Care*,
https://doi.org/10.1007/978-3-032-02200-4_19

Navigation Vignette

JB is a 65-year-old woman diagnosed with non-small cell lung cancer. Her medical history includes COPD, diabetes, stroke, hepatitis C (treated), and a remote history of IV drug use. JB lives alone on a rural, mountainous property 50 miles from the clinic and does not drive; she hitch-hiked to the clinic for her first visit with the oncology team. JB has very few friends or family in the area, and no one she thinks could be her caregiver. Her oncologist recommended an intense regimen of chemotherapy with radiation.

Follow the ongoing assessment and reassessment of JB's palliative, supportive, and hospice care needs throughout her clinical course, provided by an Advanced Practice Provider Navigator and other key personnel throughout this chapter.

Planning from the Beginning: Initial Meetings and Assessment

During initial meetings, lung cancer patients and caregivers will formalize a care plan with their medical team. For most, this discussion is the beginning of primary palliative care. The cancer treatment team will discuss options for anticancer therapy, including the anticipated effectiveness in improving quality and length of life. Clinicians will also discuss the option "best supportive care" or symptom management without anticancer treatment [1, 12].

When choosing a treatment plan, it can be helpful to recall that the overarching goal of oncology medical teams is to provide care that improves patients' length and quality of life. The challenge is that predicting an individual patient's tolerance of a treatment plan and prognosis is inexact [25]. To improve shared decision-making and patient experience, we propose that initial meetings involve assessing and discussing six areas, including the intent of therapy, medical and functional status, prognosis, coping skills/distress, patient values/goals, and resource needs.

Intent of Therapy

The intent of therapy refers to whether the cancer is curable or not. Unfortunately, there are times when patients think their cancer is curable when it is, in fact, incurable [14, 32]. Ideally, the team will discuss the intent of therapy before initiating treatment so that patients can make informed decisions about whether to proceed with anticancer therapy [7]. Knowing the intent of anticancer therapy helps patients evaluate whether they want to receive toxic therapies that have a low probability of controlling cancer. It also helps patients decide if the side effects they experience are in balance with potential for cancer control.

Physical Health, Function, and Comorbidities

A full understanding of the patient's comorbidities and baseline function assists clinicians in predicting individual treatment tolerance. Some patients can experience improvement in their cancer-related symptoms, like cough or pain, after initiating treatment. However, patients with several medical problems, weight loss, and advanced age inherently have a greater risk of physical decline from anticancer treatments and a shorter life expectancy compared to a younger patient with no health problems [22]. An aggressive oncology plan in a fragile patient with limited function will often result in deterioration of function, hospitalization, and potentially hasten death. Hence, the oncology team is likely to recommend a less intense treatment regimen to fragile patients, as the best course to achieve a balance between improving length and quality of life, even if the cancer is potentially curable [12].

Prognosis

Treatment planning often includes discussion about prognosis and the patient's life expectancy. Given the emotional impact of estimating prognosis and to respect the individual patient's desire to know this type of sensitive information, it is best practice for clinicians to ask permission before the discussion. Clinicians can also disclose the inexact nature of predictions and discuss prognosis as time ranges (i.e., years, months, weeks, days, hours) [1]. Understanding a provider's estimation of prognosis with and without treatment can help patients decide what care they prefer. Though emotionally difficult, this discussion can be helpful for patients and families to prioritize activities in case their time is short, or their projected function is limited [7].

Distress and Grief

Nearly all people with lung cancer experience an emotional response to their diagnosis and grieve the loss of their planned future. Up to 50% of cancer patients experience significant distress [26]. Elevated levels of distress impact quality of life, result in longer hospital stays, impact patients' ability to participate in cancer treatment, and shorten survival [15, 18]. Given the impact of distress on patients and their families, it is standard to screen all cancer patients for distress prior to initiating cancer-directed therapies [4]. When a patient's distress is significant enough to impact their function, care teams can consider delaying treatments anticipated to cause more symptoms. When lifesaving treatment must begin, the team can support patients by seeing or speaking to them frequently to provide ongoing screening for psychiatric and behavioral health needs and by referring for mental health and other supportive services as needed.

Caregiver, Community, and Financial Support

Cancer therapy is expensive and time-consuming. Many patients have remarkable caregivers and community support. However, some patients do not have the support necessary to complete recommended oncology care, and many can no longer work. Given that the out-of-pocket cost of care for a single month of uncomplicated medical care can easily reach $2600 US dollars, resources for food, transportation, and medications can become sparse and may not be sufficient to allow for completion of recommended medical care [10]. Providers should regularly inquire about support needs and refer to social work, financial counseling, or charitable organizations if needed [7] (see Chap. 2).

Communication and Learning Needs

Many patients have difficulty understanding the complexities of cancer planning, goals of therapy, and medical terminology [7]. Care teams should create an environment where patients and caregivers feel comfortable asking questions and requesting support. Ideally, teams will provide time for questions and respond in easy-to-understand terms.

Performing a basic assessment of patients' learning needs, language barriers, and communication preferences represents a quality care standard and is critical when meeting a patient for the first time [30]. Patients who do not share a common language with their providers should have access to a certified medical interpreter and written materials in their native language to facilitate discussions about care [30]. Finally, it is important to assess patients' informational preferences. For example, while some patients desire all information, want to review imaging, and consult many providers, others want their providers to synthesize information for them [7].

Patient Goals and Advance Care Planning

Discussing what is important to patients is the cornerstone of patient-centered care and cancer treatment planning [6]. Patients' goals include their definition of an acceptable quality of life [24]. Common patient goals include living as long as possible, control of symptoms, and limiting time in hospitals/clinics. Other goals may consist of activities that bring value to their lives or achieving important life events. Celebrations of the birth of a child, marriage, or graduation are common examples. While clinicians and patients strive to create a plan that achieves all goals, most patients' journeys with lung cancer include decision points where patients must prioritize one goal over others. Providers should anticipate that these conversations can be emotional and often require more than one meeting [24, 29].

Most Americans have not completed advance care planning [33]. Choosing a durable power of attorney and completing an advance directive enables patients to legally formalize their goals, preferences, and values and share them with their care team and caregivers [24]. A durable power of attorney is a person or group of people that a patient chooses to make decisions for them if they cannot [24]. An advanced directive or living will is a legal document summarizing goals for future medical care and often states what care patients would like to avoid should they become sicker and are unable to participate in care discussions [24]. The primary team should introduce both durable power of attorney and advance directives early in the course of illness and reaffirm their choices regularly during cancer care. Specialty palliative care (discussed later in this chapter) can help with complex advance care planning.

Navigation Vignette: Initial Supportive Care Assessment

Recall that JB is a 65-year-old woman with lung cancer, significant comorbidities, little social support, and sparse resources. After discussion, her oncologist recommended curative intent therapy. Using the Palliative Care Wheel (refer to Fig. 19.1)

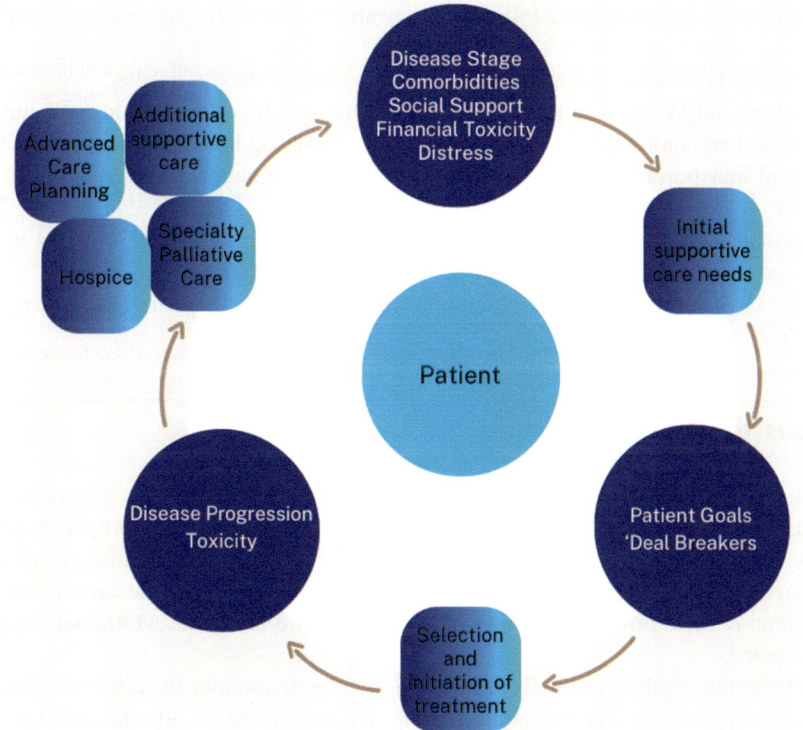

Fig. 19.1 Palliative care wheel: initial assessment and ongoing reassessment of the patient's palliative care needs

to conduct the initial supportive care assessment of JB and her needs, the Advanced Practice Provider Navigator's assessment reveals the following:

- *Intent of therapy:* Curative (chance of cure is estimated to be less than 20%).
- *Functional and medical comorbidities:* Stable and adequate currently, but at risk of deteriorating with treatment. She has no symptoms from lung cancer currently.
- *Prognosis:* Difficult to predict with her medical problems, but cancer cure is possible.
- *Coping:* Currently coping adequately but has a history of maladaptive coping.
- *Caregiver, community, and financial support:* Very limited, placing her at risk of not completing curative intent therapy.
- *Communication and learning needs:* Prefers written materials.
- *Patient goals:* JB states her goal is to cure her cancer. If this is not possible, she would like to live until the following summer to give her time to sell her property. Remaining physically active and independent is critical to achieving this goal. She has not completed advance care planning and defers any further discussion regarding this.

Following this comprehensive needs assessment, the Advanced Practice Provider Navigator recommends the following referrals:

- To the patient navigator who assists with monetary needs/services.
- To Social Work, who helps JB contact a friend who offers to house JB during treatment and to assist with transportation. Ensuring housing close to the clinic and transportation increases the chance of her completing planned cancer therapy safely.
- Financial counselors who assist JB in enrolling in a subsidized medical insurance plan to help reduce out-of-pocket costs of medications.
- To Cancer Pain Medicine for anticipated radiation-related pain in the setting of a history of IV drug use.

Reassessment

Once a treatment plan is initiated, reassessment begins (Fig. 19.1). The oncology team monitors pain, fatigue, shortness of breath, nutritional status, and other symptoms impacting quality of life. The team also reevaluates coping, learning, and supportive care needs. Regular reassessment will help determine if the cancer therapy maintains or improves an acceptable quality of life and what additional support is needed.

Periodically, the team will recommend imaging to monitor the effect of anticancer therapy on the size of visible tumors. Because there are life-threatening side effects of some cancer treatments, when there is significant functional decline or increase in symptoms caused by anticancer therapy, the team may recommend pausing anticancer treatments, and/or initiating best supportive care, even if the cancer looks smaller [12].

Navigation Vignette: Reassessment of JB

Chemotherapy worsens JB's chronic diabetic nerve pain, which contributes to a fall. She reports feeling depressed about pain and fatigue since treatment started. She has spoken to her roommate, who has agreed to be her durable power of attorney and is helping her sell her property. She wants to continue treatment to try to cure the cancer but is concerned she will not be able to. Palliative reassessment of JB and her needs reveals the following:

- *Intent of therapy:* Curative (chance of cure is estimated to be less than 20%).
- *Functional and medical comorbidities:* Impaired but can be improved with supportive care.
- *Prognosis:* Difficult to predict, but a cure is possible.
- *Coping:* Worsened but can be maximized with supportive care.
- *Caregiver, community, and financial support:* No needs identified.
- *Communication and learning needs:* Written materials about her new medication and DPOA were provided.
- *Patient goals:* JB wants to continue therapy to try to cure her cancer. Her roommate is helping her sell her property. She is pleased about this. She wants to complete the durable power of attorney form designating her roommate.

Following this comprehensive needs reassessment, the Advanced Practice Provider and Pain Medicine specialist recommended the following referrals:

- Referral to physical therapy/occupational therapy for training and recommended equipment to support her activity.
- A nonopioid medication that can help with pain and depression.
- Revisit with social work for counseling.
- Completion of the DPOA form in the clinic and referral to a notary to finalize.

Multidisciplinary Team: Supportive and Palliative Care

A multidisciplinary team can optimize the quality of life for lung cancer patients. A comprehensive ongoing assessment will uncover patient needs, resulting in referrals to supportive care services. Providing written education about supportive care services will empower patients and caregivers to request care they feel may be helpful.

Supportive care, palliative care, and hospice are terms often used interchangeably but are distinctly different. The following further defines and discusses the nuanced differences of supportive, palliative, and hospice care.

Supportive Care

Supportive care services include an array of specialists who can help people with lung cancer live better lives (Table 19.1). Patients may benefit from referral to one or more services. Some patients have complex issues where a multidisciplinary approach is imperative. For example, patients with substance use disorder and cancer-related pain often require support from pain medicine and addiction medicine specialists to continue cancer therapy, safe pain management, and to provide optimal end-of-life care [19].

Palliative Care

Palliative care is a type of supportive care appropriate for patients with a serious illness and can be delivered together with anticancer therapies. Palliative care helps with symptom management, psychosocial–spiritual needs, and advance care planning [3]. Because palliative care can help lung cancer patients live longer and with better quality of life, it is ideal to start soon after diagnosis [28]. Palliative care becomes the focus of care when cancer-directed therapies are no longer effective, appropriate, or desired [3]. Most patients are unfamiliar with palliative care or may

Table 19.1 Supportive care services

Supportive care service	Common reason for referral
Addiction medicine	Substance use disorder in the setting of cancer pain
Child life specialist	Support children of cancer patients
Medical nutrition	Optimize nutrition
Naturopath/integrative medicine	Herbal or naturopathic approaches to symptoms associated with cancer/anticancer therapies
Pain medicine	Continuous assessment and management of complex pain
Patient navigators and financial counselors	Assistance with durable needs (transportation, resources for high-cost care)
Pharmacists	Monitor and assess for medication interactions
Physical and/or occupational therapy	Optimize mobility and fall prevention
Physiatry/physical medicine	Assist patients with functional disability
Psychiatry/psychology	Ongoing monitoring and psychoanalysis for depression/anxiety and other behavioral disorders and medication management
Social work	Provide supportive counseling
Speech/language therapists	Evaluate impaired swallowing/speaking
Spiritual health	Assess spiritual distress
Support groups	Connect with patients through support groups including with other cancer patients
Wound/ostomy care	Assess for and manage chronic wounds and ostomies

equate palliative care with hospice or end-of-life care. Discussing and defining palliative care and its benefits helps patients consider the value of this service.

Primary Palliative Care

The oncology team provides primary palliative care, including medical oncology physicians and advanced practice providers. Primary palliative care is summarized by the assessment and reassessments described in this chapter. Essential elements of primary palliative care include building therapeutic relationships, symptom management, discussions of patients' values and goals, advance care planning, introducing specialty palliative care, prognosis discussions, and transition to hospice care [21].

Specialty Palliative Care

Studies suggest a survival benefit for patients who receive subspecialty palliative care concurrent with oncologic care [13, 20, 28]. Therefore, routine referral to subspecialty palliative care is considered for every patient with advanced cancer [11]. Specialty palliative care teams often include physicians, advanced practice providers, and nurses. These teams provide additional time and expertise, work alongside the oncology team, and support lung cancer patients with complex needs [13, 20, 28].

Hospice

Hospice is medical care for patients near the end of life who do not desire or are not eligible for anticancer therapy [8]. Patients enrolled in hospice often have a prognosis of 6 months or less. Multidisciplinary hospice teams often provide care in the patient's home. Depending on patients' needs and community resources, hospice care can be provided in hospice centers, hospitals, and skilled care facilities. Hospice provides medicines, equipment, and expertise to help families care for their loved ones at home with around-the-clock telephone support.

The decision to enroll in hospice can be agonizing for patients and caregivers. Care teams can help ease the stress of the transition with appropriately timed and open discussions about hospice services. Patients are often reassured that hospice care goals are aligned with the oncology team goals: life prolongation, improved quality of life, caregiver support, and reduction of suffering. Discussing how hospice helps with the expected symptoms of clinical decline can be helpful. Offering an introductory hospice meeting and continuing supportive care visits with the primary oncology team (telemedicine or the telephone) can also help bridge the transition. Learning how hospice can provide support often helps patients consider enrollment when services may offer the greatest support to the patient and their caregivers [8].

End-of-Life Discussions and Care

Initiating and normalizing discussions related to end-of-life is part of holistic care for patients with lung cancer [24, 27]. Most Americans do not have firsthand experience with death and dying and the mystery of this can be a barrier to informed decision-making [9]. Patient goals should be reassessed regularly and particularly when patients face growing cancer, a decline in function, or hospitalization [12]. Longitudinal assessment of physical decline, knowledge of patient goals combined with trusted recommendations from clinical providers can help patients and loved ones recognize and plan for the end of life. Including caregivers in conversations about the end of life and the natural dying process may allay concerns about symptoms that may be distressing to witness but are not an indication of suffering (like discontinuation of eating and drinking).

Navigation Vignette: Palliative Care Reassessment and End-of-Life Discussion with JB

Unfortunately, JBs' neuropathy and fatigue worsen. She is hospitalized for COPD exacerbation, failure to thrive, and pain. Her breathing and pain continue to be problematic following hospitalization. Her difficulties are attributed to treatment and are not expected to improve. JB decides to stop therapy. Curing her cancer is no longer within her goals of care. She would like to focus on improving her symptoms and does not want to return to the hospital. Her roommate says she can stay until she feels better. Palliative reassessment of JB and her needs reveals the following:

- *Intent of therapy:* noncurative.
- *Functional and medical comorbidities:* At risk for rehospitalization, especially without support at home. Living independently is not possible.
- *Prognosis:* Difficult to predict but likely measured in months.
- *Coping:* Impaired. Related to symptoms that are unlikely to improve.
- *Caregiver, community, and financial support:* Limited.
- *Communication and learning needs:* Prefers written materials.
- *Patient goals:* She has been able to sell her property and would like to be at her roommate's house at the end of her life. She would like to complete advance care planning to avoid hospitalization and for estate planning.

Following this comprehensive needs reassessment, the Advanced Practice Provider Navigator respects JB's informed decision and, with permission, discusses an uncertain but shortened prognosis. The Advanced Practice Provider Navigator reintroduces palliative care services and the support they can provide for patients who forgo cancer therapy. They also discussed the difference between palliative care and hospice. JB expresses interest in an introductory meeting with the hospice team and getting more help with advance care planning. The Advanced Practice Provider Navigator and team recommend:

- Referral to specialty Palliative Care.
- Referral for an introductory visit with members of the hospice team.

Conclusion

Lung cancer remains a challenging disease that significantly impacts patients and their care teams. Designing a successful supportive treatment plan includes a structured, comprehensive assessment, ongoing reassessment, and referral to supportive care services as needed. Clinicians and medical teams aim to create a trusted, therapeutic, hopeful yet realistic environment where patients can ask for clarification, support, and openly discuss their quality of life, fears, and goals while often preparing for the end-of-life.

Key Takeaways

- Patients living with lung cancer have complex symptoms and require an ongoing, comprehensive, structured assessment.
- The primary goal of lung cancer therapy is to help patients live as long as possible with a quality of life that is acceptable to the patient.
- All patients with lung cancer should receive primary palliative care and receive referrals to specialty services as needed.
- Introducing and revisiting advanced care planning, hospice services, and end-of-life care are standards of care for patients living with serious illness.

Key Readings and Resources

- Serious illness conversation guide [2]
- National Comprehensive Cancer Network patient resources for lung cancer [16]
- National Comprehensive Cancer Network guidelines for patients' palliative care [17]
- Vital Talk [31]

Conflict of Interest There are no conflicts of interest.

References

1. Arai D. Longitudinal assessment of prognostic understanding in patients with advanced lung cancer and its association with their psychological distress. Oncologist. 2021;26(12):e2265–73.
2. Ariadne Labs. Ariadnelabs.org. 2023, May. Retrieved from Serious illness conversation guide. https://www.ariadnelabs.org/wp-content/uploads/2023/05/Serious-Illness-Conversation-Guide.2023-05-18.pdf

3. Center to Advance Palliative Care. About palliative care. 2025. Retrieved May 3, 2025, from https://www.capc.org/about/palliative-care/
4. Commission on Cancer. Cancer Program Standards: ensuring patient-centered care. 2016. Retrieved from https://www.facs.org/media/t5spw4jo/2016-coc-standards-manual_interactive-pdf.pdf
5. Covey S. The seven habits of highly effective people. Franklin Covey; 1989.
6. Furber L, Cox K, Murphy R. Investigating communication in cancer consultations: what can be learned from doctor and patient accounts of their experience? Eur J Cancer Care. 2013;22:653–62.
7. Gilligan T, Coyle N, Frankel R, Berry D. Patient-clinician communication: American Society of Clinical Oncology consensus guideline. J Clin Oncol. 2017;35(31):3618–32.
8. Hospice Foundation of America. What is hospice? 2024. Retrieved May 3, 2025, from https://hospicefoundation.org/what-is-hospice/#:~:text=Hospice%20is%20medical%20care%20for,%2C%20pets%2C%20and%20valued%20possessions.
9. Institute of Medicine. Approaching death: improving care at the end of life. National Academy Press; 1997.
10. Iragorri N. The out-of-pocket cost burden of cancer care-a systematic literature review. Curr Oncol. 2021;28(2):1216–48.
11. Justin J. Sanders et al. Palliative Care for Patients With Cancer: ASCO Guideline Update. JCO. 2024;42:2336–2357. https://doi.org/10.1200/JCO.24.00542.
12. Kondo Y, Michiko Nakajima M, Nakajima G. When should anticancer treatment be ended? Why and when to discontinue palliative chemotherapy. J Clin Oncol. 2018;36(34 suppl):41.
13. Lee Y. Association between the duration of palliative care service and survival in terminal cancer patients. Support Care Cancer. 2015;23:1057–62.
14. Mack J. Patient beliefs that chemotherapy may be curative and care received at the end of life among patients with metastatic lung and colorectal cancer. Cancer. 2015;121:1891.
15. Mehert A. One in two cancer patients is significantly distressed: prevalence and indicators of distress. Psychoncology. 2018;27:75–82.
16. National Comprehensive Cancer Network. 2023a. Everything lung cancer. Retrieved May 3, 225, from NCCN: https://www.nccn.org/patientresources/patient-resources/guidelines-for-patients/lung-cancer-resources
17. National Comprehensive Cancer Network. Palliative Care. 2023b. Retrieved May 3, 2025, from chrome-extension://efaidnbmnnnibpcajpcglcefindmkaj/https://www.nccn.org/patients/guidelines/content/PDF/palliative-patient.pdf
18. Nipp R. The relationship between physical and psychological symptoms and health care utilization in hospitalized patients with advanced cancer. Cancer. 2017;123:4720–7.
19. Portnoy R, Zankhana M, Ahmed E. Cancer pain management: general principles and risk management for patients receiving opioids. 2024, April. Retrieved May 4, 2025, from https://www.uptodate.com/contents/cancer-pain-management-general-principles-and-risk-management-for-patients-receiving-opioids?search=cancer%20pain%20management%20with%20opioids&source=search_result&selectedTitle=2~150&usage_type=default&display_rank=2#H2.
20. Rugno F, Paiva B, Paiva C. Early integration of palliative care facilitates the discontinuation of anticancer treatment in women with, vol. 135. Gynecol Oncol; 2014. p. 249–54.
21. Schenker Y. Primary palliative care. Up To Date. 2024, October. https://www.uptodate.com/contents/primary-palliative-care.
22. Shi S, Wang HL. Prediction of overall survival of non-small cell lung cancer with bone metastasis: an analysis of the Surveillance, Epidemiology and End Results (SEER) database. Trasl Cancer Res. 2021;10(12):5191–203.
23. Sigel R, Giaquinto A, Jemal A. Cancer statistics. Cancer J Clin. 2024;74(1):12–49.
24. Silveira M.. Advance care planning and advance directives. 2024, December. Retrieved from UpToDate: https://www.uptodate.com/contents/advance-care-planning-and-advance-directives?search=advance%20care%20planning&source=search_result&selectedTitle=1%7E150&usage_type=default&display_rank=1.

25. Stone P, Chu C, Todd C. The accuracy of clinician predictions of survival in the Prognosis in Palliative care Study II: a prospective observational study. PLoS One. 2022;17(4):e0267050.
26. Sun H. Distress thermometer in breast cancer: systematic review and meta-analysis. BMJ Support Palliat Care. 2022;12(3):245–52. Retrieved from NCCN.org: https://www.nccn.org/professionals/physician_gls/pdf/distress.pdf.
27. Sutherland R. Dying well-informed: the need for better clinical education surrounding facilitating end-of-life conversations. Yale J Biol Med. 2019;92(4):757–64.
28. Temel J, Greer J, Muzikansky A, et al. Early palliative care for patients with metastatic lung cancer. N Engl J Med. 2010;363:733–42.
29. Temel J, Jackson V, El-Jawahri A, Rinaldi S, Petrillo L, Kumar P, et al. Stepped palliative care for patients with advanced lung cancer: a randomized clinical trial. JAMA. 2024;332(6):471–81.
30. The Joint Commission. Language access and interpreter services- understanding the requirements. 2017. Retrieved May 3, 2025.
31. VitalTalk. VitalTalk resources. 2025. Retrieved May 3, 2025, from https://www.vitaltalk.org/resources/quick-guides/
32. Weeks J. Patients expectations about the effects of chemotherapy for advanced cancer. N Engl J Med. 2012;367:161–1625.
33. Yadav K. Approximately one in three adults completes any type of advanced directive for end-of-life care. Health Aff. 2017;36:1244.

Open Access This chapter is licensed under the terms of the Creative Commons Attribution-NonCommercial 4.0 International License (http://creativecommons.org/licenses/by-nc/4.0/), which permits any noncommercial use, sharing, adaptation, distribution and reproduction in any medium or format, as long as you give appropriate credit to the original author(s) and the source, provide a link to the Creative Commons license and indicate if changes were made.

The images or other third party material in this chapter are included in the chapter's Creative Commons license, unless indicated otherwise in a credit line to the material. If material is not included in the chapter's Creative Commons license and your intended use is not permitted by statutory regulation or exceeds the permitted use, you will need to obtain permission directly from the copyright holder.

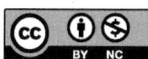

Best Practice Standards and Models of Care for High-Quality Survivorship

20

Christina R. Crabtree-Ide and Tessa Flores

Contents

Navigation Vignette.	270
Introduction.	271
Understanding the Physical and Psychosocial Effects of Lung Cancer.	272
Survivorship Guidelines.	272
Survivorship Care Plans.	275
Follow-Up Care and Cancer Surveillance.	276
Health Promotion and Disease Prevention Following Cancer Treatment.	278
Use of Telehealth and Project ECHO for Highly Effective Survivorship Programs.	279
Key Takeaways.	279
Key Readings and Resources.	279
References.	280

Abbreviations

ASCO American Society of Clinical Oncology
COPD Chronic obstructive pulmonary disease
CT   Computed tomography
ECHO Extension for Community Healthcare Outcomes
EORTC European Organization for Research and Treatment of Cancer
IR   Interventional radiology

Christina R. Crabtree-Ide and Tessa Flores contributed equally with all other contributors.

C. R. Crabtree-Ide (✉) · T. Flores
Department of Medicine, Roswell Park Comprehensive Cancer Center, Buffalo, NY, USA
e-mail: Christina.Crabtree-Ide@RoswellPark.org; TessaFaye.Flores@RoswellPark.org

© The Author(s) 2026
J. T. Fathi, M. F. Mortman (eds.), *Lung Cancer Navigation and Care*,
https://doi.org/10.1007/978-3-032-02200-4_20

LDCT   Low-dose computed tomography
NCCN   National Comprehensive Cancer Network
NSCLC   Non-small cell lung cancer
PCP   Primary care provider
PET   Positron emission tomography
RUL   Right upper lobe
SOB   Shortness of breath
SCLC   Small cell lung cancer

Navigation Vignette

Cancer Survivorship requires coordinated care and management of complex sequelae. Lung cancer Survivorship includes, but goes well beyond, lung cancer surveillance for recurrence. In this vignette, we focus primarily on one component of Survivorship care: surveillance. Comprehensive lung cancer Survivorship includes coordination between and across teams, management of late- and long-term effects, and screening for other cancers. In this vignette, navigation was critical throughout the patient journey and included coordination between navigators as well as healthcare teams. Our navigators and Survivorship team use Survivorship Care Plans as a tool that can be valuable when used well to coordinate care.

The patient was 67 years old when she was diagnosed with stage IB squamous cell carcinoma of the lung. She underwent left upper lobectomy with mediastinal lymph node sampling and required no further treatment. She was followed by thoracic surgery every 6 months with a chest CT with contrast for the first 2 years. After completing active surveillance, she met with the Thoracic Surgery Nurse Navigator (navigator) to discuss transferring to the Survivorship for continued surveillance and Survivorship care.

The navigator reviewed the recommended surveillance schedule, including an annual history and physical, and a low-dose chest CT (LDCT) with the patient. The patient agreed to transition to Survivorship. Before her first Survivorship appointment, the navigator reviewed the chart to verify that the correct imaging was ordered and scheduled. The navigator also reviewed the local health exchange to ensure that she was participating in other cancer screenings not related to her primary cancer. At her initial Survivorship visit, the navigator introduced the concept of Survivorship care—comprehensive medical care, surveillance of her lung cancer, monitoring of possible late effects of treatment, encouragement of participating in other cancer screenings, and routine visits with her PCP, along with documentation and communication to facilitate coordination between her medical teams.

She was seen by the Survivorship provider, who reviewed her personalized Survivorship Care Plan with her. The components of her care plan included timing of surveillance, type of imaging for surveillance, signs and symptoms of recurrence, possible late effects or complications of her treatment, recommended lifestyle choices, and lung cancer-specific resources. Per protocol in the Survivorship Clinic, the EORTC QLQ Core Questionnaire was administered with her to assess her quality of life. She answered 30 questions regarding functional, emotional, and global health. Upon provider review and further interview, she admitted to shortness of breath (SOB) and difficulty with long walks. Since she complained of SOB, a referral to pulmonary rehabilitation was placed. The Survivorship evaluation visit was reviewed by the navigator, who followed up with the patient to coordinate her care, including the referral to pulmonary rehab. A few days after the initial Survivorship visit, the navigator contacted the patient to see if she had any concerns or questions.

She was seen annually at the Survivorship Clinic with a history and physical, and an LDCT. Four years after transitioning to Survivorship, her surveillance LDCT revealed a new large RUL nodule. The Survivorship provider saw her and discussed obtaining a PET scan for further evaluation. The PET scan was highly suspicious for recurrent metastasis in the right upper lobe. The Survivorship provider informed the patient of the results and arranged an interventional radiology-guided biopsy, coordinated by the navigator. The navigator called a few days before the biopsy to review instructions, answer questions, and offer support. The biopsy confirmed recurrence of squamous cell carcinoma of the lung, and she was referred back to thoracic surgery.

The Survivorship navigator ensured two-way communication throughout the surveillance process and in communication with the PCP team and other providers, including rehabilitation. Navigation is critical when working through complex disease states with multidisciplinary care teams and helps patients successfully access patient-centered care.

Introduction

In the United States, there are an estimated 18.1 million cancer survivors, and that number is projected to grow due to improvements in screening, early detection, treatment, and access to care [1]. Of those cancer survivors, lung cancer is the most commonly occurring new cancer, with approximately 384,000 lung cancer survivors in the United States, which represents 4% of persons alive with cancer [1–4]. Globally, there are 2.5 million new cases of lung cancer each year, or 12.4% of the total new cases, and in 2021, there were 209,500 new cases of lung and bronchus cancer diagnosed in the United States [2, 4, 5].

In March 2021, the United States Preventive Services Task Force expanded its lung cancer screening guidelines to include a significantly larger population of screening-eligible patients, with a wider age range, which increased the number of individuals eligible for screening. These expanded guidelines especially impacted the eligibility of women (50.1% vs 44.1%) and Black individuals (9.2% vs 6.6%) since there is evidence that even though Black people and women smoke less cigarettes than White men, they are still at an increased risk for lung cancer [6, 7].

Lung cancer survivors often have a high burden of comorbidities, which lead to more complex late and long-term effects [8]. For those with tobacco and chemical exposure, lung cancer survivors suffer a disproportionate burden of chronic obstructive pulmonary disease (COPD) and cardiovascular complications [9]. In addition, the treatment for the cancer itself is often invasive, which can compound the Survivorship physical, psychosocial, and financial impacts. For example, pulmonary resection is an effective intervention for early-stage disease, yet it often leads to pain, SOB, cough, and fatigue associated with the treatment [9]. Chemotherapy can affect patients' late and long-term quality of life, including contributing to cardiopulmonary toxicities and neuropathy [9].

Understanding the Physical and Psychosocial Effects of Lung Cancer

Lung cancer survivors often experience heavy disease-related burdens, including physical, psychosocial, and financial effects. As with many cancer survivors, fatigue is a major physical effect of lung cancer and its treatment. Other common physical concerns among lung cancer and other cancer survivors are sleep disturbance, memory and concentration difficulties, weakness, and cancer-related chronic pain [8]. Shortness of breath, cough, and chronic cancer-related pain are significant symptoms more specific to lung cancer survivors. In addition, cognitive impairment resulting from chemotherapy is a concern, particularly associated with cisplatin chemotherapy and cranial radiation for brain metastasis in both SCLC and NSCLC [8].

Approximately 80% of lung cancer survivors report experiencing psychological distress, three times higher rates, compared to survivors of other cancer types [9]. These emotional concerns include fear of recurrence, living with uncertainty, accepting a new normal, and handling difficult emotions [10]. Anxiety leading up to intensive surveillance is common; patients often need to return for a visit and/or scan every 3–6 months for 1–2 years, then annually [11]. Stigma also remains a significant concern among lung cancer survivors and negatively impacts quality of life and seeking medical treatment [12, 13] (see Chap. 1: *Stigma of Lung Cancer*). Sexual health and sexual dysfunction are under-addressed and understudied among lung cancer survivors and may persist well beyond completion of treatment. In addition, due to intensive treatments, financial toxicity and socioeconomic issues often arise [8, 14].

Survivorship Guidelines

In 2006, the Institute of Medicine published a consensus report that included recommendations to address the health needs of cancer survivors. Currently, there are four main organizations and societies attempting to address the needs of survivors: National Comprehensive Cancer Network (NCCN), The Children's Oncology Group, American Society of Clinical Oncology (ASCO), and The American Cancer Society (ACS) [11, 15–18].

ASCO's clinical practice Survivorship guidelines focus on chemotherapy-induced and peripheral neuropathy, fatigue, anxiety and depressive symptoms, and fertility preservation in adult survivors. Additionally, there are specific disease site guidelines on colorectal and breast cancers [11]. The Children's Oncology Group focuses on childhood, adolescent, and young adult cancer survivors [19]. Their clinical guidelines are risk-based, exposure-related recommendations for screening and management of late effects and possible complications in pediatric cancer survivors. The ACS has nutrition and physical activity guidelines and specific disease site guidelines for breast, colorectal, head and neck, and prostate cancers [17]. The NCCN guidelines have recommendations on evaluation and management of anthracycline-induced cardiotoxicity, anxiety and depression, cognitive function, exercise, fatigue, healthy lifestyle, immunizations, menopause-related symptoms, pain, sexual function, and sleep disorders [15, 16, 20].

Multidisciplinary Care

Clinical services for lung cancer survivors include lung cancer surveillance, screening for second primary cancers, and supportive services since lung cancer survivors experience a high burden of psychosocial and physical effects after their treatment. Cancer Survivorship care includes care for and around the whole person, including prevention, health promotion, management of late and long-term effects, screening for other cancers, surveillance, and navigation through the system again should a recurrence or second primary arise (Fig. 20.1). Currently, there are no standardized roles or models of care for Survivorship, and the core functions listed above may be situated within a centralized or dedicated Survivorship program, PCP, Specialty Care, or Oncologist and others (see Chap. 4). This variation in models of care is one reason for the challenge in implementation and evaluation of Survivorship care, but at present, it leaves much room for innovations in healthcare delivery.

Prevention and Health Promotion

Prevention of late and long-term effects of cancer-related treatment and health promotion to prevent recurrence and second primary malignancies is an ongoing process in the *360° Survivorship Services and Model of Care;* it is the opinion of these authors that health promotion should be infused throughout. There are interventions to prevent some of the late and long-term effects of cancer treatment, and additional interventions and strategies to prevent recurrence and second primary malignancies.

Supportive Care Services

Lung cancer survivors need additional services to help people prepare for treatment, to regain function, and improve quality of life across the continuum in Survivorship.

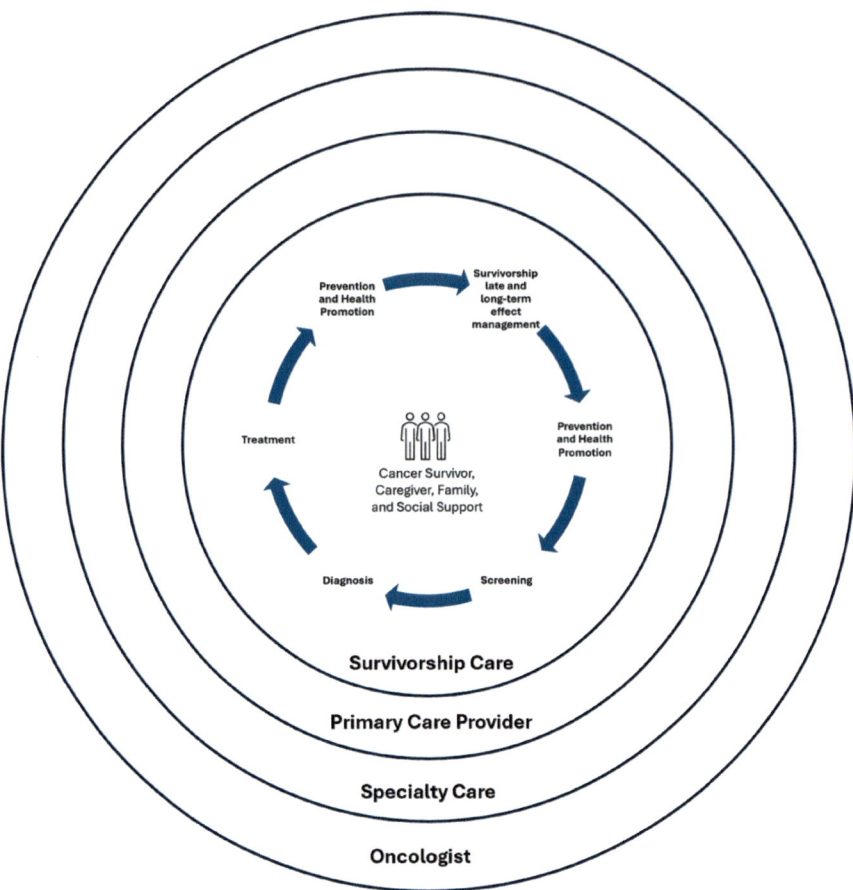

Fig. 20.1 360° Survivorship services and multidisciplinary model of care. (Adapted with permission from Flores et al. [24])

Other recommendations include respiratory muscle therapy, prehabilitation and rehabilitation, respiratory therapy, and nutrition. Connections with tobacco treatment specialists and tobacco cessation resources are recommended for people who currently or formerly smoked cigarettes. Due to the high burden of mental health and quality of life impacts, particularly for small cell lung cancer, referrals to social work and psychology are often recommended. Similarly, financial assistance and financial resources are often needed and made available through healthcare systems, and clinical support staff and/or navigators can often facilitate these connections. Wellness programs aimed at improving social support, physical activity, relaxation, and sleep quality techniques may be available to patients and often provide valuable assistance to patients, families, and caregivers.

Many lung cancer-specific survivor resources are available, and for cancer survivors in general. Navigating to these resources is critical and can be facilitated by a named "navigator" (nurse-led or patient navigator) or by a scheduler whose role includes connecting to supportive services, a clinic liaison, community health worker, or other named person whose role is to enumerate and connect with resources that are specific to the patient, the diagnosis, and their treatment. Where lung-specific resources are unavailable, community resources that are not specific to lung cancer can be readily adapted to fit the needs of patients.

Survivorship Care Plans

When Survivorship was being developed as a field, the goal of Survivorship care plans was to enhance Survivorship care by facilitating the transition from treatment to posttreatment care by way of a tool to help communication between primary providers and the patient and oncology care team. Survivorship care plans were intended to engage patients and primary care teams in the knowledge of what treatments the patient received, patients' current and historical treatments, the risk of potential late effects and complications, recommended cancer surveillance, other cancer screenings, and cancer-specific resources, including the management of late and long-term effects and prevention of recurrence and second primary malignancies.

Unfortunately, the implementation of care plans was more focused on delivering a document to the patient, rather than ensuring accurate information was reliably and consistently shared more broadly for high-quality care of the cancer survivor; therefore, the roll-out of care plans fell short of the intended goal. Challenges continue to persist in cancer survivors receiving an up-to-date Survivorship care plan, with a maximum of 43% of patients, but as little as 12% of cancer survivors receiving a care plan [31]. A major challenge is Survivorship care plans are time-intensive to create and place a significant nonreimbursable burden on the clinical team to collate past data and populate the plan. With this, long-standing tension and lack of clarity around who will initiate, maintain, and disseminate the Survivorship plan remain. Finally, ongoing controversy surrounding their utility and implementation, and dissemination barriers to providing care plans persist.

The connections between a myriad of providers and services may be reinforced in a care plan for the patient and caregiver, but they do not always include a formal care plan. Models of Survivorship care vary by health system and clinic; data and evaluation of models of care and effectiveness of the different models are limited to date. Despite these barriers, Survivorship care plans can be a valuable resource for patients and primary care teams and provide a roadmap of the care provided, expectant guidance, and recommendations. The Survivorship Care Plans are just one facet of Survivorship care, but the summary of the care and treatment recommendations must be provided to the patient and the provider team. It is critical that the provider team includes the PCP and that there is a designated staff member (e.g., navigator) who will help to coordinate and schedule follow-up care specific to oncology follow-up, supportive care, and specialty follow-up appointments.

Follow-Up Care and Cancer Surveillance

There are two main guidelines for surveillance of lung cancer recurrence. ASCO guidelines are recommendations for stage I–III lung cancer (Table 20.1). NCCN guidelines further delineate their surveillance by the type of lung cancer—small cell vs non-small cell—the staging, and the treatment received (Tables 20.2 and 20.3). Much of the medical field uses ASCO guidelines, whereas the National Cancer Institute-designated Cancer Centers use NCCN for patients with stage IV disease [1, 2, 12].

ASCO guideline recommendations apply to patients who have had curative treatment of Stage I–III non-small cell lung cancer and small cell lung cancer. According to ASCO guidelines, survivors should be seen more frequently in the first 2 years after treatment since most recurrences occur within this time frame. At 3 years posttreatment, follow-up visits are spaced out to annual visits. Follow-up consists of a history, physical, and imaging [12].

NCCN has similar guidelines. However, their guidelines differentiate between non-small and small cell lung cancer and further delineate with staging and treatment. Since these guidelines address stage IV disease, there are recommendations for surveillance of brain metastasis. Like ASCO guidelines, patients are seen more frequently within the first 3 years posttreatment, with follow-ups spaced out when further from completion of treatment [1, 2].

Table 20.1 ASCO guidelines [12]

ASCO			
Staging/pathology	Posttreatment years	Follow-up	Time interval
Stage I–III NSCLC	<2 years	History Physical Diagnostic chest CT with adrenals	Every 6 months
Stage I–III SCLC			
Stage I–III NSCLC	>2 years	History Physical LDCT	Annually
Stage I–III SCLC			

Table 20.2 NCCN Non-small cell lung cancer guidelines [2]

NCCN			
Staging/treatment	Posttreatment years	Follow-up	Time interval
Non-small cell lung cancer			
Stage I–II primary *without* radiation	<3 years	History Physical Contrast CT chest	Every 6 months
Stage I–II primary treatment *with* radiation			Every 3–6 months
Stage III–IV			Every 3–6 months
Stage I–II primary treatment *without* radiation	>3 years	History Physical LDCT	Annually
Sage I–II primary *with* radiation	3–5 years	History Physical Contrast CT chest	Every 6 months
Stage III–IV			
All NSCLC	>5 years	History Physical LDCT	Annually

Table 20.3 NCCN small cell lung cancer guidelines [1]

NCCN			
Staging	Posttreatment years	Follow-up	Time interval
Small cell lung cancer			
Limited stage	1 year	History Physical Surveillance CT Brain MRI/CT	Every 3 months
	2 years	History Physical Surveillance CT Brain MRI/CT	Every 3 months Every 6 months
	3 years	History Physical Surveillance CT	Every 6 months
	>3 years	History Physical Surveillance CT	Annually

(continued)

Table 20.3 (continued)

NCCN Staging	Posttreatment years	Follow-up	Time interval
Extended stage	1 year	History Physical Surveillance CT Brain MRI/CT	Every 2 months Every 3–4 months
	2 years	History Physical Surveillance CT Brain MRI/CT	Every 3–4 months Every 6 months
	3 years	History Physical Surveillance CT	Every 3–4 months
	4–5 years	History Physical Surveillance CT	Every 6 months
	>6 years	History Physical Surveillance CT	Annually

Health Promotion and Disease Prevention Following Cancer Treatment

Tobacco cessation and referral to smoking cessation programs are imperative for lung cancer survivors who continue to smoke after being diagnosed with lung cancer. Stigma and shame impact care-seeking behaviors and have been linked to negative mental and physical health outcomes and may be associated with delayed care seeking, premature termination of treatment, and a perception of the disease that it is self-inflicted and high mortality rates [12]. Thus, psychosocial and tobacco cessation support are important supportive services as needed.

The NCCN and World Cancer Research Fund have exercise and healthy lifestyle recommendations for cancer survivors [21]. All survivors are encouraged to maintain a healthy weight, strive for 150 min of weekly activity, consume a nutrient-rich plant-based diet, limit consumption of red meats, processed meats, and ultraprocessed foods, and reduce alcohol consumption. These recommendations are foundations for improved health for everyone, and asynchronous resources and support are also available to support these behaviors, including the 30-day cancer prevention checklist and the Healthy 10 challenge [21, 22]. The World Cancer Research Fund recommends specifically that lung cancer survivors should avoid high-dose beta-carotene supplements since these supplements can increase lung cancer in people who currently or formerly smoked [23].

Use of Telehealth and Project ECHO for Highly Effective Survivorship Programs

ProjectECHO® was developed to increase specialty medical knowledge of community providers in remote and underserved areas. The ECHO model is a telementoring model where the community providers manage their patients' complex diseases with the guidance of specialists. Educational programs for clinical care teams have successfully improved health outcomes for a host of chronic diseases, particularly where specialty care is scarce. Recently, the Centers for Disease Control and Prevention have funded several learning series supporting patient navigation and cancer Survivorship. New York State teams and others have successfully implemented ProjectECHO® programs to educate rural primary care provider teams about cancer Survivorship needs [19, 24–29].

Key Takeaways

- Lung cancer Survivorship is multidisciplinary, and navigation plays a critical role in the coordination of whole-person care.
- Structured plans provided to patients and community providers are imperative in coordinating multidisciplinary care and can help empower patients and providers to successfully manage complex care.
- Reminders and navigation through follow-up care are beneficial, particularly for lung cancer survivors with a heavy burden of comorbidities, poor mental health outcomes, and shame and stigma that may impact care-seeking and timeliness of care.
- Survivorship is an opportunity to fill gaps in care, including screening for other cancers, surveillance for recurrence, health promotion/prevention, and connection with supportive care services.

Key Readings and Resources

- Lung Cancer Surveillance After Definitive Curative-Intent Therapy: ASCO Guideline [11]
- NCCN Guidelines: Small Cell Lung Cancer [15]
- NCCN Guidelines: Non-Small Cell Lung Cancer [16]
- NCCN Guidelines: Lung Cancer Screening [20]
- American Institute for Cancer Research: Lung Cancer [30]
- Cancer Prevention Recommendations: World Cancer Research Fund [23]

Conflict of Interests Dr. Crabtree-Ide owns Danaher Corp, Fortive Corp, Vontier Corp, Veralto Corp, and Marriott stock.

References

1. National Institutes of Health (NIH) National Cancer Institute Division of Cancer Control & Population Sciences. Statistics and Graphs 2025 [cited 2025 2/13/2025]; Available from: https://cancercontrol.cancer.gov/ocs/statistics.
2. Yates P, et al. Supportive and palliative care for lung cancer patients. J Thorac Dis. 2013;5(Suppl 5):S623–8.
3. Shapiro CL. Cancer survivorship. N Engl J Med. 2018;379(25):2438–50.
4. Centers for Disease Control and Prevention. U.S. Cancer Statistics Lung Cancer Stat Bite. 2024; Available from: https://www.cdc.gov/united-states-cancer-statistics/publications/lung-cancer-stat-bite.html
5. World Health Organization. Global cancer burden growing, amidst mounting need for services. 2024 [cited 2025 2/13/2025]; Available from: https://www.who.int/news/item/01-02-2024-global-cancer-burden-growing%2D%2Damidst-mounting-need-for-services.
6. Pinheiro LC, et al. Analysis of eligibility for lung cancer screening by race after 2021 changes to US preventive services task force screening guidelines. JAMA Netw Open. 2022;5(9):e2229741.
7. Yell N, et al. Comparison of the characteristics of the population eligible for lung cancer screening under 2013 and population newly eligible under 2021 US Preventive Services Task Force recommendations. Cancer Causes Control. 2024;35(9):1233–43.
8. Rajapakse P. An update on survivorship issues in lung cancer patients. World J Oncol. 2021;12(2–3):45–9.
9. Pozo CLP, Morgan MAA, Gray JE. Survivorship issues for patients with lung cancer. Cancer Control. 2014;21(1):40–50.
10. Yun YH, et al. Prognostic value of quality of life score in disease-free survivors of surgically-treated lung cancer. BMC Cancer. 2016;16:505.
11. Schneider BJ, et al. Lung cancer surveillance after definitive curative-intent therapy: ASCO guideline. J Clin Oncol. 2020;38(7):753–66.
12. Chambers SK, et al. A systematic review of the impact of stigma and nihilism on lung cancer outcomes. BMC Cancer. 2012;12:184.
13. Siwik CJ, et al. Depressive symptoms among patients with lung cancer: elucidating the roles of shame, guilt, and self-compassion. J Health Psychol. 2022;27(5):1039–47.
14. Flynn KE, et al. Sexual functioning along the cancer continuum: focus group results from the patient-reported outcomes measurement information system (PROMIS®). Psychooncology. 2011;20(4):378–86.
15. National Comprehensive Cancer Network. NCCN Guidelines: Small Cell Lung Cancer. NCCN National Comprehensive Cancer Network; 2025.
16. National Comprehensive Cancer Network. NCCN Guidelines: Non-small cell lung cancer. NCCN National Comprehensive Cancer Network; 2025.
17. American Cancer Society. American cancer Society 2025; Available from: https://www.cancer.org/
18. Children's Oncology Group. Children's Oncology Group 2025 [cited 2025 2/17/2025]; Available from: https://www.childrensoncologygroup.org/
19. Etling MA, et al. The continuing evolution of a cancer prevention, screening, and survivorship ECHO: a second year of implementation. Cancer Med. 2023;12(6):7398–405.
20. National Comprehensive Cancer Network. NCCN Guidelines: Lung Cancer Screening. NCCN National Comprehensive Cancer Network; 2025.
21. American Institute for Cancer Research. Healthy 10 Challenge. 2025 [cited 2025 2/17/2025]; Available from: https://healthy10challenge.org/
22. American Institute for Cancer Research. 30 Day Cancer Prevention Checklist. 2020 [cited 2025 2/17/2025]; Available from: https://www.aicr.org/resources/media-library/30-day-cancer-prevention-checklist/.

23. World Cancer Research Fund. Our Cancer Prevention Recommendations. 2025 [cited 2025 2/13/2025]; Available from: https://www.wcrf.org/preventing-cancer/cancer-prevention/our-cancer-prevention-recommendations/.
24. Flores T, et al. The cancer screening and survivorship program at Roswell Park Comprehensive Cancer Center. J Cancer Surviv. 2024;18(1):11–6. http://creativecommons.org/licenses/by/4.0/.
25. Agley J, et al. Reflections on project ECHO: qualitative findings from five different ECHO programs. Med Educ Online. 2021;26(1):1936435.
26. Davenport AP, et al. Analysis of a pilot study delivering cancer survivorship education to community healthcare professionals utilizing the project ECHO model. J CME. 2024;13(1):2433916.
27. Pariser AC, et al. Delivery of cancer survivorship education to community healthcare professionals. J Cancer Educ. 2023;38(2):625–31.
28. Rohan E, et al. Pairing project ECHO and patient navigation as an innovative approach to improving the health and wellness of cancer survivors in rural settings. J Rural Health. 2022;38(4):855–64.
29. Severance TS, et al. Cancer prevention, screening, and survivorship ECHO: a pilot experience with an educational telehealth program. Cancer Med. 2022;11(1):238–44.
30. AICR American Institute for Cancer Research. Lung Cancer. 2020 4/20/2020; Available from: https://www.aicr.org/cancer-survival/cancer/lung-cancer/.
31. Birken SA, et al. Survivorship care planning: why is it taking so long? J Natl Compr Cancer Netw. 2017;15(9):1165–9.

Open Access This chapter is licensed under the terms of the Creative Commons Attribution-NonCommercial 4.0 International License (http://creativecommons.org/licenses/by-nc/4.0/), which permits any noncommercial use, sharing, adaptation, distribution and reproduction in any medium or format, as long as you give appropriate credit to the original author(s) and the source, provide a link to the Creative Commons license and indicate if changes were made.

The images or other third party material in this chapter are included in the chapter's Creative Commons license, unless indicated otherwise in a credit line to the material. If material is not included in the chapter's Creative Commons license and your intended use is not permitted by statutory regulation or exceeds the permitted use, you will need to obtain permission directly from the copyright holder.

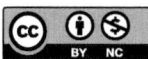

Integrative, Complementary, and Alternative Therapies in Lung Cancer Care

21

Rose Wai-Yee Fok and Gary Deng

Contents

Introduction	284
Navigator Vignette	284
Lung Cancer and CAM	285
Avoid Harmful Alternative Therapies	286
Risks of Harmful Alternative Therapies	287
Integrate Beneficial Complementary Therapies	288
CAM: Upon Diagnosis	290
CAM: Acute Treatment	291
CAM: Survivorship	293
CAM: Palliative Care	293
Steps in Advising on CAM	294
Conclusion	294
Key Takeaways	295
Key Readings and Resources	295
References	296

Abbreviations

ASCO   American Society of Clinical Oncology
CAM   Complementary and alternative medicine
CBT   Cognitive behavioral therapy

R. W.-Y. Fok
Division of Medical Oncology, National Cancer Centre Singapore, Singapore, Singapore
e-mail: rose.fok.w.y@singhealth.com.sg

G. Deng (✉)
Integrative Oncology, UCI Health, University of California, Irvine, Irvine, CA, USA
e-mail: garyd2@hs.uci.edu

© The Author(s) 2026
J. T. Fathi, M. F. Mortman (eds.), *Lung Cancer Navigation and Care*,
https://doi.org/10.1007/978-3-032-02200-4_21

CBT-I   Cognitive behavioral therapy for insomnia
CINV   Chemotherapy-induced nausea and vomiting
EORTC   European Organisation for Research and Treatment of Cancer
ESAS   Edmonton Symptom Assessment System
HCP   Healthcare professionals
IP   Integrative physicians
MBI   Mindfulness-based interventions
MYCAW   Measure Yourself Concerns and Wellbeing
PCC   Patient-centered care
SIO   Society for Integrative Oncology

Introduction

Many cancer patients are interested in complementary and alternative therapies, therapies that have not been provided by mainstream Western medical care. Patient navigators and allied health professionals are uniquely positioned to help patients navigate this complex landscape. This chapter will give an overview of integrative, complementary, and alternative medicine (CAM) related to lung cancer, showcase the current state of science, and empower you to give evidence-informed advice to guide patients in their cancer journey. The fundamental knowledge and skills discussed here will help you direct patients to beneficial treatments while avoiding harm.

Navigator Vignette

Mr. D., a 60-year-old manager, was recently diagnosed with metastatic, non-small cell lung cancer (stage IV). He is undergoing chemotherapy with cisplatin, pemetrexed, and bevacizumab.

Mr. D. has done much reading on the internet about cancer and cancer treatment since his diagnosis. He read that hyperthermia, Gerson's diet, intravenous vitamin C, coffee enema, and soursop juice could help treat cancer. He also experiences nausea and neuropathy, side effects from chemotherapy. He worries a lot about the progression of cancer and has a hard time staying asleep at night. Mr. D. and his wife dislike taking medications and want "something natural" that can help his cancer treatment and relieve some of the side effects. They heard about acupuncture, yoga, and meditation but have no experience with them.

They asked his oncologist for advice. The oncologist feels ill-equipped to answer those questions, as they are not part of the standard medical training curriculum. Fortunately, Mr. D. also works closely with a lung cancer navigator. With Mr. D. and his wife, the team identifies his goals of care and health priorities. His oncologist shares treatment-related priorities: (1) Mr. D. should not be doing anything that may cause harm; (2) If there is anything safe that can help him tolerate chemotherapy better so that he can benefit the most from it, which would be very welcome. The lung cancer navigator patiently listened to Mr. D. and his wife and further inquired about their values, current health-related goals, and alternative therapies they've researched and are seriously interested in using to combat Mr. D.'s lung cancer. The navigator gently guided Mr. D. and his wife in navigating the myriad of complementary and alternative therapies in this scenario.

Lung Cancer and CAM

To help patients navigate the treatment of lung cancer vis-à-vis CAM, one needs to know about CAM in general, what it entails, and the pros and cons.

Lung cancer is one of the deadliest forms of cancer worldwide, significantly impacting patients and their families. Because advanced lung cancer has a poor prognosis, despite current standard treatment, patients want to explore all and any possibilities, including those traditionally not used in mainstream Western medical care—collectively called CAM. According to the National Center for Complementary and Integrative Health (NCCIH), more than 30% of adult Americans and 12% of children use CAM [1]. There is a difference between "complementary," which implies a nonmainstream approach used with conventional medicine to help with cancer treatment, and "alternative," when a nonmainstream approach is used instead of conventional medicine to treat cancer [2]. NCCIH Strategic Plan FY 2021–2025 has worked to advance the position that evidence-based complementary therapies should be "integrated" with and not used as an "alternative" to conventional medicine [3]. Safe and beneficial complementary therapies can be integrated into regular cancer care to improve patient quality of life and outcomes—leading to integrative oncology [4]. Integrative oncology is defined as a patient-centered, evidence-informed field of cancer care that utilizes mind and body practices, natural products, and/or lifestyle modifications from different traditions alongside conventional cancer treatments [5, 6].

Meanwhile, there is a paradigm shift toward patient-centered care (PCC), which has led to a fundamental change in cancer care, from a purely disease-centered approach, measuring survival-related outcomes, to recognizing the importance of quality-of-life outcomes. In this context, patients' values, preferences, and expectations are important factors in making medical decisions, rather than the care centered mainly on health care professionals (HCP) [7]. Having the patient engaged in shared decision making may facilitate the chances of success [8–11]. Shared decision-making is the pinnacle of PCC by addressing decisional conflicts weighing benefits and risks of treatment options [12–14]. A national survey by the National Cancer Institute showed that PCC impacts cancer patients' quality of care and enhances trust in healthcare professionals by addressing feelings, understanding the next steps, clearly explaining, spending adequate time with the patients, and managing uncertainty and involvement in shared decision-making [15]. Therefore, patients' interests in CAM should be addressed instead of being brushed aside.

An initial encounter between a navigator and the patient should focus on "learning about the patient as a person"—their value system, upbringing, cultural background, belief system, and preferences and priorities in treatment. Only with this information can we provide patient-centered care and offer further advice accordingly.

Avoid Harmful Alternative Therapies

What are the alternative therapies that are harmful or counterproductive? They are therapies promised and promoted as effective cancer treatments, while there is no evidence supporting such claims. They can be roughly grouped into three categories.

Fallacious Theories

(1) Those based on fallacious theories. For example, some proponents claim that parasites cause cancer. Therefore, antiparasitics, such as ivermectin or fenbendazole, are promoted as valid cancer treatment. Another example is "ozone therapy," where blood is removed from the body, exposed to ozone, then infused back into the body, purportedly because "cancer cells do not like oxygen." Obviously, other than causing oxidative stress and harm to the blood cells, no ozone will be delivered to the tumor tissue in a sufficient amount to cause any harm to cancer cells.

No Scientific Plausibility

(2) Those with no scientific plausibility as an effective cancer treatment. For example, "hydrogen water" is being sold and promoted by some as a cancer treatment. Unbeknownst to lay people (the end users), very little hydrogen can be dissolved in water (around 1.6 mg/L). Drinking a few drops of this water offers no biological activity against cancer cells.

Active In Vitro but Not in Clinical Use

(3) Those with activity against cancer cells in vitro (in petri dishes) but are not potent enough to cause cancer shrinkage in the human body. For example, dozens of papers are published each year about a natural product's ability to cause apoptosis (cell death). This jargon makes a casual reader think it can make it a powerful anticancer agent. However, upon closer reading of the Methods section of the paper, you will find the concentration needed is in the mM range,

far more than what can be achieved by oral ingestion of the said natural product (usually in the nanoM or low microM range). Many dietary supplements or herbal extracts belong to this "active, but not potent enough for clinical use" category.

Risks of Harmful Alternative Therapies

False Sense of Effectiveness and Foregoing Effective Cancer Therapy

A patient has a false sense of effectiveness and forgoes truly effective cancer therapy, risking disease progression that turns a curable condition into an incurable one. For example, a patient with stage 1 lung cancer could have been cured by surgical resection. Instead, the patient feared surgery and chose to use an ineffective alternative therapy. Months later, unchecked cancer growth led to the cancer spreading to the brain and the bones—a stage 4 disease which cannot be cured.

Costly Ineffective Therapies

Many alternative therapies are expensive, promoted, and marketed by entrepreneurs. Some cost thousands of dollars or tens of thousands of dollars. Using them can deplete a patient's already-stretched financial resources without offering any health benefits, further contributing to and even compounding patient and family suffering.

Ineffective Placebo Dosing

Although many alternative therapies are low risk because the purported active ingredients are in minuscule dosage to cause benefit or harm—the promoter would rather give people placebos than assume legal risk of liabilities; some are high risk and can cause serious harm. One example is the "alkaline therapy" with cesium chloride. The story goes: cancer cells like an acidic environment. Inducing systemic alkalinity by taking cesium chloride would kill and treat cancer cells. To a layperson, this is quite intuitive. However, anyone with a basic understanding of physiology would know that the body maintains a near-neutral environment for cells to function properly. Making the body too alkaline creates a condition—alkalosis, which causes a myriad of dysfunctions. Indeed, cesium chloride used as an alternative cancer treatment has been shown to induce torsades de pointes, a potentially fatal cardiac arrhythmia [16].

Potential Danger of Unregulated Dietary Supplements and Herbal Products

The quality of dietary supplements and herbal products varies tremendously and is not regulated. They also have their toxicities, which can interfere with other medications. For example, an herbal product, PC-SPES, was promoted as a natural treatment for prostate cancer. However, synthetic estrogen, DES, and ethinyl estradiol were detected in this supposedly totally natural product [17]. Kava kava, a herb that has been used to help with stress and anxiety, may cause liver damage [18, 19]. St. John Wort, which some people use for depression, may reduce the plasma level of certain chemotherapy drugs, so patients are, in effect, not getting an adequate dose [20, 21].

To help the public and healthcare professional to learn about those alternative therapies, our institution (Memorial Sloan Kettering Cancer Center) built and has been maintaining a freely available online database listing close to 300 entries on specific complementary and alternative therapies, showing what they are, what we know about them, and the evidence or lack thereof on each entry (aboutherbs.com), all backed by peer-reviewed publications. This website serves as a clearinghouse of data and valuable resource for finding evidence-based information.

The number of alternative cancer therapies is large and ever-evolving. Cancer patients learn about them from internet searches, social media, newsletters, word-of-mouth within their communities, and well-meaning friends and family members. Open discussion with patients about their interest in, reasons for, and usage of alternative therapies is essential for a navigator and allied health professional to help them navigate this area. If a patient does not have confidence that you are genuinely interested in what they feel is important to them, approaches to health that are aligned with their cultural background, belief system, and personal preference, they will be less likely to fully disclose what they are using or follow your advice on those therapies. A patient-centered approach is critical here.

Integrate Beneficial Complementary Therapies

Complementary therapies, such as acupuncture, mindfulness meditation, massage therapies, yoga, etc. (see below), are low-risk, nonpharmacological interventions that can reduce side effects and improve quality of life during treatment of lung cancer. Over the years, there has been much research on many complementary therapies, so much so that some have enough scientific evidence to warrant their incorporation into evidence-based clinical practice.

After a rigorous review of the state of the science, several evidence-based clinical practice guidelines have been formulated and published by professional organizations. The American College of Chest Physicians produced guidelines for treating patients with lung cancer [22]. More recently, the Society of Integrative Oncology

(SIO), in collaboration with the American Society of Clinical Oncology (ASCO), have jointly published clinical practice guidelines for integrative modalities in managing anxiety/depression, pain. and fatigue [23–27]. Other resources include systematic reviews of lung cancer clinical practice guidelines and updates [28, 29].

Many cancer centers have established integrative oncology programs to guide patients in the use of CAM. As part of palliative and supportive care, the pragmatic models of integrative physician (IP) treatment programs have been studied for lung cancer patients in a real-world clinical setting. In one model, at 6 weeks following the initial IP consultation, patients with high adherence to weekly integrative medicine treatments reported a significant improvement in pain, sleep, emotional functioning (on EORTC), depression (ESAS), and well-being (MYCAW) [30].

Specific complementary modalities have been shown to be helpful during the lung cancer journey. Different stages of a patient's treatment course present different clinical issues and priorities (Table 21.1). These evidence-based recommendations are summarized according to the stage of treatment as follows. Knowing these recommendations gives patient navigators and allied health professionals confidence in discussing with patients how complementary therapies can be incorporated into their care.

Table 21.1 Integrating CAM into traditional therapeutic regimens in the cancer journey with areas of focus

Cancer journey				
Diagnosis	Treatment	Survivorship	Recurrence/advanced disease	End-of-life
Anxiety/mood issues	Postsurgical pain	Immunity	Depression/mood issues	Best supportive care (symptom control, QOL)
Sleep	Chemo/RT-induced nausea	Nutrition	Sleep	Nutrition
Exploring ALL treatment options, including alternative therapies, which we steer patients away from	CIPN	Stress reduction	Similar treatment issues	Anticipatory care (spiritual needs)
	Fatigue	Sleep	Fatigue	
		Prevent recurrence	Experimental treatment, e.g., IV vitamin C, mistletoe…	
		Physical activity		

CAM: Upon Diagnosis

At diagnosis, many patients will experience an adjustment reaction, anxiety, and even depression as they cope with accepting the life-threatening disease, reset their priorities, and adjust goal setting. Insomnia commonly accompanies most cancer patients as they cope with information overload and emotional turmoil. HCPs can recommend the following complementary therapies that help mitigate specific symptoms.

Anxiety and Depression

SIO-ASCO recommendations for treating symptoms of anxiety during active treatment include mindfulness-based interventions (MBIs), yoga, relaxation, music therapy, reflexology, and aromatherapy (using inhalation) and for treating anxiety symptoms after cancer treatment include MBIs, yoga, acupuncture, tai chi and/or qigong, and reflexology [24]. For depression symptoms during treatment, recommended modalities include MBIs, yoga, music therapy, relaxation, and reflexology, and for posttreatment, recommendations include MBIs, yoga, tai chi, and/or qigong (Table 21.2) [25].

Table 21.2 SIO-ASCO guidelines for management of anxiety and depression symptoms with integrative therapies

Active treatment	Active treatment-related diagnostic and treatment procedures	Post treatment
Anxiety		
Mindfulness-based therapies	Hypnosis	Mindfulness-based therapies
Yoga	Lavender essential oil inhalation	Tai chi/Qigong
Relaxation therapies		Reflexology
Music therapy		
Reflexology		
Depression		
Active treatment		*Post treatment*
Mindfulness-based therapies		Mindfulness-based therapies
Yoga		Yoga
Music therapy		Tai chi/qigong
Relaxation therapies		
Reflexology		

Adapted from Ref. [25]

Exploring Alternative Therapies

There may be a time when some patients want to explore alternative therapies, especially when they are told that standard therapy is not curative or has undesirable side effects. An important role for the HCP is to support the patient to undergo conventional cancer treatment with the best potential for cure. HCPs should update and provide clarifications to patients with the latest evidence of risk/benefits/precautions and steer away from harmful interventions (see section "Avoid harmful alternative therapies"). If an HCP feels ill-equipped to provide detailed and nuanced discussions, referral to an HCP properly trained in integrative oncology who is knowledgeable about alternative therapies and skilled in patient-centered communication would be warranted. Many major cancer centers provide such services.

CAM: Acute Treatment

Pain

SIO-ASCO guidelines recommend acupuncture, reflexology, massage therapies, music therapies, and mind–body practices for the management of pain symptoms. The types of pain amenable to various complementary therapies are summarized in Table 21.3 [26].

Chemotherapy-Induced Nausea and Vomiting

Multinational Association of Supportive Care in Cancer/European Society for Medical Oncology consensus antiemetic guidelines 2023 recommend if a nonpharmacological intervention is considered, it should be used in addition to

Table 21.3 SIO-ASCO guidelines for management of pain symptoms with integrative therapies

Pain				
General pain or musculoskeletal pain	CIPN	Procedural pain	Surgical pain	Pain during palliative and hospice care
Acupuncture	Acupuncture		Acupuncture	
Reflexology	Reflexology			
Massage				Massage
Yoga				
Guided imagery with progressive muscle relaxation				
		Hypnosis		
			Music	

Adapted from Ref. [26]

guideline-directed recommendations when feasible and based on patient preference [31]. Acupuncture or electroacupuncture was recommended for chemotherapy-induced nausea and vomiting (CINV), particularly acute vomiting, but effects may be short-lived. Another recommendation is that adjunctive progressive muscle relaxation training (alone or with guided imagery) be used to manage CINV.

Fatigue

Fatigue is a multifactorial symptom. Many lung cancer patients experience fatigue during active treatment, cancer recurrence, or advanced disease [32]. At various stages of cancer treatment, exercise, cognitive behavioral therapy (CBT), mindfulness-based programs, tai chi or qigong, yoga, moxibustion, psychoeducation and American ginseng, etc., can be considered, as per SIO-ASCO guidelines (Table 21.4) [27].

Sleep

Insomnia is underrecognized and undermanaged among patients with cancer throughout the cancer journey, with prevalence rates of 30–70% [33–38]. Prevalence of insomnia generally improved over time but remained pervasive in a significant proportion of patients [39]. In patients receiving chemotherapy, the incidence is about three times higher than in the general population [40].

Table 21.4 SIO-ASCO guidelines for management of cancer fatigue with integrative therapies

Fatigue		
Active treatment	After active treatment	Post treatment
Exercise (aerobic, resistance, combination)	Exercise (aerobic, resistance, combination)	Cognitive behavioral therapy
Cognitive behavioral therapy with/ without hypnosis	Cognitive behavioral therapy	Corticosteroids
Mindfulness-based program (MBSR, MBCT)	Mindfulness-based program (MBSR, MBCT, MAPS)	
Tai chi or qigong	Yoga	
Psychoeducation	Acupressure	
American ginseng	Moxibustion	
Interventions NOT recommended		
Active treatment	After active treatment	Post treatment
Wakefulness agents	Wakefulness agents	Wakefulness agents
Psychostimulants	Psychostimulants	Psychostimulants
L-carnitine		
Antidepressants		

Adapted from Ref. [27]

Cognitive-behavioral therapy for insomnia (CBT-I) is the "gold standard" non-pharmacologic treatment for insomnia in cancer and non-cancer patients, with medium-to-large effect sizes for sleep outcomes and associated with sustained effects [41, 42]. There is emerging evidence for acupuncture and moxibustion for the management of cancer-related insomnia [43–45]. A secondary analysis among cancer survivors with comorbid pain and insomnia, acupuncture led to rapid pain reductions, which contributed to improvement in insomnia, whereas CBT-I had a delayed effect on pain, likely achieved by insomnia improvement [52]. Auricular acupuncture can potentially address cluster symptoms like pain and insomnia [46]. Massage therapy may help improve sleep outcomes for cancer survivors, but current evidence regarding relaxation therapy remains low [47]. An Asian practice guideline recommended acupuncture and herbal treatment to address insomnia in both cancer patients and survivors [48, 49]. Exercise has shown multiple benefits in cancer patients with improved physical functioning and decreased fatigue, with limited evidence on sleep outcomes [50–52].

CAM: Survivorship

Cancer survivors often have to self-navigate cancer care after the active treatment phase, given the reduced clinical touchpoints [52, 53]. Furthermore, the prevalent use of novel treatments has been associated with new toxicities [54, 55]. Care guidelines and decision aids have been developed to provide evidence-based resources to cancer survivors to understand possible late and long-term toxicities of treatment [56–59].

Cancer survivors have keenly sought CAM to boost immunity, prevent recurrence, and promote health [60, 61]. None of those can be achieved with a single intervention. Comprehensive lifestyle changes that focus on optimizing diet, exercise, stress management, sleep, and circadian rhythms, a supportive social environment, and positive elements in a patient's life would help improve a patient's overall wellness.

CAM: Palliative Care

Lung cancer patients are living longer with the advancement of supportive care and newer drug options but continue to cope with burdensome symptoms like pain, coughing, and SOB. Moreover, conventional palliative and supportive care is limited in its ability to address many of these symptoms adequately. Palliative care may be best suited to discuss ongoing symptom management, advanced care planning, and complex end-of-life conversations [62, 63]. There is emerging evidence supporting the inclusion of an integrative healthcare approach within supportive care services to improve value and enhance holistic patient care of patients with lung cancer [64, 65]. Integrative palliative care is a new transformative field that aims to alleviate suffering, leveraging the shared values of healing, well-being, patient-centered care, and whole-person care [66].

This new field can incorporate nonpharmacologic strategies, such as acupuncture or mindfulness meditation, into standard palliative care for pain management. Besides providing holistic symptom management and helping patients to engage more meaningfully in daily living and relationships, integrative palliative care can also reduce medication dependence [67].

Patients with very advanced lung cancer and running out of treatment options may want to explore unconventional therapies. Helping patients accept the futility of further treatment is challenging. Referring to trained integrative oncology professionals for an in-depth and convincing discussion of what those therapies can and cannot offer assists patients tremendously in transitioning from active cancer treatment to focusing on palliation.

Steps in Advising on CAM

Below is a step-by-step algorithm to incorporate CAM in a routine clinical consultation:

1. Open the conversation by acknowledging the patient's interest in CAM.
2. Reassure the patient that the HCP role is to support and work together to achieve the best outcome.
3. Provide ample opportunity for patients to voice any questions or concerns.
4. Explore psychosocial and cultural context, then analyze patients' areas of priority.
5. Demonstrate your understanding that patients want low-toxicity therapies that help their cancer journey and that some such therapies are available.
6. Introduce the broader concept of integrative medicine, an approach to health that promotes the well-being of the body, mind, and spirit.
7. Offer a comprehensive lifestyle assessment and recommend changes.
8. Discuss specific mainstream and complementary therapies that are appropriate for the patient's clinical concerns, considering their situation and needs.
9. Explain why some therapies are either without scientific merit or potentially harmful.
10. Summarize the key points and confirm their understanding.
11. Document the encounter, arrange follow-up visits to monitor adverse reactions and responses to treatment, and adjust the treatment plan as required [68].

Conclusion

Unmet symptom needs and a desire for holistic health approaches or even cures are among the motivations patients have for seeking out CAM. Integrative oncology is a patient-centered, evidence-informed field of comprehensive cancer care that prioritizes safety and the best available evidence to offer safe and effective complementary therapies and conventional cancer treatments [69].

Patient navigators and allied health professionals have an important role in building trust and engaging in open and informed conversations with their patients to understand their needs, set realistic expectations, and dispel myths regarding natural cancer cures. They are also instrumental in working with the oncological team to support conventional cancer treatment, guide patients toward evidence-informed complementary therapies, and steer away from harmful practices. This approach will respect patients' choices, improve adherence, and empower self-management toward positive health outcomes.

Key Takeaways

- As new therapies for lung cancer have significantly improved the length and quality of survival after diagnosis, we need to explore new care models that incorporate CAM along with conventional cancer treatments.
- Seeing cancer in the context of a patient's life helps facilitate patient-centered care.
- Integrative oncology focuses on treating the whole person, not just the disease. It addresses physical, emotional, and psychological needs to provide holistic care and improve quality of life.
- A personalized, open, and informed conversation will foster trust and empower patients in shared decision-making.
- The goal is to create a comprehensive and personalized approach that enhances treatment outcomes and supports the overall health of cancer patients.
- Integrative oncology is a developing field with emerging evidence, and healthcare professionals need to equip themselves with the latest update.
- Despite the benefits, challenges include the need for more rigorous research to establish the efficacy of certain complementary therapies, as well as access and cost barriers for some patients.

Key Readings and Resources

- National Cancer Institute. Office of Cancer Complementary and Alternative Medicine [70]
- National Center for Complementary and Integrative Health. What does NCCIH do [71]
- Memorial Sloan Kettering Cancer Center. About Herbs, Botanicals & Other Products [72]
- Deng and Cassileth [68]
- SIO-ASCO Guidelines: The Society for Integrative Oncology-American Society of Clinical Oncology Joint Guidelines on Integrative Therapies for Symptom Management-Overview and Key Recommendations [24]

- SIO-ASCO Guidelines: Integrative Oncology Care of Symptoms of Anxiety and Depression in Adults With Cancer: Society for Integrative Oncology–ASCO Guideline [25]
- SIO-ASCO Guidelines: Integrative Medicine for Pain Management in Oncology: Society for Integrative Oncology–ASCO Guideline [26]
- SIO-ASCO Guidelines: Management of Fatigue in Adult Survivors of Cancer: ASCO–Society for Integrative Oncology Guideline Update [27]

Conflicts of Interest No conflicts of interest.

References

1. National Center for Complementary and Integrative Health. Complementary, alternative, or integrative health: what's in a name? [Internet]. Bethesda (MD): National Institutes of Health; [cited 2025 Apr 27]. Available from: https://www.nccih.nih.gov/health/complementary-alternative-or-integrative-health-whats-in-a-name.
2. Institute of Medicine Committee on the Use of Complementary Alternative Medicine by the American, Public. Complementary and Alternative Medicine in the United States. Washington (DC): National Academies Press (US); 2005.
3. National Center for Complementary and Integrative Health. Strategic plan FY 2021–2025 [Internet]. Bethesda (MD): National Institutes of Health; [cited 2025 Apr 27]. Available from: https://www.nccih.nih.gov/about/nccih-strategic-plan-2021-2025.
4. Mao JJPG, Andrade CJ, Ligibel JA, Basu P, Cohen L. Integrative oncology: addressing the global challenges of cancer prevention and treatment. CA Cancer J Clin. 2022;72(2):144–64.
5. Witt CM, Balneaves LG, Cardoso MJ, Cohen L, Greenlee H, Johnstone P, et al. A comprehensive definition for integrative oncology. JNCI Monographs. 2017;2017(52):lgx012. https://doi.org/10.1093/jncimonographs/lgx012.
6. Semeniuk G, Bahadini B, Ahn E, Zain J, Cheng J, Govindarajan A, et al. Integrative oncology and the clinical care network: challenges and opportunities. J Clin Med. 2023;12(12):3946. https://doi.org/10.3390/jcm12123946.
7. Kennedy BM, Rehman M, Johnson WD, Magee MB, Leonard R, Katzmarzyk PT. Healthcare providers versus patients' understanding of health beliefs and values. Patient Exp J. 2017;4(3):29.
8. Balogh EP, Ganz PA, Murphy SB, Nass SJ, Ferrell BR, Stovall E. Patient-centered cancer treatment planning: improving the quality of oncology care. Summary of an Institute of Medicine workshop. Oncologist. 2011;16(12):1800–5. https://doi.org/10.1634/theoncologist.2011-0252.
9. Ben-Arye E, Samuels N. Patient-centered care in lung cancer: exploring the next milestones. Transl Lung Cancer Res. 2015;4(5) https://doi.org/10.3978/j.issn.2218-6751.2015.03.07.
10. Hibbard JH, Mahoney E, Sonet E. Does patient activation level affect the cancer patient journey? Patient Educ Couns. 2017;100(7):1276–9. https://doi.org/10.1016/j.pec.2017.03.019.
11. Hibbard JH. Patient activation and the use of information to support informed health decisions. Patient Educ Couns. 2017;100(1):5–7. https://doi.org/10.1016/j.pec.2016.07.006.
12. Elwyn G, Frosch D, Thomson R, Joseph-Williams N, Lloyd A, Kinnersley P, et al. Shared decision making: a model for clinical practice. J Gen Intern Med. 2012;27(10):1361–7. https://doi.org/10.1007/s11606-012-2077-6.
13. Barry MJ, Edgman-Levitan S. Shared decision making—the pinnacle of patient-centered care. N Engl J Med. 2012;366(9):780–1. https://doi.org/10.1056/NEJMp1109283.
14. Légaré F, Adekpedjou R, Stacey D, Turcotte S, Kryworuchko J, Graham ID, et al. Interventions for increasing the use of shared decision making by healthcare professionals. The. Cochrane Database Syst Rev. 2018;2018(7):CD006732. https://doi.org/10.1002/14651858.CD006732.pub4.

15. Elkefi S, Asan O. The impact of patient-centered care on cancer patients' QOC, self-efficacy, and trust towards doctors: analysis of a National Survey. J Patient Exp. 2023;10:23743735231151533. https://doi.org/10.1177/23743735231151533.
16. Wiens M, Gordon W, Baulcomb D, Mattman A, Mock T, Brown R. Cesium chloride-induced torsades de pointes. Can J Cardiol. 2009;25(9):e329–e31.
17. Oh WK, Kantoff PW, Weinberg V, Jones G, Brian IR, Derynck MK, Bok R, Smith MR, Bubley GJ, Rosen RT, DiPaola RS, Small EJ. Prospective, multicenter, randomized phase II trial of the herbal supplement, PC-SPES, and diethylstilbestrol in patients with androgen-independent prostate cancer. J Clin Oncol. 2004;22(18):3705–12.
18. Clouatre DL. Kava: examining new reports of toxicity. Toxicol Lett. 2004;150(1):85–96. https://doi.org/10.1016/j.toxlet.2003.07.005.
19. Perez JHJ. Altered mental status and ataxia secondary to acute Kava ingestion. J Emerg Med. 2005 Jan;28(1):49–51.
20. Mathijssen RH, Verweij J, de Bruijn P, Loos WJ, Sparreboom A. Effects of St. John's wort on irinotecan metabolism. J Natl Cancer Inst. 2002 Aug 21;94(16):1247–9.
21. Werneke U, Earl J, Seydel C, Horn O, Crichton P, Fannon D. Potential health risks of complementary alternative medicines in cancer patients. Br J Cancer. 2004;90(2):408. https://doi.org/10.1038/sj.bjc.6601560.
22. Deng GE, Rausch SM, Jones LW, Gulati A, Kumar NB, Greenlee H, et al. Complementary therapies and integrative medicine in lung cancer: diagnosis and management of lung cancer, 3rd ed: American College of Chest Physicians Evidence-Based Clinical Practice Guidelines. CHEST. 2013;143(5):e420S–e36S. https://doi.org/10.1378/chest.12-2364.
23. Society for Integrative Oncology and the American Society of Clinical Oncology. SIO-ASCO Guideline Proposes Evidence-Based Approaches to Pain Management Incorporating Integrative Medicine Interventions 2022. Accessed 27 Apr 2025.
24. Carlson LE, Tripathy D, Zick SM, Balneaves LG, Lee RT, Greenlee H. The Society for Integrative Oncology-American Society of Clinical Oncology Joint Guidelines on Integrative Therapies for Symptom Management-Overview and Key Recommendations. J Integr Complement Med [Internet] [cited 2024 Nov 2]. 2024;30(7):596–601.
25. Carlson LE, Ismaila N, Addington EL, Asher GN, Atreya C, Balneaves LG, et al. Integrative oncology care of symptoms of anxiety and depression in adults with cancer: Society for Integrative Oncology–ASCO guideline. J Clin Oncol. 2023;41(28):4562–91. https://doi.org/10.1200/JCO.23.00857.
26. Mao JJ, Ismaila N, Bao T, Barton D, Ben-Arye E, Garland EL, et al. Integrative medicine for pain management in oncology: society for integrative oncology–ASCO guideline. J Clin Oncol. 2022;40(34):3998–4024. https://doi.org/10.1200/JCO.22.01357.
27. Bower JELC, Alici Y, Barton DL, Bruner D, Canin BE. Management of Fatigue in adult survivors of cancer: ASCO–Society for Integrative Oncology Guideline Update. JCO. 2024;42:2456.
28. Gowin KMM, Zick SM, Lee RT, Lacchetti C, Mehta A. Integrative therapies in cancer care: an update on the guidelines. Am Soc Clin Oncol Educ Book. 2024 Jun;44(3):e431554.
29. Ng JY. Complementary and integrative medicine mention and recommendations: a systematic review and quality assessment of lung cancer clinical practice guidelines. Integrative medicine. Research. 2021;10:100452.
30. Ben-Arye E, Gressel O, Lifshitz S, Peled N, Keren S, Samuels N. Integrative oncology for patients with lung cancer: a prospective pragmatic controlled trial. Lung Cancer. 2024;193:107857. https://doi.org/10.1016/j.lungcan.2024.107857.
31. Herrstedt J, Clark-Snow R, Ruhlmann CH, Molassiotis A, Olver I, Rapoport BL, et al. 2023 MASCC and ESMO guideline update for the prevention of chemotherapy- and radiotherapy-induced nausea and vomiting. ESMO Open. 2024;9(2):102195. https://doi.org/10.1016/j.esmoop.2023.102195.
32. Robbins-Welty GA, Chammas D, Silverman EJ, Lowry MF, Hale E, Martinez C, et al. Top ten tips palliative care clinicians should know about diagnosing, categorizing, and addressing fatigue. J Palliat Med. 2024;28:jpm.2024.0232. https://doi.org/10.1089/jpm.2024.0232.

33. Savard J, Morin CM. Insomnia in the context of cancer: a review of a neglected problem. J Clin Oncol. 2001;19(3):895–908. https://doi.org/10.1200/JCO.2001.19.3.895.
34. Mercadante S, Girelli D, Casuccio A. Sleep disorders in advanced cancer patients: prevalence and factors associated. Support Care Cancer. 2004;12(5):355–9. https://doi.org/10.1007/s00520-004-0623-4.
35. Sela RA, Watanabe S, Nekolaichuk CL. Sleep disturbances in palliative cancer patients attending a pain and symptom control clinic. Palliat Support Care. 2005;3(1):23–31. https://doi.org/10.1017/S1478951505050042.
36. Le Guen Y, Gagnadoux F, Hureaux J, Jeanfaivre T, Meslier N, Racineux J-L, et al. Sleep disturbances and impaired daytime functioning in outpatients with newly diagnosed lung cancer. Lung Cancer. 2007;58(1):139–43. https://doi.org/10.1016/j.lungcan.2007.05.021.
37. Romito F, Cormio C, De Padova S, Lorusso V, Ma B, Fimiani F, et al. Patients attitudes towards sleep disturbances during chemotherapy. Eur J Cancer Care. 2014;23(3):385–93. https://doi.org/10.1111/ecc.12106.
38. Davidson JR, MacLean AW, Brundage MD, Schulze K. Sleep disturbance in cancer patients. Soc Sci Med. 2002;54(9):1309–21. https://doi.org/10.1016/S0277-9536(01)00043-0.
39. Savard JIH, Villa J, Caplette-Gingras A, Morin CM. Natural course of insomnia comorbid with cancer: an 18-month longitudinal study. JCO Clin Cancer Inform. 2011;29(26):3580–6.
40. Palesh OG, Roscoe JA, Mustian KM, Roth T, Savard J, Ancoli-Israel S, et al. Prevalence, demographics, and psychological associations of sleep disruption in patients with cancer: University of Rochester Cancer Center–Community Clinical Oncology Program. J Clin Oncol. 2009;28(2):292. https://doi.org/10.1200/JCO.2009.22.5011.
41. Howell D, Oliver TK, Keller-Olaman S, Davidson JR, Garland S, Samuels C, et al. Sleep disturbance in adults with cancer: a systematic review of evidence for best practices in assessment and management for clinical practice. Ann Oncol. 2014;25(4):791–800. https://doi.org/10.1093/annonc/mdt506.
42. Qaseem A, Kansagara D, Forciea MA, Cooke M, Denberg TD. For the clinical guidelines Committee of the American College of P. Management of Chronic Insomnia Disorder in adults: a clinical practice guideline from the American College of physicians. Ann Intern Med. 2016;165(2):125–33. https://doi.org/10.7326/M15-2175.
43. Choi T-Y, Kim JI, Lim H-J, Lee MS. Acupuncture for managing cancer-related insomnia: a systematic review of randomized clinical trials. Integr Cancer Ther. 2017;16(2):135–46. https://doi.org/10.1177/1534735416664172.
44. Lee B, Kim B-K, Kim M, Kim A-R, Park H-J, Kwon OJ, et al. Electroacupuncture for treating cancer-related insomnia: a multicenter, assessor-blinded, randomized controlled, pilot clinical trial. BMC Complement Med Ther. 2022;22(1):77. https://doi.org/10.1186/s12906-022-03561-w.
45. Chen L, Li J, Xu S, Liu Z, Jiao Y, Zhou Z. Efficacy of acupuncture therapy on cancer-related insomnia: a systematic review and network meta-analysis. Front Neurol. 2024;15:15. https://doi.org/10.3389/fneur.2024.1342383.
46. Garner BK, Hopkinson SG, Ketz AK, Landis CA, Trego LL. Auricular acupuncture for chronic pain and insomnia: a randomized clinical trial. Med Acupunct. 2018;30(5):262–72. https://doi.org/10.1089/acu.2018.1294.
47. Samuel SR, Gururaj R, Kumar KV, Vira P, Saxena PUP, Keogh JWL. Randomized control trial evidence for the benefits of massage and relaxation therapy on sleep in cancer survivors—a systematic review. J Cancer Surviv. 2021;15(5):799–810. https://doi.org/10.1007/s11764-020-00972-x.
48. Lam WCZL, Liu Y, Shi N, Ng B, Ziea E, et al. Hong Kong Chinese medicine clinical practice guideline for cancer palliative care: pain, constipation, and insomnia. Evid Based Complement Alternat Med. 2019;22:1038206. https://pmc.ncbi.nlm.nih.gov/articles/PMC6362507/
49. Haddad NE, Palesh O. Acupuncture in the treatment of cancer-related psychological symptoms. Integr Cancer Ther. 2014;13(5):371–85. https://doi.org/10.1177/1534735413520181.

50. Mercier J, Savard J, Bernard P. Exercise interventions to improve sleep in cancer patients: a systematic review and meta-analysis. Sleep Med Rev. 2017;36:43–56. https://doi.org/10.1016/j.smrv.2016.11.001.
51. Campbell KL, Winters-Stone KM, Wiskemann J, May AM, Schwartz AL, Courneya KS, et al. Exercise guidelines for cancer survivors: consensus statement from international multidisciplinary roundtable. Med Sci Sports Exerc. 2019;51(11):2375. https://doi.org/10.1249/MSS.0000000000002116.
52. Halpern MT, McCabe MS, Burg MA. The cancer survivorship journey: models of care, disparities, barriers, and future directions. Am Soc Clin Oncol Educ Book. 2016;35:231–9. https://doi.org/10.1200/EDBK_156039.
53. Nekhlyudov LGP, Arora NK, Rowland JH. Going beyond being lost in transition: a decade of Progress in cancer survivorship. J Clin Oncol [Internet]. 2017;35(18):1978.
54. Carbone DP, Gandara DR, Antonia SJ, Zielinski C, Paz-Ares L. Non–small cell lung cancer: role of the immune system and potential for immunotherapy. J Thorac Oncol. 2015;10(7):974. https://doi.org/10.1097/JTO.0000000000000551.
55. Patrinely JR, Young AC, Quach H, Williams GR, Ye F, Fan R, et al. Survivorship in immune therapy: assessing toxicities, body composition and health-related quality of life among long-term survivors treated with antibodies to programmed death-1 receptor and its ligand. Eur J Cancer. 2020;135:211–20. https://doi.org/10.1016/j.ejca.2020.05.005.
56. O'Brien MA, Whelan TJ, Villasis-Keever M, Gafni A, Charles C, Roberts R, et al. Are cancer-related decision aids effective? A systematic review and meta-analysis. J Clin Oncol. 2009;27(6):974–85. https://doi.org/10.1200/JCO.2007.16.0101.
57. McAlpine K, Lewis KB, Trevena LJ, Stacey D. What is the effectiveness of patient decision aids for cancer-related decisions? A systematic review subanalysis. JCO Clinical Cancer Informatics. 2018;2:1–13. https://doi.org/10.1200/CCI.17.00148.
58. Ke Y, Zhou H, Chan RJ, Chan A. Decision aids for cancer survivors' engagement with survivorship care services after primary treatment: a systematic review. J Cancer Surviv. 2022;18(2):288. https://doi.org/10.1007/s11764-022-01230-y.
59. National Comprehensive Cancer Network. NCCN Guidelines for patients: survivorship care for cancer-related late and long-term effects. 2024.
60. Amichai T, Grossman M, Richard M. Lung cancer patients' beliefs about complementary and alternative medicine in the promotion of their wellness. Eur J Oncol Nurs. 2012;16(5):520–7. https://doi.org/10.1016/j.ejon.2012.01.004.
61. Choi JY, Ji W, Choi C-M, Chung C, Noh JM, Park C-K, et al. Awareness and use of Complementary and alternative medicine in Korean lung cancer patients. Tuberculosis Respir Dis. 2020;84(2):105. https://doi.org/10.4046/trd.2020.0098.
62. Orstad S, Fløtten Ø, Madebo T, Gulbrandsen P, Strand R, Lindemark F, et al. "The challenge is the complexity"—a qualitative study about decision-making in advanced lung cancer treatment. Lung Cancer. 2023;183:107312. https://doi.org/10.1016/j.lungcan.2023.107312.
63. Presley CJ, Dalal N, Davenport AP, Gounden A, Ramchandran K, Tonorezos E. Survivorship in advanced lung cancer: understanding a new landscape and opportunities. Am Soc Clin Oncol Educ Book. 2024;44 https://doi.org/10.1200/EDBK_433298.
64. Wojtacki J, Pawlowski L, Pawlowska I, Lichodziejewska-Niemierko M. Complementary and alternative medicine (CAM) use among patients with cancer undergoing palliative care: a pilot study of a single institution in Poland. J Clin Oncol. 2017;35(5_suppl):178. https://doi.org/10.1200/JCO.2017.35.5_suppl.178.
65. Balboni TA, Hui K-KP, Kamal AH. Supportive care in lung cancer: improving value in the era of modern therapies. Am Soc Clin Oncol Educ Book. 2018;38:716–25. https://doi.org/10.1200/EDBK_201369.
66. Chiaramonte DR, Adler SR. Integrative palliative care: a new transformative field to alleviate suffering. J Altern Complement Med. 2020;26(9):761–5. https://doi.org/10.1089/acm.2020.0366.

67. Adler SR, Marchand LR, Heap N. Integrative palliative care: enhancing the natural synergy between integrative health and palliative medicine. J Altern Complement Med. 2019;25(3):257–9. https://doi.org/10.1089/acm.2019.29063.sra.
68. Deng G, Cassileth B. Complementary or alternative medicine in cancer care—myths and realities. Nat Rev Clin Oncol. 2013;10(11):656–64. https://doi.org/10.1038/nrclinonc.2013.125.
69. Latte-Naor S, Mao JJ. Putting integrative oncology into practice: concepts and approaches. J Oncol Pract. 2019;15(1):7–14. https://doi.org/10.1200/JOP.18.00554.
70. National Cancer Institute. Office of Cancer Complementary and Alternative Medicine. https://cam.cancer.gov/. Accessed 2025.
71. National Center for Complementary and Integrative Health. What does NCCIH do? https://www.nccih.nih.gov/. Accessed 2025.
72. Memorial Sloan Kettering Cancer Center. About Herbs, Botanicals & Other Products. https://www.mskcc.org/cancer-care/diagnosis-treatment/symptom-management/integrative-medicine/herbs. Accessed 2025.

Open Access This chapter is licensed under the terms of the Creative Commons Attribution-NonCommercial 4.0 International License (http://creativecommons.org/licenses/by-nc/4.0/), which permits any noncommercial use, sharing, adaptation, distribution and reproduction in any medium or format, as long as you give appropriate credit to the original author(s) and the source, provide a link to the Creative Commons license and indicate if changes were made.

The images or other third party material in this chapter are included in the chapter's Creative Commons license, unless indicated otherwise in a credit line to the material. If material is not included in the chapter's Creative Commons license and your intended use is not permitted by statutory regulation or exceeds the permitted use, you will need to obtain permission directly from the copyright holder.

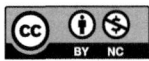

Policy and Advocacy in Lung Cancer

22

Angela M. Barry and Laurie Fenton Ambrose

Contents

Navigation Vignette.. 302
Introduction... 302
The Meaning of Policy... 303
The Evolving Lung Cancer Policy Environment........................ 304
Policy Advocacy and You... 305
Conclusion... 307
Key Takeaways... 307
Key Readings and Resources.. 308
References... 308

Abbreviations

ACA	Affordable Care Act
CDMRP	Congressionally Directed Medical Research Program
CMS	Centers for Medicare and Medicaid Services
HHS	US Department of Health and Human Services
LCA	Lung Cancer Alliance
LCS	Lung cancer screening
LCRP	Lung Cancer Research Program
LDCT	Low-dose computed tomography
MSA	Master Settlement Agreement
MEDCAC	Medicare Evidence Development & Coverage Advisory Committee

A. M. Barry (✉) · L. F. Ambrose
GO2 for Lung Cancer, Washington, DC, USA
e-mail: abarry@go2.org; lfambrose@go2.org

© The Author(s) 2026
J. T. Fathi, M. F. Mortman (eds.), *Lung Cancer Navigation and Care*,
https://doi.org/10.1007/978-3-032-02200-4_22

NCCN   National Comprehensive Cancer Network
NCD   National coverage determination
NLST   National Lung Screening Trial
OOPC   Out-of-pocket costs
USPSTF   United States Preventive Services Task Force

Navigation Vignette

Navigator A. works within a busy lung cancer screening (LCS) program, providing patient care across the comprehensive screening process. A's experiences with patient outreach, education and follow-up have revealed many barriers and burdens in the LCS process, including specific CMS reimbursement requirements that hinder provider referral and patient uptake for their patients at high risk of lung cancer.

When CMS releases a new draft national coverage determination (NCD) for LCS, Navigator A. notices several important changes in screening eligibility that will create access for new populations. However, the draft NCD retains several onerous reimbursement requirements that will continue impacting referral and uptake. Navigator A. also notes CMS has opened a 30-day public comment period for this draft NCD.

After consulting with their health system leadership, Navigator A. takes several steps to advocate for additional regulatory policy change. First, they contact a trusted lung cancer patient advocacy organization for talking points and template language to help them craft a public comment submission. Second, they gather aggregate program data that shows their program's early detection impact as well as the uptake gap among their estimated eligible population. Third, they compile specific examples of how CMS's reimbursement rules contribute to low referral rates among their system's primary care physicians and make the screening process time-consuming and complicated for their patients. Finally, they draft a public comment for review by their leadership and, once approved, submit it through the CMS public comment webpage.

Introduction

It is perhaps fitting that the topic of "policy" comes at the conclusion of this *Lung Cancer Navigation and Care* comprehensive guide—first, because policy is most relevant and meaningful when it is built on a strong foundation of evidence, which all of the preceding chapters have helped us gather. When erected on such a foundation, policy can create structure and consistency in how evidence-based practice is implemented for optimal population impact. Second, many people are wary of policy considerations and policy-related involvement due to a dislike of *politics*, so hopefully, the preceding chapters have created momentum that will inspire the reader to overcome any initial reluctance toward the policy topic.

This chapter aims to demystify policy as an appropriate and necessary arena in which lung cancer navigators should actively and confidently engage. We will explore various ways in which policy shapes the vital work that navigators do, and how, in turn, navigators can draw upon their experience and expertise to shape policy for the betterment of their patients, their peers, and the broader population of those at risk for or living with lung cancer.

The Meaning of Policy

When considering the word "policy," many people immediately associate it with "law." Black's Law Dictionary defines policy as "the general principles by which a government is guided in its management of public affairs, or the legislature in its measures," with the purpose to benefit the state or community [1]. This can mean laws formally passed through a legislative process (e.g., Congressional passage of the Affordable Care Act), but it can also mean regulations that a government agency enacts through the rulemaking authority the legislature has delegated to it (e.g., CMS coverage determinations). Indeed, while we readily recognize the potential to influence policymaking by advocating to Congress about particular laws, regulatory policy is a similarly important but nonetheless underrated arena where public input opportunities are not only allowed but often mandated through a public comment process [2]. For example, when the United States Preventive Services Task Force (USPSTF) prepares to consider a new or revised recommendation, they solicit public comments at several steps along the way—from the design of their proposed evidence review, to their initial draft decision and ultimately the final recommendation statement. These recommendations determine whether preventive services such as LCS must be covered by commercial insurance, and if so, for whom—a momentous consideration for navigators and their patients at high risk of lung cancer.

Furthermore, thanks to the US system of federalism, policymaking doesn't just happen in Washington, D.C., where the levers of power may be remote from our daily lives, but at the state and local level as well. Through state legislatures and agencies, local councils, and elected officials, much meaningful policymaking occurs "close to home" for those most directly impacted by it [3]. The lessons learned and successes realized through state policy may eventually be magnified through adoption nationally by Congress. As Supreme Court Justice Brandeis noted, when states enact new policies constituting "novel social and economic experiments," they may "serve as a laboratory" from which the rest of the country may learn and inform their future state and national policy choices [4]. So, for instance, as states begin to address prior authorization reform, their experiences may guide Congress toward similar steps in the future to minimize care delays associated with the prior authorization process.

It is also important to recognize that policy extends beyond formal government legislation and rulemaking. Organizational policies within a healthcare system that guide clinical workflows, or within a commercial payer that determine medical necessity for clinical services coverage, are potentially important factors to consider when evaluating a community's health policy environment and public health needs [5]. For example, when a commercial payer's coverage policies impose step therapy, restricting lung cancer patient access to the range of medications recommended within current National Comprehensive Cancer Network (NCCN) clinical guidelines and limiting provider discretion in choosing among clinically recommended therapies, the impact of policy decisions ripple through the patient community as treatment pathways narrow and become harder to navigate.

Finally, while the making and influencing of policy is a political process, and politics is an arena that many find uncomfortable and wish to avoid, it is useful to consider the seminal definition of politics coined by political scientist Harold Lasswell: "who gets what, when, and how" [6]. At the most fundamental level, politics is a component of all human behavior. We are all involved in it every day, regardless of how much we believe ourselves to be nonpolitical.

The Evolving Lung Cancer Policy Environment

Laurie Fenton Ambrose, coauthor of this chapter, recalls that when Sheila Ross, an original founder of the groundbreaking patient advocacy organization ALCASE, reached out in 2003 to enlist her help with the movement that became the Lung Cancer Alliance (LCA, one of two legacy organizations that later merged to become GO2 for Lung Cancer), Sheila pointedly stated: "Lung cancer is a political problem, not a science problem. Unless we change federal health policies, the status quo will remain." This stark insight serves as a call to action, revealing that scientific advancement is necessary *but not sufficient* to transform lung cancer survival rates. Policy shapes the arena in which much scientific research is funded and conducted and its results disseminated and implemented. For lung cancer, this arena has historically been politically charged and stigmatized.

The evidence linking smoking and lung cancer, for instance, long faced an uphill battle in the face of tobacco industry interests that blocked and/or co-opted scientific studies, controlled the resulting messaging and poured money into political access to derail unfavorable policy [7]. Some key legal/policy developments helped turn the tide and begin pulling back the curtain on tobacco industry manipulation of the scientific evidence on smoking-related illnesses. For instance, the 1998 Master Settlement Agreement (MSA) signed between 52 US state and territory attorneys general and, eventually, over 45 tobacco companies [8], and then ultimately the considerable public attention generated by a US Department of Justice federal suit against the nation's largest cigarette manufacturers and tobacco trade organizations. This landmark case culminated in a 2006 ruling by US District Judge Gladys Kessler that the tobacco companies had violated antiracketeering laws and the imposition of numerous remedies requiring these companies to truthfully inform the public of the health risks associated with use of their product [9].

Within Congress, the tide was similarly turning at this time, with 2006 marking the first ever bipartisan, bicameral (support from members of the House and Senate representing both political parties) concurrent resolutions designating lung cancer a national health priority [10, 11]. Three years later, the first lung cancer-specific federal research pipeline was created through the Fiscal Year 2009 congressional appropriation, providing $20 million in the FY09 budget for the Department of Defense Lung Cancer Research Program (LCRP) within the Congressional Directed Medical Research Program (CDMRP) [12]. This is far from a comprehensive description of federal policy developments, but the intent is to demonstrate how lung cancer began to attain greater public and policymaker awareness, the recognition of tobacco industry exploitation gained traction, and the desire for evidence-based solutions ultimately created opportunities to prioritize lung cancer research funding.

This is not to say that policy progress eliminated the scourge of lung cancer stigma. In 2014, as the CMS Medicare Evidence Development & Coverage Advisory Committee (MEDCAC) held a public hearing to consider a request to recommend Medicare coverage for LCS with low-dose CT (LDCT) given the evidence of a 20% lung cancer mortality benefit in the National Lung Screening Trial (NLST), one committee member nonetheless questioned whether this was a "prudent use of resources," noting that this amounted to "writing a check…to reduce deaths from lung cancer that we know are largely caused by tobacco" when those funds could be better used to support tobacco control efforts [13]. Notably, among the members of the public who spoke in support of Medicare coverage for LCS were several healthcare professionals in frontline LCS implementation roles who shared firsthand insights into early detection's impact for their patients—two of these speakers specifically represented roles now recognized as clinical and lay navigation [13]. While MEDCAC voted that day not to recommend coverage, CMS nonetheless issued an NCD less than a year later to begin covering this screening service for Medicare beneficiaries.

Shortly thereafter, harnessing an opportunity created by public excitement at the rapid pace of medical advancements in lung cancer including low-dose CT (LDCT) screening and new targeted therapies and immunotherapies for those diagnosed, LCA drove the 2015 creation of a bipartisan Congressional Lung Cancer Caucus, providing a vital gateway to convene and educate members of Congress and their staff on emerging scientific advancements and opportunities to improve access and capacity for patient-centered, high-quality early detection, treatment, and care [14]. This caucus, which must be re-formed every 2 years with each new Congress, promotes sustained Congressional awareness and attention to lung cancer and has served as the engine for the introduction and cosponsor recruitment of key legislative priorities, including the Women and Lung Cancer Research and Preventive Services Act [15].

Policy Advocacy and You

Opportunities for policy involvement by navigators and other healthcare professionals abound. At the federal level, advocates can encourage their member of Congress to join the Congressional Lung Cancer Caucus and support legislation that addresses current identified needs of the lung cancer population, such as prior authorization reform, coverage for biomarker testing, access to telehealth, preservation of preventive services coverage mandates, and numerous other vital issues.

State legislatures are increasingly demonstrating successful passage, implementation, and impact of lung cancer-related policies. In 2022, Kentucky passed a law creating a state Lung Cancer Screening Program and Lung Cancer Screening Advisory Committee with an initial appropriation of $500,000 and a statutory purpose to increase lung cancer screening, reduce morbidity and mortality, and reduce treatment costs for the Commonwealth [16]. Furthermore, multiple states, including Kentucky, have passed laws requiring all state-regulated insurance plans to cover biomarker testing [17]. The story does not end with the passage of these laws, however. There is still a need for policy engagement to help monitor implementation and identify necessary, future policy revisions.

Recent research has revealed multiple ways in which policy gaps create hurdles and barriers for patient access and uptake of preventive care, including cancer screenings. Out-of-pocket costs (OOPC) associated with follow-up testing can hinder patients from moving forward through the diagnostic process following an initial positive screening exam. While many states have begun eliminating such cost-sharing for diagnostic testing following screening mammography, this should be implemented consistently across the USPSTF recommended cancer screenings [18]. Notably, in 2024, Maryland's legislature passed a bill limiting copayment, coinsurance, and imposition of deductibles for lung cancer screening and follow-up diagnostic imaging for those whose screening is recommended by the USPSTF, to be consistent with their state's coverage requirements for mammography and breast cancer diagnostic services. This law also prohibits the imposition of prior authorization for these covered services, which helps address a significant workflow complication and time burden for ordering providers and screening programs, thereby easing an access barrier for their patients [19].

On a more granular level, a 2024 study revealed a troubling pattern of increased claims denials for preventive care services among particular at-risk populations, including those with low incomes, low education levels, or who represent racial and ethnic minorities. Billing errors were the second most common denial type overall, and two-thirds of denied claims were not resubmitted by the physician. While some claims were likely written off by the provider, the cost of many of these denials was undoubtedly borne by the patients least able to bear them. The study publication noted the policy implications and the need for solutions at multiple levels, including organizational/system-level policy changes such as uniform billing standards and regulatory efforts to create greater billing and claims clarity [20]. While LCS was not included among the seven specific preventive services included in this study's analysis, breast and colorectal cancer screenings were included, and one can reasonably anticipate that at-risk patients within the LCS population are similarly disadvantaged, if not more so.

What is one to do? A 2020 Viewpoint editorial published in JAMA laid out a moral argument for healthcare professionals to expand their "lane" to include proactive and systematic involvement in necessary social change to secure the health of the community. Even if one does not agree with the specific policy areas the author identified as morally compelling, their philosophical framing is worth noting: "Science and knowledge can guide action; they do not cause action" [21]. If the scientific truths that guide a navigator's clinical life are to have a broader impact, the navigator has to proactively extend them with action beyond the narrow clinical lane. For further justification to be policy savvy and engaged, one need only consult the American Nurses Association 2025 Code of Ethics, which in Provision 7.4 notes that "Nurses are engaged in sharing institutional, community and social policies. Given their ethical commitments and body of knowledge, nurses have important contributions to make in health-related policy" [22].

Conclusion

Healthcare policies exist at multiple levels, from the national level to the local and even health system/organizational level, providing multiple pathways for navigator policy involvement and advocacy. These policies shape "who gets what, when, and how"—from which research topics are prioritized for funding, to which patients have access to particular treatments, and even how clinical workflows impact navigator capacity to address the needs of high-risk, vulnerable patients.

While policy can seem intimidating and the problems to be addressed are vast and complex, lung cancer navigators are uniquely positioned to recognize and represent the needs of patients facing many hurdles and barriers and to identify policy solutions that can help ensure their consistent access to the high-quality, patient-centered care they deserve. Opportunities for policy change abound, and the need is vast. It is therefore fitting to close with the words of Churchill: "Never give in, never give in, never, never, never—in nothing, great or small, large or petty—never give in except to convictions of honour and good sense" [23].

Key Takeaways

- Opportunities to impact policy occur at multiple levels, both inside and outside formal government structure.
- While lung cancer has historically been under-prioritized, there are many examples of successful policy impact in the lung cancer arena, revealing momentum to be harnessed and replicated.
- Navigators have vital perspectives to bring to the policy arena and an obligation to lend their voice on behalf of the patients they serve and their professional community.

Key Readings and Resources

- State of Lung Cancer Report [24]
- GO2 for Lung Cancer Advocacy Toolkit [25]
- GO2 for Lung Cancer Policy Priorities [26]
- GO2 for Lung Cancer Voices Summit [27]
- American Cancer Society Cancer Action Network [28]
- American Lung Association Policy & Advocacy [29]
- LUNGevity Public Policy for Supporters & Advocates [30]

Conflicts of Interest
Angela M. Barry—reports no financial or nonfinancial conflicts of interest.
Laurie Fenton Ambrose—reports no financial or nonfinancial conflicts of interest.

References

1. Black HC, Nolan JR, Holan-Haley JM, et al. Black's law dictionary. 6th ed. St. Paul: West Publishing Co.; 1990. p. 1157.
2. Dudley SE, Brito J. Regulation: a primer. 2nd ed. Washington, DC: The George Washington University Regulatory Studies Center; 2012. p. 25–30.
3. Madison J. Federalist No. 46. In: Brock W, editor. The Federalist. London: Everyman J.M. Dent; 1996.
4. New State Ice Co. V. Liebmann. 285 U.S. 262 (1932). Brandeis dissenting, para 51. Available from: https://www.law.cornell.edu/supremecourt/text/285/262
5. Brownson R, Baker E, Leet T, et al. Evidence-based public health. 2nd ed. New York: Oxford University Press; 2011.
6. Lasswell HD. Politics: who gets what, when, how. New York: McGraw-Hill; 1936.
7. Berridge V. The policy response to the smoking and lung cancer connection in the 1950s and 1960s. Hist J. 2006;49(4):1185–209. https://doi.org/10.1017/S0018246X06005784.
8. National Association of Attorneys General: The Master Settlement Agreement. https://www.naag.org/our-work/naag-center-for-tobacco-and-public-health/the-master-settlement-agreement/. Accessed 23 Apr 2025.
9. United States v. Philip Morris USA Inc., 449F. Supp. 2d 1 (2006). Available from: https://www.justice.gov/sites/default/files/civil/legacy/2014/09/11/amended%20opinion_0.pdf
10. S. Res. 408: A Resolution expressing the sense of the Senate that the President should declare lung cancer a public health priority and should implement a comprehensive interagency program that will reduce lung cancer mortality by at least 50 percent by 2015, 109th Congress, 2nd Session (2005–2007), 02 May 2006. Available from: https://www.congress.gov/bill/109th-congress/senate-resolution/408/text?s=4&r=1&q=%7B%22search%22%3A%22S.+Res.+408%22%7D
11. H. Res. 739: Expressing the sense of the House of Representatives that the President should declare lung cancer a public health priority and should implement a comprehensive interagency program that will reduce lung cancer mortality by at least 50 percent by 2015, 109th Congress (2005–2006), 28 March 2006. Available from: https://www.congress.gov/bill/109th-congress/house-resolution/739/text

12. Department of Defense Lung Cancer Research Program (LCRP) Funding for Fiscal Year 2009 (FY09). Congressionally Directed Medical Research Program, 6 August 2009. Gale Academic OneFile [available from: https://cdmrp.health.mil/pubs/press/2009/09lcrppreann].
13. Centers for Medicare and Medicaid Services: Medicare Evidence Development & Coverage Advisory Committee, pp. 116–120, 124–128, 295–296. Baltimore, MD. 30 April 2014. [Posted meeting transcript available from: https://www.cms.gov/Regulations-and-Guidance/Guidance/FACA/downloads/id68c.pdf].
14. Congress Brings Heightened Focus on Lung Cancer. PR Newswire, 27 August 2015. Available from: https://link.gale.com/apps/doc/A426825339/AONE?u=anon~df3733a3&sid=sitemap&xid=e2ec45bf
15. Boyle & Fitzpatrick Introduce Bill to Study and Prevent Lung Cancer Among Women. Boyle. House.Gov Media Center, 11 July 2023. Available from: https://boyle.house.gov/media-center/press-releases/boyle-fitzpatrick-introduce-bill-study-and-prevent-lung-cancer-among
16. HB 219: An Act Relating to Lung Cancer Screening. 2022 Regular Session, Kentucky General Assembly, 31 March 2022. Available from: https://apps.legislature.ky.gov/recorddocuments/bill/22RS/hb219/bill.pdf
17. American Cancer Society Cancer Action Network: Access to Biomarker Testing. https://www.fightcancer.org/what-we-do/access-biomarker-testing (July 2024). Accessed 22 Apr 2025.
18. Taylor CD, Fendrick AM, Dossett LA. Redefining cancer screening coverage—screening to diagnosis. JAMA Health Forum. 2024;5 https://doi.org/10.1001/jamahealthforum.2024.2814.
19. HB 1259/CH0868: An Act Concerning Health Insurance—Breast and Lung Cancer Screening—Coverage Requirements. 2024 Regular Session, Maryland General Assembly, 16 May 2024. Available from: https://mgaleg.maryland.gov/2024RS/Chapters_noln/CH_868_hb1259t.pdf
20. Hoagland A, Yu O, Horný M. Social determinants of health and insurance claim denials for preventive care. JAMA Netw Open. 2024;7 https://doi.org/10.1001/jamanetworkopen.2024.33316.
21. Berwick DM. The moral determinants of health. JAMA. 2020;324 https://doi.org/10.1001/jama.2020.11129.
22. American Nurses Association. Code of Ethics for Nurses, Provision 7.4 Contributions through Nursing, Health, and Social Policy Development. (2025). Available from: https://codeofethics.ana.org/provision-7-4
23. Churchill W. Harrow School Speech October 29, 1941. https://www.nationalchurchillmuseum.org/never-give-in-never-never-never.html (1941). Accessed 24 Apr 2025.
24. American Lung Association. State of Lung Cancer Report. 2024. https://www.lung.org/research/state-of-lung-cancer. Accessed 24 April 2025.
25. GO2 for Lung Cancer. Lung Cancer Advocacy Toolkit. 2025. https://go2.org/advocacy/lung-cancer-advocacy-toolkit/. Accessed 25 Apr 2025.
26. GO2 for Lung Cancer. Policy Priorities. 2025. https://go2.org/advocacy/policy-priorities/. Accessed 25 April 2025.
27. GO2 for Lung Cancer. Lung Cancer Voices Summit. 2025. https://go2.org/advocacy/lung-cancer-advocacy-toolkit/. Accessed 8 May 2025.
28. American Cancer Society Cancer Action Network: What we do. 2025. https://www.fightcancer.org/landing-pages/what-we-do. Accessed 25 Apr 2025.
29. American Lung Association. Policy & Advocacy. 2025. https://www.lung.org/policy-advocacy. Accessed 8 May 2025.
30. LUNGevity. Public Policy for Supporters & Advocates. 2025. https://www.lungevity.org/for-supporters-advocates/public-policy. Accessed 8 May 2025.

Open Access This chapter is licensed under the terms of the Creative Commons Attribution-NonCommercial 4.0 International License (http://creativecommons.org/licenses/by-nc/4.0/), which permits any noncommercial use, sharing, adaptation, distribution and reproduction in any medium or format, as long as you give appropriate credit to the original author(s) and the source, provide a link to the Creative Commons license and indicate if changes were made.

The images or other third party material in this chapter are included in the chapter's Creative Commons license, unless indicated otherwise in a credit line to the material. If material is not included in the chapter's Creative Commons license and your intended use is not permitted by statutory regulation or exceeds the permitted use, you will need to obtain permission directly from the copyright holder.

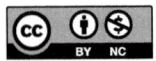

GPSR Compliance

The European Union's (EU) General Product Safety Regulation (GPSR) is a set of rules that requires consumer products to be safe and our obligations to ensure this.

If you have any concerns about our products, you can contact us on ProductSafety@springernature.com

In case Publisher is established outside the EU, the EU authorized representative is:

Springer Nature Customer Service Center GmbH
Europaplatz 3
69115 Heidelberg, Germany

Batch number: 09745535

Printed by Printforce, the Netherlands